The Vaccine Book Parents Deserve

Empowering and Reliable Evidence to Make an Informed Choice for Your Children

By Scott A. Johnson

The Vaccine Book Parents Deserve: Empowering and Reliable Evidence to Make an Informed Choice for Your Children / Scott A. Johnson

ISBN-13: 978-0997548778 / ISBN-10: 0997548770

Cover design: Scott A. Johnson
Cover Copyright: © Scott A. Johnson 2020

Discover more books by Scott A. Johnson at authorscott.com

Published by Scott A. Johnson Professional Writing Services, LLC: Orem, UT

*To parents everwhere that are seeking
to do what is best for their children.*

*To my wife and children who tirelessly support me in my
desire to help raise healthier generations naturally.*

Contents

Preface

The idea of vaccinations is a noble one—to spare children and adults from infectious illnesses, some of which cause significant permanent harm or death. Since their inception, vaccines have reduced disease, disability, and death from a variety of infectious diseases. Today, many people believe that few medical interventions can compare with the impact vaccines have had on lives. The World Health Organization estimates that vaccines prevented at least ten million deaths between 2010 and 2015 alone.[1] Although improved sanitation and hygiene certainly contributed to a reduced incidence of infectious illnesses, they can't explain reductions in some infectious illnesses that coincide with the introduction of a vaccine for that illness. Nor the reduction in vaccine-preventable illnesses in developing countries with current poor sanitation and hygiene. Many consider vaccines the greatest success story in medical history.

But as with all things medicine, no therapy is used without risks, and the benefits-to-risks must be weighed before agreeing to the treatment or intervention. The number of recommended vaccines has dramatically increased since only a handful were recommended in the 1960s and 1970s making many people question the safety of this untested practice. The intention of this book is to provide the risks and benefits of current vaccinations so parents, caregivers, and medical professionals can make informed decisions. It will provide insights into vaccine ingredients, the manufacturing process, and reported adverse effects as well as explanations of the infection, its prevalence, and the complications that can occur. In the end, the goal is to provide crucial knowledge so individuals can be empowered to make important decisions regarding vaccination based on a deeper understanding of them.

No parent wants to be responsible for harming their child, whether from refusing vaccination or the side effects of vaccinations. Years ago, virtually all parents simply followed their doctor's advice and indiscriminately consented to the recommended vaccination schedule. However, in the information age, parents are becoming more knowledgeable about the risks and possible side effects of vaccinations, particularly in certain groups of children. These parents don't want their children to catch any serious infection, but they also don't want their children to potentially be harmed by the vaccination either. This leaves parents in a Catch-22 and faced with very difficult choices. Yet many parents feel ill-equipped to make these decisions because so much conflicting information is available. The internet made information vastly more accessible, but it also provided an open forum for throngs of people to pontificate opinions and unverified information. Extremists on both sides of the debate use scare tactics, preying on the emotions of concerned parents, to persuade parents to their side of the argument. Parents are left to decipher who they should trust and believe.

Lest someone think people who choose to decline one or more vaccines are uneducated, antiscience "antivaxxers," research shows that parents who refuse vaccines are highly educated, value scientific information, and are capable researchers.[2,3,4,5,6,7] The data suggests that mothers with a college degree and higher incomes were the least likely to fully vaccinate their children, while mothers with a high school diploma and lower incomes often fully vaccinate their children. The most common reasons cited for delaying or refusing vaccination include safety concerns, personal or religious beliefs, and a desire for more transparency in information shared by healthcare providers. The latter reason is a desire for more information and education. For many reasons, including time and knowledge, this is difficult to get from many healthcare professionals. To fill in the gap, this book presents research and pertinent information to educate interested parents and healthcare professionals who prefer to hear both sides of the issue.

While almost all pediatricians vaccinate their children, some doctors do not vaccinate their children in accordance with recommended vaccination schedules. A survey of 582 pediatricians found that 10 percent of general pediatricians and 21 percent of subspecialist pediatricians (e.g., pediatric cardiologist or pediatric endocrinologist) planned to reject at least one vaccine for their children.[8] The most commonly rejected vaccines were measles, rotavirus, meningococcal, and hepatitis A. Other research shows that 8 percent of pediatricians don't fully vaccinate their children and 34 percent deviate from the recommended timing of vaccination for their own children.[9] Pediatricians themselves even reject vaccines—meningococcal, pneumococcus, and influenza—they are personally recommended to receive.[10] Why do these pediatricians choose not to vaccinate according to recommended schedules? Most often, they expressed concerns about safety, giving too many vaccines at once, or a desire for natural immunity through infection.

This book is pro-information and pro-informed choice. Parents and individuals have a right to know and understand the risks of any treatment or preventive measure recommended by their healthcare professional. Pros and cons of the treatment recommendation should be thoroughly discussed before treatment is administered. The Association of American Physicians and Surgeons (AAPS) agreed in a statement to legislators that reads the AAPS "strongly opposes federal interference in medical decisions, including mandated vaccines."[11] Furthermore, they emphasize the right to be fully informed "of the risks and benefits of a medical procedure" and that "patients [or parents] have the right to reject or accept that procedure." There are three possible choices when it comes to vaccinations: (1) all vaccinations, (2) no vaccinations, and (3) selective (partial) vaccination. It is not an all-or-nothing decision, and parents, individuals, and healthcare professionals should each be informed before recommending or receiving vaccinations.

There is a concerted effort to suppress information that suggests vaccines deserve careful consideration. From Google to Facebook and Amazon to YouTube, giant corporations have developed algorithms or established policies that censor any information that's critical of or questions the prescribed vaccination schedules and their safety and efficacy.[12,13] If you don't think this is true, try searching for the information yourself, and you'll have trouble finding it unless you use alternative search engines. It has even been proposed to use social media and computer models to monitor and identify individuals who are critical of vaccines.[14,15,16,17] In addition, it has been proposed to "partner with influential individuals on social media to disseminate" mainstream vaccine views and subdue antivaccine sentiment.[18] This book seeks to bring this information to the light, not so people will choose not to vaccinate but so people can make informed choices. Without this information, parents are unable to balance the risks and benefits of the various vaccines.

Some proponents of vaccines believe that anyone who questions vaccines cannot be credible. Even worse, some vaccine proponents aggressively abuse, threaten, and censor anyone who questions the dominant views and generally accepted narrative about vaccines. Doctors or scientists who question vaccines are at the greatest risk. They threaten the public perception that all experts support vaccination and may be subject to harassment, attempts to discredit or harm their professional reputation, and even a loss of licensing or livelihood.[19] Proponents of vaccines imply there are no legitimate scientific concerns about vaccination and therefore brand parents, researchers, physicians, and citizen activists as "antiscience." Scientific advancement requires novel ideas and the challenging of existing mainstream ideas. Suppression of these challenges and new ideas impedes the evaluation of all available evidence and has a detrimental effect on research. Indeed, bias against new ideas can threaten the careers of scientists who put forward new theories or interpretations, this despite the fact that doing so under the right circumstances and in the right way can lead to major advances and innovations.

Readers are encouraged to review the information contained in this book through a new and unbiased lens. Admittedly, a very difficult task. Indeed, the theory of cognitive dissonance causes us to fight against ideas that contradict currently accepted beliefs. We feel uncomfortable when new information challenges a deeply held belief and either seek to justify our existing belief or accept the new information. Many of us have preconceived notions about vaccines that introduce a significant bias that causes us to accept information that supports our current beliefs and reject information that doesn't. We tend to see only what we want to believe and what supports our rigid and predetermined notions. The hope is that this book will foster critical thinking, understanding, and respect to diminish biases that impede clear and rational thinking.

All vaccines are not equally important. Some infections are more common or more deadly, while others are fairly harmless. While pediatricians and other doctors that administer vaccinations regularly should be the most informed about them, this simply isn't the case. Very little time is spent on vaccination education in medical schools and postgraduate training. The busy schedules of doctors also leave little time to debate the pros and cons with each parent who requests more information during a doctor's visit. Most doctors simply don't have sufficient time to answer all the questions parents may have about vaccination. These facts make a book like this of great importance for parents to receive the necessary information to make an informed choice. You, as a parent, are entitled to reliable, evidence-based information to know what treatment your child receives. Empowered with this knowledge, you will be well equipped to make an informed decision about vaccinations.

How to Use This Book

....
....

To begin, the infection will be discussed, including general information, symptoms, and how it is transmitted. Prevalence refers to how common the infection is. In general, worldwide statistics will be provided when available. Many of the infections are rare in developed countries that have good hygiene, adequate medical care, satisfactory sanitation, and aggressive vaccine programs. Less developed countries generally experience higher incidence of the infections and, with that, higher mortality rates. Next, complications and health risks associated with the infection will be discussed, including mortality rates where available.

Vaccines are first described along with their recommended schedule. The manufacturing process for each vaccine is included to show how many of the controversial ingredients end up in the vaccine and to allow parents and healthcare professionals to evaluate possible risks involved. This information can be a bit technical, so if you just want to see the end results, the ingredients, and controversial ingredients, skip to those sections. Ingredients as provided by the manufacturers are included with amounts of specific ingredients when reported. The controversial ingredients section informs parents of the ingredients within the vaccine that people seek to avoid, may potentially cause harm, or are associated with health risks. More detailed information on these controversial ingredients and their potential to cause harm is found in chapter 1.

Next, common adverse reactions and serious adverse reactions identified by the vaccine manufacturer and listed on the vaccine's package insert are listed. Typically documented in clinical trials of the vaccine, these reactions are generally considered vaccine related and often mild or related to injection-site reactions. Frequency of the adverse reactions is reported when provided. The Vaccine Adverse Events Reporting System (VAERS) was established for healthcare providers and parents to report adverse reactions they believe are associated with vaccines. Vaccine inserts list these as postmarketing surveillance reactions when a specific reaction is reported enough times. These reactions are not conclusively related to the vaccine and may be coincidental but can help identify a pattern or increased occurrence of certain adverse events after vaccination. The last section summarizes published studies—many of which are observational—that have identified an association with a possible harm or reaction and the vaccine.

Parents are encouraged to evaluate all the information and prayerfully consider how to proceed. Involving your child's pediatrician or other healthcare professional is always a good idea. If he doesn't agree with your decision, get a second opinion or find another physician who respects your parental rights. Every parent is entitled to engage healthcare professionals they trust to help them make the right choice for their child—no matter the decision.

2019 Recommended Vaccination Schedule[20]

 = Range of recommended ages for children

	Birth	1 month	2 months	4 months	6 months	12 months	15 months	18 months	19-23 months	2-3 years	4-6 years
HepB	HepB	Hep B				HepB					
RV			RV	RV	RV						
DTaP			DTaP	DTaP	DTaP		DTaP	DTaP			DTaP
Hib			Hib	Hib	Hib	Hib					
PCV13			PCV13	PCV13	PCV13	PCV13					
IPV			IPV	IPV		IPV					
Influenza (Yearly)					Influenza (Yearly)						
MMR						MMR					MMR
Varicella						Varicella					Varicella
HepA						HepA (two doses, 2nd 6 mo. after 1st)					

	7-8 years	9-10 years	11-12 years	13-15 years	16-18 years
Influenza (Yearly)			Influenza (Yearly)		
HPV (if at increased risk)		HPV (if at increased risk)			
Tdap, Tetanus, Diphtheria, Pertussis			Tdap, Tetanus, Diphtheria, Pertussis		
HPV			HPV		
MenACWY			MenACWY		MenACWY
MenB					MenB (Children not at increased risk with provider recommendation)
Pneumococcal (if at increased risk)					
Hepatitis A (if at increased risk)					
HepB, Polio, MMR, Chickenpox Varicella (if catching up on missed vaccines)					

15

1

Controversial Vaccine Ingredients

Several aspects of vaccine production and the ingredients they contain worry parents. Vaccines may contain remnants of the manufacturing process and ingredients that the modern informed consumer seeks to avoid. They range from toxic metals used as adjuvants and preservatives to foreign DNA from animals, insects, and other humans. Before discussing each of the recommended vaccines, we will briefly review the controversial components that vaccines contain. This is important because as the ingredients come up, you will already have an idea why they are controversial and why some might choose to avoid them.

Human DNA from Aborted Fetuses

In order to develop mass-produced vaccines, researchers must grow bacteria or viruses in cultures. Unlike bacteria, which grow well in a laboratory environment in a suitable growth medium, viruses must infect living cells—animal, insect, or human—to produce vaccines. This is because viruses are not living organisms. Instead, they are complicated collections of proteins, lipids, carbohydrates, and nucleic acids. Without a living cell to infect, viruses would not be able to spread. Viruses use a host cell's own components to produce more copies after they infect a live cell. Cell-based vaccines are grown in cultured cells of animal, insect, or human origin, which inevitably leaves traces of the cultured cell in the end vaccine. Moreover, the potential presence of latent DNA viral contaminants—some associated with cancer—is a major public safety concern.

As you read through this book, you will find a number of vaccines that use cells from aborted fetuses, which introduces traces of foreign human DNA into those who receive these vaccines. The use of aborted fetal tissue cell lines raises serious religious, personal, moral, and ethical issues. To be clear, newly aborted fetuses are not necessary to maintain a supply of these cells. Instead, the original cells obtained from a fetus or embryo are used to grow a continuous supply of cells for research and scientific purposes in a lab. Many are opposed to using aborted fetal cells because they disagree with the practice of abortion alone, but the consequences of mixing our DNA with foreign (not from self) DNA from other humans is also of concern. We don't fully know that happens when the DNA of one human being is inserted into the DNA of another human being. Because the DNA is human, it is possible, though not likely, that the fetal DNA fragments will be incorporated into the recipient's DNA, including the brain.[21,22] This process is called homologous recombination and occurs when a segment of a cell's DNA is substituted by another segment of similar DNA. The human genome naturally contains regions that are susceptible to the insertion of DNA to create genetic diversity in our offspring. Some experts are concerned that vaccines that inject fragments of foreign fetal DNA may be acting as a "Trojan horse" to initiate childhood neurological disorders. As the new genetic material (foreign DNA) is inserted into a normal gene, it is possible for it to initiate abnormal immune and inflammatory responses.

Injection of fragments of foreign human fetal DNA into infants and children could trigger an immune response that may cause the child's own DNA to cross-react. Cross-reactivity describes when antibodies produced against a specific foreign agent (antigen) recognize antigens from benign sources as invading substances and inappropriately mount an immune response against them. Think of this like playing a game of laser tag. You are on the blue team and assigned to shoot the targets of all red team members. However, a mix up occurs and some of your blue team members have red targets. You shoot and eliminate those with red targets, including some of your own team members. In a similar manner, when cross-reactivity occurs, both healthy and abnormal cells are targeted for destruction.

If sufficient levels (about 5 ng/mL) of foreign fetal DNA are present in the body, it can activate toll-like receptors (TLRs) and lead to autoimmune attacks. Toll-like receptors play a key role in immune responses—both innate and adaptive. Activating these receptors causes increased expression of multiple inflammatory genes that play a role in protecting against infectious agents. Inappropriate triggering of TLR pathways may initiate autoimmune reactions and damage to healthy tissue.[23] Research in mice suggests that activation of TLRs during early developmental stages—like the age that many vaccines are given—impairs brain development and increases the risk of neurological disorders like schizophrenia and autism.[24] Researchers hypothesize that responses to fetal DNA, and the subsequent genetic defects and inflammation of the brain, may cause autism in susceptible individuals.[25] This hasn't been proven, but exhaustive study on how fetal DNA fragments affect immune responses and DNA sequences should have been completed before using them in the manufacturing process and certainly before introducing them into an infant's body.

The health consequences of vaccine-introduced fetal cell DNA does appear to have a minor association with autism rates in humans. One study concluded that vaccines manufactured in fetal cell lines contain unacceptably high levels of foreign DNA fragments.[26] Enough DNA that they could form double-strand breaks—when both strands of the DNA are severed—or insertional mutagenesis. Considered the most dangerous of all DNA lesions, double-strand DNA breaks can result in chromosomal rearrangements and the death of the cell. Insertional mutagenesis may occur if foreign fetal DNA incorporates into the child's DNA, causing genetic mutations. Same species DNA easily inserts itself into the recipient's (the child receiving the vaccine) DNA and can alter genetic function. The presence of this foreign DNA deserves more study to determine its implications and dangers for individuals receiving vaccines manufactured with aborted fetal cells.

Animal Cells in Vaccines

Animal cells have been used for the production of human vaccines since vaccine farms were established to harvest lymph from calves infected with the cowpox virus in the late 1800s. The close resemblance of cowpox to a mild form of smallpox and the observation that dairy farmers were immune to smallpox led to the production of the first smallpox vaccine. From this point to the first half of the twentieth century, many vaccines were produced using animals—either by growing the pathogen in live animals or in embryonated chicken eggs.

Derived from the kidney tissue of an adult female cocker spaniel, the MDCK (Madin-Darby Canine Kidney) cell line has been used for research purposes since 1958. Dog kidney cells are not as much of a concern as fetal cells because they are nonhuman and highly unlikely to be incorporated into human DNA. However, MDCK proteins may shuttle adventitious viruses—from contaminated MDCK cells—into our cells. Such was the case from 1955 to 1963, when monkey kidney cells (called VERO, from African green monkeys) used to produce polio vaccines (oral and injected) and the adenovirus vaccine (used for military personnel) were found to be contaminated with polyomavirus simian virus 40, or SV-40. This virus is associated with human cancers including brain tumors, non-Hodgkin's lymphoma, bone cancer, and mesothelioma.[27] Millions of people (perhaps more than one hundred million) were injected with this cancer-causing virus during this eight-year period. Observational research has documented an increased incidence of certain cancers among the people exposed to SV-40 contaminated vaccines.[28,29,30] Other research refutes this claim and suggests that there is inadequate evidence to confirm that exposure to SV-40 via the contaminated vaccines increases cancer rates.[31,32,33]

Years later, improved processes and screening were implemented to exclude viral contaminants in live-cell vaccines. Despite these efforts, the introduction of SV-40 and other contaminants has continued to a small degree. In 1980, 150 newborns were injected with a hepatitis A vaccine contaminated with SV-40 virus.[34] Another recent example is when it was discovered that a rotavirus vaccine (Rotarix) contained porcine circovirus 1 (PCV1).[35] Porcine circoviruses are divided into three types: PCV1, PCV2, and PCV3. An enzyme derived from pig tissue called trypsin was blamed as the source of contamination. This contaminant is still listed on the vaccine package insert today. In fact, another rotavirus vaccine (RotaTeq) states that DNA from porcine circoviruses (PCV-1 and PCV-2) have been detected in the vaccine. Although PCVs can infect and replicate in human cells, they are not known to cause illness in humans.[36,37]

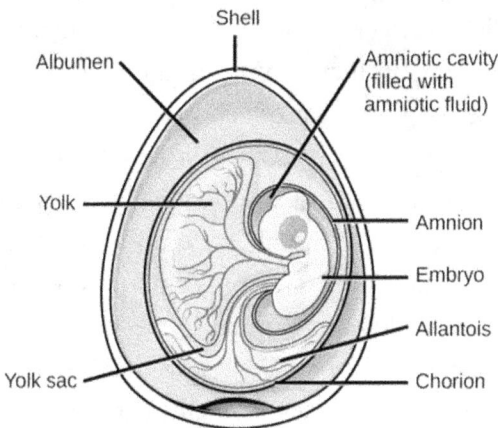

Image Credit: CNX OpenStax / CC BY

In addition to human and dog kidney cells, vaccine viruses are also grown in chick cells. Today, embryonated chicken eggs (ECEs) are primarily used to grow influenza virus. To grow the virus in ECEs, pathogen-free eggs are used eleven to twelve days after fertilization. The eggs are nicked and a hole drilled for insertion of the virus into the allantoic cavity—a sac-like structure filled with clear fluid that helps the embryo exchange gases and manage liquid waste—just below the air sac. The virus then replicates during the incubation period and is later harvested for use during vaccine production.

Based on the formation of tumors in rodents injected with cell lines used during vaccination, the US Food and Drug Administration concluded in a report that certain cell lines used in vaccine production might cause cancer.[38] According to the FDA report, "Some of these tumor-forming cell lines may contain cancer-causing viruses that are not actively reproducing" and that the viruses "are hard to detect using standard methods." The tumor-forming cells include MDCK (used for influenza vaccines), Chinese hamster ovary (CHO; utilized to make hepatitis B vaccines used in China), aborted human fetal retina (PER.C6; used for poliovirus vaccines), and aborted human embryonic kidney (HEK293; used for influenza vaccines) cells. They further stated that these latent (not currently replicating) viruses pose a potential threat to human health because they could "become active under vaccine manufacturing conditions," which would allow them to replicate and potentially cause illness. Obviously, better detection methods need to be developed to identify viral contaminants in cell cultures used for vaccine production to reduce the health threat of latent viruses.

Viral vaccines are also grown in insect cell cultures from the cabbage looper and fall armyworm. Growing influenza viruses in insect cells speeds the production process, allowing for the production of flu vaccines in about ten weeks. Baculoviruses are pathogenic DNA viruses that infect insect cells. They have been used as natural pest control agents, but their slow speed of kill and the narrow number of insects they kill limits their agricultural applications. Baculoviruses are used in vaccine production by cloning hemagglutinin—surface proteins important to the viral entry and infection of a cell—genes from influenza or HPV viruses into baculoviruses. This genetic information provides the cell instructions to infect insect cells and grow the viral antigens (recombination proteins) that are used in influenza and HPV vaccines.[39] There is always a possibility that adventitious pathogens contaminating the insect cells used during vaccine production could end up in the vaccines. Some also question the safety of foreign insect DNA particles inside our blood and tissues and what health effects this might have, although no adverse effect on human health has been observed in investigations of baculoviruses.[40]

Mercury (Thimerosal)

From the 1930s, the mercury-containing preservative, thimerosal (49.55 percent mercury by weight), was extensively used in childhood vaccines

(DTaP, Hib, HepB) to prevent the growth of microbes during the manufacturing process. Because of increasing concern and pressure, the US Public Health Service recommended removing thimerosal from vaccines in 1999 to reduce mercury exposure in infants as much as possible. Vaccine manufacturers did just that and removed thimerosal from many vaccines by about 2002. Today, the tetanus only and some influenza vaccines still contain thimerosal, as do many vaccines used in developing countries.

There are two different compounds that contain mercury: methylmercury and ethylmercury. Methylmercury is found in the environment and formed by mercury metal. It is the type consumed by humans when they eat contaminated fish. Ethylmercury is formed when the body metabolizes thimerosal. It readily crosses the blood-brain barrier where it largely converts to highly toxic inorganic mercury-containing compounds that persist in brain tissues for years.[41]

Research with newborn monkeys suggests that ethylmercury and methylmercury are initially absorbed and distributed to tissues similarly, but ethylmercury clears the blood 5.4 times faster than methylmercury.[42] In a comparison of the distribution and excretion of mercury forms, brain concentrations of thimerosal were three to four times lower than the methylmercury group—half-lives of 24.2 days and 59.5 days, respectively. However, the proportion of inorganic mercury in the brain of the thimerosal group was significantly higher (21%–86%) than the methylmercury group (6%–10%). This is troubling since inorganic mercury remains in the brain much longer—estimated to be more than a year before half of it is cleared. While laboratory studies show a similar toxicity between the two forms of mercury for cardiovascular, immune, and neural cells, the toxicity of ethylmercury appears to be lower when tested in animals.[43] Based on all available animal and epidemiological evidence, the CDC states that there isn't "any evidence that thimerosal causes harm."[44]

At any rate, mercury isn't healthy for any brain, especially those still developing or undernourished, or for premature infants. Low-level exposure to inorganic mercury in the developing brain is associated with excessive activation of microglia (brain cells that act as the first and primary form of defense in the central nervous system) in the brain, a phenomenon also observed in children with autism spectrum disorder (ASD).[45,46,47,48] In addition, low brain levels of inorganic mercury causes brain-cell death and motor deficits (poor movement and coordination), according to animal research.[49] Similar neurological impairment and motor deficits have been documented in humans exposed to ethylmercury.[50] This same study concluded that "the high order of toxicity from thimerosal and its ethylmercury breakdown product has been known and published for decades" and its use in pharmaceutical products "represents a medical crisis in the modern day." Indeed, the FDA recognized the potential hazards of thimerosal in a range of pharmaceutical products—like topical antiseptics and ointments—and began eliminating it from them during the 1980s. The totality of this evidence suggests that methylmercury is not an adequate reference to determine the health effects of ethylmercury, and ethylmercury and its breakdown products represent a source of potential harm to humans, especially unborn and newborn children.

Emerging evidence indicates that thimerosal does indeed pose a health risk. There are almost two hundred studies that have associated thimerosal with harmful effects—ADHD, autism, death, emotional disturbances, allergic reactions, malformations, acrodynia (irritability, sensitivity to light, pink discoloration of the hands and feet, and nerve inflammation due to chronic exposure to mercury), autoimmune conditions, Well's syndrome, developmental delay, and neurodevelopmental disorders.[51,52,53,54,55] Observational studies have consistently revealed a link between ethylmercury exposure and neurodevelopmental disorders.[56] Despite this consistency, vaccine proponents refuse to accept the link between thimerosal exposure and neurodevelopmental disorders because correlation does not prove causation.

Unsurprisingly, neurodevelopmental disorders are among the most commonly reported adverse effects of thimerosal-containing vaccines because many are given during key brain development periods in a child's life. The greatest risk was observed among infants who received these vaccines during their first month of life. Interestingly, infants in the Amazon with low exposure to methylmercury from fish but the highest exposure to ethylmercury from vaccines had worse cumulative neurodevelopmental—the ability of the brain to develop normal pathways for healthy nervous system function—scores when compared to infants with lower ethylmercury exposure.[57] It is well known that consumption of fish that are frequently contaminated with methylmercury during childhood may harm a child's neurodevelopment.[58,59] However, this research suggests that ethylmercury exposure through vaccination is also relevant to neurobehavioral outcomes, particularly when accounting for the combined effects of dietary and pharmaceutical exposure to mercury.

Utilizing data from the Vaccine Safety Datalink (VSD), which contains vaccination and demographic data reported by participating healthcare organizations, the relationship between thimerosal-containing HepB vaccines and neurodevelopmental delays was assessed. Children who were diagnosed with developmental delays—speech, coordination, hearing, or reading—were significantly more likely to have received thimerosal-containing vaccines during the first, second, and sixth months of life as recommended by the CDC.[60] In total, these children were three times more likely than children who did not receive thimerosal-containing vaccines to be diagnosed with developmental delays. An additional study that looked at the thimerosal-containing HepB vaccine found that infants who received this vaccine showed poorer psychomotor development—muscle control involved in the ability to sit, crawl, stand, walk, run, and jump—at 12 and 24 months of age when compared to children unexposed to thimerosal.[61] These psychomotor deficits persisted through the three-year follow-up period. Additional research revealed that boys who received the HepB vaccine with thimerosal were nine times more likely to require special education services than unvaccinated boys were.[62] Remember: these are associations and do not prove causation, but the evidence cannot be ignored that infants who receive thimerosal vaccines are significantly more likely to experience neurodevelopmental delays.

In order to assess the association between thimerosal-containing vaccines and autism, researchers analyzed data in VAERS (Vaccine Adverse Events Reporting System) database, which is jointly maintained by the CDC and FDA. Comparing children who received thimerosal-containing vaccines to children who received thimerosal-free vaccines, scientists concluded that there "was a significantly increased risk [of] ASD" among children who received the thimerosal version of the DTaP (twice the risk) and HepB (triple the risk) vaccines.[63] Other research has associated giving the MMR vaccine or Rho(D)-immune globulin injections that contain thimerosal during fetal growth with higher autism rates.[64,65,66] Another group of CDC researchers evaluated data from the VSD that included over 400,000 infants. The conclusion of the CDC researchers was that the risk of developing a neurodevelopmental disorder was almost twice as high (1.8 times) in infants who received greater than 25 mcg of ethylmercury from thimerosal-containing vaccines during the first month of life when compared to infants not exposed to thimerosal.[67] One-month-old infants with the highest cumulative exposure to thimerosal were 7.6 times more likely to develop autism, five times more likely to develop a sleep disorder, and twice as likely to develop a speech disorder. Another review of VSD data for more than 1.9 million infants found that infants exposed to the most mercury (37.5 mcg) were significantly more likely to develop pervasive developmental disorder (three times more likely), specific developmental delay, hyperkinetic syndrome—a behavioral disorder associated to ADHD, or tic disorder.[68] The risk of vaccine-related autism appears to be more common in boys (five times more likely), particularly non-Caucasian boys.[69] A meta-analysis of forty-four studies revealed that mercury is an important causal factor in the development of autism because people diagnosed with autism have an impaired ability to detoxify and excrete mercury.[70] It is possible that

26

some children are at an increased risk of mercury toxicity that could predispose them to autism.

Atypical autism—some symptoms of autism are present, but the level of symptoms is insufficient to diagnose autism—is also associated with thimerosal-containing vaccines. Children diagnosed with atypical autism were significantly more likely to have been exposed to ethylmercury through thimerosal-containing vaccines.[71] The same researchers point out that abnormal brain connectivity is experienced more frequently by children administered thimerosal-containing vaccines.[72] This suggests thimerosal may cause neurological damage that is below the threshold of an official diagnosis of autism.

However, other researchers disagree with the conclusions of the studies above. A meta-analysis of case-control cohort studies concluded that vaccines and their components (including thimerosal) are "not associated with the development of autism or autism spectrum disorder."[73] Another review concluded that "epidemiologic studies continue to provide evidence that there is no association between thimerosal exposure and autism."[74] Part of this discrepancy among researchers analyzing data could be the complexity of the data being analyzed and what data they include.[75] Whereas infants younger than six months in 1999 may have been exposed to 200 mcg of mercury, infants today are exposed to 25 mcg or less of thimerosal through the annual flu shot during the first six months of life.

Although vaccine-related autism has been a focus of researchers and parents, it is not the only potentially debilitating developmental disorder associated with vaccines. An association between thimerosal-containing vaccines and mental retardation, speech disorders, ADHD, personality disorders, and abnormal thinking has also been observed.[76,77,78,79] Remarkably, one study found that every 1 mcg of thimerosal injected into a child via vaccine increases the risk of mental retardation 4.8 percent, autism 2.9 percent, and speech disorders 1.4 percent.[80] This is remarkable since some of the flu vaccines approved for use in children contain 25 mcg of thimerosal. A review evaluating VAERS data found the incidence of autism and mental retardation was six times higher among children who received DTaP vaccines preserved with thimerosal.[81] A review of 5,591 adverse events from VAERS determined that children who received thimerosal-containing DTaP vaccines were at a greater risk of mental retardation, autism, and neurodevelopmental delays when compared to children who received DTaP without thimerosal.[82] Premature infants and infants who receive thimerosal from vaccines who are of a lower weight than their peers or who are exposed to multiple neurological toxins—including aluminum adjuvants in vaccines—along with thimerosal, are likely at greater risk of harm.[83] The fact that ethylmercury preferentially accumulates in the brain and persists for months should be sufficient to avoid thimerosal-containing vaccines during the first two years of life when a significant amount of neurodevelopment is taking place.

Another risk of exposure to mercury is premature puberty (called precocious puberty: puberty that begins before age 8 in girls and before age 9 in boys). Mercury is a known endocrine system disruptor that may interfere with sex hormone production and increase the risk of premature puberty. The available data suggests that infants that receive thimerosal from vaccines during the first month of life or an additional 100 mcg of mercury from vaccines during their first seven months of life are five times more likely to experience premature puberty.[84,85] Premature puberty may stunt the child's growth, cause self-esteem issues, increase the risk of breast cancer in girls later in their lives, and increase the risk of diabetes, heart disease, and premature death.[86,87] Given children's unprecedented exposure to endocrine-disrupting chemicals—BPA, phthalates, n-nonyl phenol, and methyl parabens—these days, it is unlikely that thimerosal exposure alone caused premature puberty. Rather, cumulative exposure to multiple toxins in personal care and household products, water, air, food, furniture, clothing, and more is a more likely cause.

28

It makes sense to avoid toxic compounds, including thimerosal, as much as possible. We are exposed to a plethora of toxins every day as it is. Preference should be given to vaccines without thimerosal and only one thimerosal-containing vaccine should be given at a time.

Aluminum

Aluminum (also spelled aluminium) is a lightweight, silvery-white metal and chemical element abundantly found in the Earth's crust. It is widely used in food packaging, aircraft, automobiles, and even mobile phones. It is used in vaccines as an adjuvant—an agent that helps create a stronger immune response—because the immune response may be insufficient to develop adequate antibodies to an antigen (e.g., influenza) without it. Therefore, adjuvants are used to trigger stronger immune responses to improve vaccine efficacy and protection against infectious illnesses. Interestingly, aluminum adjuvants are often used in vaccine safety studies as placebos, which yields false confounding data for adverse reactions because aluminum adjuvants are known to cause adverse reactions by themselves.

Adjuvanted vaccines are known to cause more local (injection-site pain, redness, and swelling) and systemic reactions (fever, body aches, general malaise, etc.) than nonadjuvanted vaccines. Injected aluminum poses a greater risk than ingested aluminum because it bypasses the protective barriers of the gastrointestinal tract, therefore producing toxicity at a lower dose. Vaccines based solely on antigens from infectious agents are largely ineffective in triggering sufficient immune responses. Indeed, the use of highly purified antigens to improve vaccine safety has reduced the immunogenicity—the ability of a foreign substance to provoke an immune response—and efficacy of vaccines. Adding adjuvants is currently necessary to make them work better.

Aluminum is a neurotoxin capable of destroying brain cells involved in cognitive and motor functions.[88,89] Even small amounts of injected aluminum can result in brain accumulation (cerebellum) and neurotoxicity.[90] Small amounts of aluminum remain throughout the

29

body, sometimes for years, in locations from the muscles to the brain.[91] Following injection, aluminum enters the bloodstream and can travel to distant tissues and organs in the body via phagocytic cells.[92,93] Aluminum causes strong innate immune responses at the site of injection.[94] Macrophages in muscle fascia sense the aluminum disturbance and alert the immune system and recruit cells that trigger an inflammatory response. In response, aluminum particles are taken up by phagocytic cells that spread the aluminum throughout the body.[95]

Furthermore, the same process that allows aluminum adjuvants to boost immunity can also result in hyperactive immune responses that are a known risk for autoimmune conditions.[96] This can result in systemic reactions to aluminum-adjuvanted vaccines. For example, people with a family history of autoimmune diseases, the presence of autoantibodies, a previous adverse reaction to vaccination, or certain genetic signatures may be more susceptible to vaccine-related autoimmunity.[97,98,99] Overstimulation of the immune system carries the inherent risk of triggering autoimmune disorders—called autoimmune/inflammatory syndrome induced by adjuvants (ASIA). Since aluminum significantly stimulates the immune system, it has the potential to cause serious immune disorders in humans.

Some evidence suggests that autism is highly heritable (transmitted from parent to offspring based on inherited genetics). Evaluation of more than two million individuals in five countries—Denmark, Finland, Sweden, Israel, and western Australia—found the heritability of autism was 80.8 percent (ranging from 50.9%–80.8%).[100] However, studies with twins indicate that environmental factors account for about 55 percent of autism risk and genetics only explains 37 percent of cases.[101] A child's brain is more permeable to toxins, and the kidneys are less able to eliminate them during early childhood. Genetic predispositions may sensitize some children to central nervous system damage caused by aluminum adjuvants. It is highly plausible that early-life assaults on the immune system caused by environmental substances foreign to the body (called xenobiotics), such as aluminum, contribute to neurodevelopmental disorders, including autism. Indeed, experimental evidence shows that simultaneous administration of as few as two to three adjuvants can overcome genetic resistance to autoimmune attacks.[102] The body is well equipped to regulate immune responses so that immune cells don't react to healthy cells or benign substances. However, when overstimulated by a foreign substance, healthy cells and tissues can become targets of the immune system. Considering that children in some developed countries receive a total of 126 antigens and significant amounts of aluminum adjuvants through routine vaccinations, rigorous evaluation of the safety of the current recommended vaccine schedule is urgently needed.

A study examined the evidence of aluminum neurotoxicity in animals and humans, particularly from vaccines in 2013. What the researchers found was that injected aluminum provokes autoimmune reactions that may partly explain the neurotoxicity that arises in some people after injection of aluminum.[103] Furthermore, they reported that aluminum exposure contributes to age-related neurological deficits resembling Alzheimer's disease and amyotrophic lateral sclerosis/Parkinson's dementia complex in adults. In young children, aluminum-adjuvanted vaccines were associated with autism. These age-related neurological deficits may occur because of increased genetic susceptibility.

Epidemiological research identified a correlation with the amount of aluminum received via vaccines, especially between 2 and 4 months of age, and autism rates.[104] Aluminum is able to cross both the blood-brain barrier and the blood-cerebrospinal fluid barriers, which may provoke immune-mediated inflammation in neural tissues. This means that aluminum can migrate to both brain tissues and the spinal cord. Studies on animals and humans have shown that aluminum adjuvants alone can cause autoinflammatory and autoimmune conditions.[105] Although they do not prove aluminum causes autism spectrum disorder, the findings conceivably implicate aluminum adjuvants as contributing factors to increased rates of autism.

Although generally well tolerated without serious systemic reactions, aluminum may cause widespread muscle pain or weakness, chronic fatigue, and cognitive dysfunction—memory impairment or attentional deficits—in a small portion of susceptible individuals.[106] Called macrophagic myofasciitis (MMF), this condition occurs when aluminum abnormally persists within macrophages at the site of previous immunization causing a lesion.[107] These lesions are frequently found at common vaccination sites, such as the deltoid muscles of adults and quadriceps in children. Biopsies of the lesions from children identified the presence of tumor-forming macrophages (CD68-positive) and abnormal periodic acid-Schiff-positive macrophages in all children tested, and aluminum hydroxide crystals in 25 percent of cases.[108] Tumor-forming macrophages are found in cancerous tumors and promote blood vessel growth to sustain the tumor. They are also involved in metastasis—travel of cancer cells to distant sites. The presence of abnormal periodic acid-Schiff-positive macrophages is a characteristic sign of MMF. Other symptoms include debilitating headache, joint pain, shortness of breath, mood disorders, and sleep disturbances. Because MMF mimics the symptoms of multiple other conditions, it is a very difficult condition to diagnose. Recently, it was proposed that Morin stain detects aluminum with high selectivity and sensitivity, which may improve MMF and vaccination lesion diagnosis.[109] Widespread muscle weakness and chronic fatigue are reported more frequently in people with a lesion in the deltoid muscle where an aluminum-containing vaccine was injected.[110] All of this is evidence that aluminum from vaccines may contribute to disrupted immune and nervous system function.

Functional magnetic resonance imaging (fMRI) using single-photon emission computerized tomography and positron emission tomography has identified a pathological pattern in the posterior brain—temporal lobes, limbic system, and cerebellum—of people with MMF.[111] These areas of the brain are involved in memory, comprehension, emotion, learning, motivation, movement, coordination, and muscular activity, all of which are affected by MMF. Scientists have also identified a distinctive pattern of poor glucose metabolism and blood distribution in the brains of people with MMF.[112] Glucose is essentially the sole fuel source for the human brain except during periods of starvation. The brain lacks areas to store glucose, so it requires a continuous supply of glucose to function efficiently. Poor blood distribution in the brain further hampers brain function. Additionally, they found that MMF is linked to altered detoxification activities. Poor aluminum detoxification could lead to abnormally high accumulation of aluminum in the brain and other tissues. Prolonged aluminum exposure in the brain could potentially initiate neurological symptoms, depending on how much is present. Together, these findings could explain the poor cognitive abilities and muscle function witnessed in people with MMF.

Researchers have discovered that people with the HLA-DRB1*01 gene—a gene that is part of a family of genes critical to immune system function and helps it distinguish the body's own proteins from proteins made by foreign invaders—are more susceptible to MMF after exposure to an aluminum adjuvant.[113] Current evidence indicates that aluminum from aluminum adjuvants persists in the body, producing an ongoing local immune reaction. In those who are genetically susceptible, abnormal immune responses could contribute to MMF or other neurological disorders, particularly since the nervous system is the most sensitive to aluminum toxicity. Whether aluminum is a cause of MMF or simply initiates a train of events that results in MMF in susceptible individuals requires further research.

Women are more likely than men to develop MMF. Why this is the case is poorly understood currently. Between 20 and 33 percent of people with MMF develop an autoimmune condition, such as multiple sclerosis-like symptoms characterized by damage to the protective covering (myelin sheath) that surrounds nerve fibers in the nervous system.[114,115,116] Half of people with MMF experience chronic fatigue and some rheumatoid arthritis.[117,118]

A muscle biopsy and diagnosis of MMF can occur from 3 months to 20 years following administration of an aluminum-containing vaccine. Even though this is not proof that aluminum adjuvants cause MMF, clinical and experimental data suggests more attention should be paid to the escalating doses of aluminum-adjuvanted vaccines given to the general population, particularly people with immature or altered blood-brain barriers or inflammatory conditions.

Veterans of the Persian Gulf War (1990–1991) received vaccinations (e.g., cholera, meningitis, rabies, tetanus, and typhoid vaccines) containing aluminum and squalene adjuvants. Some veterans of the war experienced a chronic and multisymptomatic disorder called Gulf War syndrome (GWS). GWS is characterized by a wide range of short-term and long-term symptoms, including muscle pain, cognitive problems, insomnia, fatigue, rashes, and gastrointestinal disturbances. Some experts hypothesize that GWS was caused by nerve gas, an agent given to protect against nerve gas (pyridostigmine bromide), psychological factors, or other chemicals (smoke from oil well fires, solvents, etc.). Nevertheless, some experts believe that GWS was predominantly a result of multiple adjuvanted vaccines given prior to deployment. Animal research correlated aluminum adjuvants—given in doses equivalent to human doses—to Gulf War syndrome.[119,120] The animal research demonstrated a significant loss of motor neurons (nerve cells that control muscles) and progressive deficits in strength after exposure to aluminum. One scientist concluded that administering multiple vaccinations containing aluminum adjuvants over a short period of time, like prior to deployment, is the primary risk factor for Gulf War syndrome.[121] It is possible that an overload of aluminum triggered a hyperactive immune response that failed to switch off, ultimately damaging the nervous system and causing GWS.

The science of aluminum toxicity associated with vaccination is not settled. The vast majority of scientists and health professionals consider the safety of aluminum adjuvants as well established.[122,123] Part of the argument from this group is that patients undergoing allergen-specific immunotherapy receive far greater amounts of injected aluminum when compared to amounts injected through routine vaccination.[124] There is good evidence that large amounts of aluminum are harmful to humans, but whether the amount used in vaccines is harmful is not conclusive in the eyes of the majority of the medical community. At the very least, the evidence suggests that a personalized vaccination schedule based on susceptibility to injury and the avoidance of multiple aluminum-adjuvanted vaccines simultaneously is prudent. More research is urgently needed to settle the matter, particularly to identify populations that may be more susceptible to vaccine injury.

There is ample evidence that large amounts of aluminum are harmful to humans, but less evidence exists that the amounts used in vaccines are harmful to humans. The observed small number of adverse events may be because of individual susceptibility. Like mercury, it is best to avoid taxing your child's immune system by giving her multiple aluminum-adjuvanted vaccines at once. The more aluminum injected into a child, particularly infants, the greater the risk of an overactive immune response. Speak with your healthcare professional about giving aluminum-containing vaccines at different appointments.

Other Adjuvants

As stated earlier, adjuvants contribute to an immune response that helps induce a protective adaptive immune response to a pathogen antigen. A growing concern about aluminum adjuvants and an increasing knowledge of the role of adjuvants in vaccines led to the creation of additional adjuvants.[125] Other adjuvants used in vaccines include monophosphoryl lipid A + aluminum salt (Cervarix), squalene oil-in-water emulsion (Fluad), monophosphoryl lipid A (MPL; anticancer vaccines and Shingrix), and QS-21—a compound extracted from the Chilean soapbark tree (Shingrix, a shingles vaccine), and cytosine phosphoguanine (Heplisav-B).

One of the concerns about any adjuvant is that the cost of immunogenicity is an accompanying inflammatory response and localized or systemic toxicity effects. Adjuvant-related inflammatory responses typically occur immediately or within the first twenty-four hours after vaccination. Local adjuvant adverse effects can cause injection-site problems or the formation of granulomas (an inflammatory response involving a collection of immune cells in an attempt to wall off a substance perceived by the immune system as foreign), noninfected abscesses, swollen lymph nodes, and chronic skin ulceration.[126,127] Abnormal immune activation caused by adjuvants—particularly those that initiate strong innate immune responses—are less common but can provoke systemic reactions including autoimmunity.[128,129,130,131] Although strong systemic inflammatory reactions to adjuvants typically self-resolve once the innate immune response subsides, they can last for several weeks after vaccination. This means that the immune system could be hyperactive for weeks after receipt of an adjuvanted vaccine.

Some systemic reactions to nonaluminum adjuvants include the following:[132]

- ✓ *Oil emulsion adjuvants*: fever, headache, diarrhea, general malaise, nausea, joint pain, muscle aches, lethargy, autoimmune conditions (arthritis, hepatitis, lupus), uveitis, and narcolepsy
- ✓ *Saponin adjuvants (and QS-21)*: red blood cell destruction, flu-like symptoms, general malaise, and fever
- ✓ *Monophosphoryl lipid A*: flu-like symptoms, headache, autoimmune conditions (arthritis, hepatitis, lupus), uveitis, enlarged spleen, damage to lymphoid tissue, and immunosuppression
- ✓ *Cytosine phosphoguanine*: autoimmune conditions (Wegener's granulomatosis, hypothyroidism, vitiligo)

The reality is that the potential toxicity of these new adjuvants and their ability to disrupt healthy immune function are poorly understood. That is not surprising given the fact that the most widely used adjuvant, aluminum, that has been given to billions of people still has unanswered questions about its connection to systemic adverse events. Given the vital importance of adjuvants in stimulating a protective immune response against infectious illnesses, more research into the mechanisms and safety of adjuvants is critically important. In reality, some vaccines would be utterly useless without an adjuvant because they simply can't trigger a sufficient immune response to provide protection from infection. Perhaps in the future, an adjuvant will be identified that improves vaccine efficacy without compromising the immune system or promoting local and systemic adverse events in susceptible individuals.

Human Serum Albumin (Blood Protein)

Human serum albumin is a protein found in human blood. As the most abundant protein in human blood plasma, it serves to transport hormones, fatty acids, and other compounds through the bloodstream. Human serum albumin is used to stabilize live, attenuated viruses and prevent vaccine antigens from adhering to the walls of injection vials. It is found in some MMR vaccines and is obtained from donors previously screened for certain viruses. The European Medicines Agency recommended the removal of all human blood-derived products from vaccine production because of the risk that it may contain infectious agents (such as HIV and hepatitis).[133] Recombinant human serum albumin may be used as an alternative in line with this recommendation. This albumin is genetically engineered by combining DNA from multiple sources in a lab and then purified to be free of viruses and bacteria. Theoretically, because human serum albumin is derived from human blood, there is a risk that it might contain infectious agents and harm humans. To date, no infectious illnesses have ever been associated with the use of human serum albumin because of the meticulous screening process.

2-Phenoxyethanol

The solvent 2-phenoxyethanol is a preservative used in personal care products, cosmetics, and vaccines, with excellent antimicrobial activity.

Chemically, 2-phenoxyethanol is a glycol ether. It is considered harmful if swallowed, absorbed through the skin (irritating and causes allergic response), or inhaled. Both Europe and Japan restrict its use in cosmetics to a 1 percent concentration, but also state that the use of multiple products containing a low dose could result in cumulative overexposure.

Comparing the toxicity of vaccine preservatives—2-phenoxyethanol, thimerosal, and benzethonium chloride—2-phenoxyethanol was found to be the least toxic to neurons.[134] Despite its lower toxicity, the study authors concluded that "none of the compounds commonly used as preservatives in US-licensed vaccine/biological preparations can be considered an ideal preservative." Other scientists disagree and call 2-phenoxyethanol a safe and effective substitute for thimerosal.[135] It certainly appears to be much safer than thimerosal, and the very small amounts used in vaccines are not expected to be toxic or cause harm to humans.

Cetyltrimethylammonium Bromide

Harmful if swallowed and irritating to the skin, cetyltrimethylammonium bromide (CB) is a chemical used as a surfactant and detergent. It is used in vaccines as an excipient, which are inactive substances that serve as vehicles—stabilize, bulk up, enhance solubility, facilitate absorption, or reduce viscosity—for active substances. CB may cause developmental toxicity at moderate doses according to animal research.[136] But the levels in vaccines are not likely to be problematic.

Formaldehyde

Also known as formalin, formaldehyde is a naturally occurring organic compound used in the manufacture of building materials and many household products. It is also used to preserve cadavers. Formaldehyde has a long history of use in vaccine manufacturing as well. It is used to inactivate viruses and detoxify bacterial toxins.

Based on data from studies in people, animals, and lab research, formaldehyde is classified as a probable human carcinogen and may cause leukemia, particularly myeloid leukemia in humans.[137,138] At body temperature, formaldehyde is oxidized to formic acid, which leads to acidosis and nerve, liver, and kidney damage.[139] Formaldehyde is a potent allergen in humans.[140] Exposure to formaldehyde can cause a multitude of adverse reactions in the cardiovascular system, nervous system, skin, gastrointestinal system, liver, and others. But this is from inhaling or ingesting it, and the risks of injected formaldehyde are not well known. A model of formaldehyde metabolism after intramuscular injection determined that a single dose of 200 mcg of formaldehyde is almost entirely removed from the site of injection within thirty minutes.[141] Assuming local metabolism only, peak blood/total water and body concentrations of formaldehyde were estimated at 22 mcg/L and 66 mcg/L, respectively. Based on the model and several assumptions, the study authors concluded that residual formaldehyde in vaccines is safe in infant vaccines. Other than years of anecdotal data, we don't have a lot of information, in the form of peer-reviewed studies, to determine the potential harmful effects of formaldehyde after injection. However, looking at levels in food and how much humans naturally produce may provide clues on its potential harmful effects.

Formaldehyde naturally occurs in many foods and beverages—grapes, apples, bananas, plums, carrots, onions, spinach, beef, poultry, seafood, and coffee. For example, you would consume about 1 mg of formaldehyde after eating a medium apple. An eight-ounce cup of coffee typically contains just under 1 mg of formaldehyde. Both of these exposures far exceed the residual amounts left in vaccines (often less than 15 mcg). Moreover, adults naturally produce about 1.5 ounces of formaldehyde as a byproduct of metabolism every day.[142] It is estimated that humans have between 1.5 and 3 mcg/mL of formaldehyde in their blood. While ingesting formaldehyde or naturally producing it in our cells is certainly different than injection into our muscles, the residual amounts of formaldehyde in vaccines likely pose little risk to humans.

Glutaraldehyde

Glutaraldehyde is an organic compound used as a disinfectant, preservative, fixative, and medication. Studies on glutaraldehyde show that it may cause respiratory issues like asthma, headache, allergic contact dermatitis, hives, diarrhea, and colitis, but like formaldehyde, this is from inhalation, skin contact, or ingestion.[143,144,145,146] Most experts consider the residual amounts of glutaraldehyde in vaccines to be harmless despite a significant lack of safety research.

Monosodium Glutamate

Better known by its acronym, MSG, monosodium glutamate is a very common food additive used to enhance the flavor of foods. It is derived from the amino acid glutamate (glutamic acid), a nonessential oil amino acid. MSG is used as a preservative and stabilizer in some vaccines. It is considered an excitotoxin—substances that overstimulate neuron receptors—that may damage or kill brain cells when exposed to it regularly and for prolonged periods.[147,148] Studies have confirmed a link between MSG consumption in foods and various side effects— nausea, headaches, flushing, or sweating—something coined as "Chinese restaurant syndrome" because it is so ubiquitously used in Chinese food.[149,150] Consuming three grams or a direct intravenous injection of 50 mg is considered sufficient to produce symptoms. It can also cause allergic reactions. While a small minority of people may suffer from temporary reactions to MSG, vaccines that contain MSG don't come anywhere near the 50 mg required to produce adverse reactions, so it poses minimal risk.

Nonylphenol Ethoxylate, Octylphenol Ethoxylate, and Octoxynol-10

Phenols, nonylphenol ethoxylate, octylphenol ethoxylate, and octoxynol-10 are surfactants used in laundry detergents, personal care products, paints, lawn care products, and automotive products. They are used to extract viral particles from the fatty membranes of chick embryos during the production of the influenza vaccine. Phenols tend to persist in the environment and are very harmful to aquatic life. They have been detected in human breast milk, blood, and urine and are associated with developmental and reproductive harm in animals.[151] Nonylphenol is distributed widely throughout the body, with extensive distribution to fatty tissues.[152] Although in trace amounts, there is insufficient data to determine the safety of these phenols, especially considering the influenza vaccine is recommended yearly, exposing humans to multiple cumulative doses.

Polysorbate 80 and Polysorbate 20

Used as surfactants in soaps, cosmetics, and eye drops and as an emulsifier in food and pharmaceutical products, polysorbates keep oil and water components of vaccines mixed together. It is used in multiple vaccines—DTaP, Tdap, influenza, HPV, and pneumococcal—to hold the ingredients together. One of the greatest concerns with polysorbates is their treatment with ethylene oxide. The problem with this practice is that the polysorbates can be contaminated with 1,4-dioxane, a potentially dangerous byproduct. The EPA classified 1,4-dioxane as likely to be carcinogenic to humans by all routes of exposure.[153] Study of polysorbate 80 implies that it is more harmful when injected as opposed to when ingested.[154] Unfortunately, evidence suggests that polysorbate 80 also actively transports metals and toxins into the brain by disrupting the function of the blood-brain barrier.[155,156,157] This is less than ideal if mercury or aluminum are also present in the vaccine since polysorbate 80 could increase accumulation of these neurotoxins in brain tissue.

Emerging evidence links polysorbate 80 to reproductive harm in females. Experimental research in newborn female rats showed that injection of polysorbate 80 disrupted reproductive function and caused damage to the ovaries and uterus that persisted months after the injection.[158] Based on this evidence scientists concluded that assurance given by vaccine proponents of "no biologically plausible" link between HPV4 vaccine and ovarian effects cannot be given."[159] Curiously, polysorbate 80 has been used as a "placebo" in HPV vaccine safety trials, which obviously can produce confounding results since it is known to cause reproductive harm. This is of particular importance since the HPV vaccine has been associated with ovarian damage, so using polysorbate 80 as a placebo could make the HPV vaccine appear safer than it really is. Polysorbate 80 has been identified as a cause of anaphylactic reaction.[160] The study authors stated polysorbate 80 "can cause severe nonimmunologic anaphylactoid reactions." Anaphylactoid reactions, more commonly called nonimmunologic anaphylaxis today, are reactions that produce similar symptoms as anaphylaxis but are not triggered by antibodies released by the immune system. Instead, these reactions are caused by the release of chemicals from mast cells or basophils. Like true anaphylaxis, they can be fatal.

Polysorbate 20 appears to be less harmful and toxic than polysorbate 80, but still has the risk of being contaminated with 1,4-dioxane.[161] Its reputation as a safer polysorbate may also be to fewer studies evaluating its potential risks than polysorbate 80. Contamination of polysorbates with 1,4-dioxane and the potential for reproductive harm is concerning.

Sodium Deoxycholate and Sodium Taurodeoxycholate

Sodium deoxycholate and sodium taurodeoxycholate are bile salts and detergents used to break down cells and solubilize—to break down and absorb into another substance—cellular and membrane components. They are used to disrupt viral particles during the manufacture of flu vaccines. Research in rats shows that both sodium deoxycholate and sodium taurodeoxycholate disrupt blood–brain barrier (BBB) function, which allowed brain damage to occur.[162,163] Lower doses caused subtle disruption of the BBB, but larger doses caused significant disruption. Disrupted BBB function is observed in neurological disorders and brain damage. Poor integrity of the BBB can also allow higher levels of toxins and pathogens to accumulate in brain tissues. Bile salts are also known to enhance the absorption of substances that have poor solubility in water.[164] The disruption of the BBB combined with an ability to improve the absorption of potentially harmful compounds is concerning.

2

Hepatitis B (HepB)

What Is Hepatitis B Infection?

Hepatitis B is a potentially life-threatening sexually transmitted liver infection caused by the hepatitis B virus (HBV). It is most commonly transmitted from mother to child during birth and delivery (perinatal transmission), but it can also be transmitted by contact with blood, semen, or other body fluids of an infected person (horizontal transmission). Mothers are tested for hepatitis B during prenatal care, and infants born to mothers who test positive are treated with an antihepatitis B antibody injection called hepatitis B immune globulin (HBIG). The virus can survive outside the body and infect others for at least seven days. Hepatitis B can be an acute (short-term) or chronic (long-term) infection. Infants who are infected are at a greater risk of chronic infection—approximately 90 percent of infected infants become chronically infected, compared with 25–50 percent of children and 2–6 percent of adults.[165,166] Infection during childhood, especially during the first year of life, has a greater risk of chronic infection and long-term health effects. Since most HBV infections occur during birth, appropriate and proactive prenatal care is vital.

Hepatitis means inflammation of the liver. Liver inflammation triggers the accumulation of genetic and epigenetic defects that cause liver damage and poor liver function. Hepatitis can be caused by three different viruses: hepatitis A, hepatitis B, and hepatitis C. Hepatitis A is spread when a person ingests fecal matter after contact with contaminated objects, food, or drinks. It usually lasts from a few weeks to several months and rarely causes lasting liver damage. Hepatitis C is spread by contact with the blood of an infected person, including from blood transfusions. Some cases result in mild symptoms that last a few weeks, but most hepatitis C infections cause serious, chronic infections—up to 85 percent of infections.[167]

Many people with hepatitis experience no symptoms, and so they don't know they are infected, which is problematic for the spread of these viruses. Symptoms of acute hepatitis generally occur two to six weeks after infection, whereas chronic hepatitis can take years (even decades) for symptoms to appear. Symptoms include fever, nausea, vomiting, abdominal pain, extreme fatigue, loss of appetite, light-colored stools, dark urine, jaundice (yellowing of the skin and eyes), and joint pain. On average, symptoms occur about ninety days after infection—range of 60–150 days. There is no treatment for acute infections, but people with chronic infections are treated with antiviral medications and monitored regularly for liver damage and liver cancer.

How Prevalent Is It?

People at greatest risk for hepatitis B infections include infants born to infected mothers, drug users that share needles or other drug equipment, people who have unprotected sex with multiple partners, or individuals that live with a chronically infected person—there is an 11–57 percent reported infection rate among family members of hepatitis B surface antigen (HBsAg) carriers.[168,169,170,171] Anyone exposed to hepatitis B–infected blood can receive an HBIG injection to reduce the risk of infection.

According to the World Health Organization, hepatitis B is most prevalent in the Western Pacific and African regions, where just over 6 percent of the population is infected.[172] Because many don't know they are infected, other estimates suggest up to 10 percent of these populations are infected.[173] The Eastern Mediterranean, Southeast Asia, and European region have a prevalence rate of 1.6–3.3 percent, while only 0.7 percent of people in the Americas are infected. Hepatitis C is more common in the United States than hepatitis B, particularly since so many baby boomers were infected prior to the discovery of hepatitis C in 1989.

What Are the Health Risks of Hepatitis B?

Chronic hepatitis can lead to serious conditions like liver cirrhosis or liver cancer. About 25 percent of people who develop chronic hepatitis B as children and 15 percent who become chronically infected after childhood die prematurely from liver cirrhosis or liver cancer.[174,175] Worldwide, HBV represents the leading cause of liver cancer, causing 60–70 percent of cases globally—about sixteen cases per one hundred people in the world.[176] In the United States, hepatitis C more commonly causes liver cancer.[177] The high incidence of end-stage liver failure caused by chronic hepatitis B infection is associated with a high rate of mortality—15–40 percent of the chronically infected die within ten to twenty-five years.[178] Worldwide, 887,000 deaths were attributed to liver cirrhosis and liver cancer caused by hepatitis B in 2015.[179]

One thing to keep in mind when considering the risk of severe illness or death from viruses and other microbes is that there are trillions of pathogenic microbes around and within us. We are literally surrounded by them and come in contact with them every single day. Normally, these microbes are present in and on the human body without causing harm or death. Microbes literally occupy all of our body surfaces (skin, gut, and mucous membranes) and reside in our cells and blood. In fact, estimates suggest that we have between 30 and 37.2 trillion human cells and from 38 to 100 trillion bacterial cells in the human body, not to mention an untold number of viruses and fungi.[180,181,182,183] Few realize just how many bacteria we carry around each and every day because we are taught to fear all bacteria beginning at a young age.

Exposure to viruses has hugely influenced the human species. Indeed, our constant relationship with viruses has long been recognized as a key driver of adaptability in humans and life itself. Viruses are responsible for many of the mutations that have resulted in changes in the human genome and greater diversity.[184] Research suggests that an astonishing 30 percent of all protein adaptations in humans have been driven by viruses.[185] We now know that virtually any type of protein that comes in contact with a virus can participate in adaptations to that virus. Because viruses hijack the function of cells they infect to replicate and spread rapidly, they can trigger cellular adaptations, maybe more so than environmental triggers. Humans have an intimate relationship with microbes that has shaped and continues to shape who we are and how our bodies function.

The majority of microbes establish themselves as persistent settlers of our bodies. Experts believe that nearly half of all human DNA originated from viruses that infected our ancestors, inserting their genetic information (nucleic acid) into our ancestor's egg and sperm cells.[186] These tiny invaders have a shared interest in our survival because a dead host means dead microbes. And though some microbes do make us sick and even kill us, this usually is limited to people who have a dysfunctional immune system caused by underlying preexisting conditions (cardiorespiratory, metabolic, immune, and others) caused by years of poor lifestyle choices and exposure to toxic chemicals. Autoimmune disorders, diabetes, heart disease, obesity, and respiratory illnesses are characterized by dysregulation of normal immune function and inflammation.[187,188,189,190,191] People with these preexisting conditions are more likely to experience severe illness or mortality after infection with a microbe.

Viruses make us sick by disrupting cell function and killing healthy cells. Bacteria do the same but can also make toxins that destroy and disrupt cells or even trigger an enormous immune reaction that is itself toxic or multiply so rapidly that they crowd out healthy cells. Fungi invade tissues and disrupt their function, consume energy and nutrients intended for the host, and also produce toxic chemicals. The presence of or infection by a microbe does not always lead to illness, however. Instead, illness strikes when an immune system is weak and unable to mount a sufficient defense against the microbe. On the other hand, the immune system could be dysfunctional and trigger an overactive immune response that damages healthy cells and tissues in your body. In a twist of fate, we are betrayed and harmed by the very system that acts as our protector, our own immune system.

When pathogens enter the body and multiply excessively to become a threat, your immune system engages its troops and defenses—white blood cells, antibodies, and other mechanisms—to rid your body of the excess foreign invaders. Many of the classic symptoms of infection, such as fever, malaise, and headache, result from your immune system's reaction to the invader. A dysfunctional immune system can contain defective natural killer cells, which hyperactivate the inflammatory response and kill off too many cells in response to microbe invasion. During this uncontrolled and overactive immune response, the microbe causes significantly more damage within the body that can lead to organ failure. Once an infection progresses to these advanced stages, the immune system response can be more harmful than helpful if it is not resolved quickly and appropriately.

Left unresolved, an immune flare-up can ensue where the immune system overproduces cytokines and chemokines—small proteins involved in cell signaling and immune-inflammatory response to infections—and a surge of activated immune cells enter affected tissues. Basically, these chemical messengers provide instructions for the immune system to respond appropriately to infections and maintain a healthy state through efficient control of invading microbes. Called a cytokine storm, the infectious microbe prompts a massive number of activated white blood cells to release inflammatory cytokines, which in turn activate more white blood cells. During this dangerous feedback loop, the immune system goes haywire, and inflammation flares out of control. The resulting tissue inflammation allows the microbe to be more aggressive, causing severe illness and increasing the risk of mortality.[192,193] In the end, death results from collateral damage caused by an overactive immune system that is attempting to clear the microbe rather than limit the virulence factors it produces, not the microbe itself. Knowing this, we can limit severe illness and mortality caused by microbes by keeping our immune systems healthy in the first place and resolving the immune and inflammatory process that launches following infection.

Reviewing our close symbiotic relationship with viruses and other microbes and their influence on human genetics and cellular function, it is clear that humans require regular exposure to pathogens to remain in a state of health. In this way, pathogens help shape human physiological functions from early development to digestion and many other functions in between. Pathogens are not the enemy. They are part of our normal daily biological experience and often assist healthy physiological function. Illness and disease occur when this delicate system of biodiversity in and on the human body is compromised.

Some people experience HBV reactivation—reappearance or increased HBV in the DNA of a person with previously inactive or resolved hepatitis B. People undergoing cancer chemotherapy, taking immunosuppressive drugs, coinfected with hepatitis C or HIV, or undergoing organ or bone marrow transplant are at a greater risk of HBV reactivation. Reactivation can cause a flare in disease activity that is often accompanied by elevated liver enzymes with or without symptoms. Severe flares can be deadly. Since hepatitis B is largely lifestyle dependent, the risks and benefits of the vaccine should be weighed.

HepB Vaccine

Description

The HepB vaccine is given in three doses, at birth, one month, and six months. Although only infants born to mothers with hepatitis B need a dose at birth, some hospitals routinely give the vaccine to newborns even without parent's consent. Parents who wish to delay HepB vaccination should make their wishes clearly known to hospital staff.

A determined effort to reduce hepatitis B transmission by vaccinating high-risk populations (sexually promiscuous adults, IV drug users, and prostitutes) occurred in the 1980s. However, low compliance among these high-risk groups resulted in this being a failed attempt to eradicate the disease from the population. Mother-to-baby transmission was significantly reduced by proactive prenatal care and administration of HBIG, but again, this tackles only a small portion of new hepatitis B cases each year. This caused researchers to vaccinate every single baby even though protection was not needed until the teen years among teens who are sexually active or people who live with a chronically infected person. Outside of mother-to-baby transmission or infected-blood exposure, there is no real evidence that hepatitis B is a childhood infectious disease.

Vaccine Manufacturing Process

The HepB vaccine does not contain the actual hepatitis B virus. Instead, it is genetically engineered by combining parts of DNA from the hepatitis B virus with DNA from yeast cells (*Saccharomyces cerevisiae*) incubated in a solution of soy, sugar, minerals, and amino acids. Using recombinant DNA technology, this is called a recombinant vaccine. The yeast creates a hepatitis B protein—hepatitis B surface antigen—that is purified from the yeast and then combined with aluminum as an adjuvant to stimulate an immune system reaction when the vaccine is injected. The protein and aluminum are then added to a saline solution. The two most common HepB vaccines currently used are Recombivax HB (uses formaldehyde to purify the vaccine) and Engerix-B (does not use formaldehyde). There is also a newly approved—in 2017—two-dose vaccine called Heplisav-B (uses polysorbate 80 instead of formaldehyde) that uses a different yeast (*Hansenula polymorpha*) to produce the hepatitis B surface antigen and is aluminum-free. Instead, the hepatitis B surface antigen is combined with a small synthetic immunostimulatory adjuvant (cytosine phosphoguanine motifs—1018 adjuvant), which binds to toll-like receptor 9 to stimulate a directed immune response to the antigen.

Ingredients

Recombivax HB[194]

- Hepatitis B surface antigen (pediatric: 5 mcg per dose; adolescents/adults: 10 mcg)
- Aluminum (approximately 0.5 mg/mL; about 250 mcg per pediatric dose)
- Saline solution
- Yeast proteins
- Formaldehyde (<15 mcg/mL)

Engerix-B[195]

- Hepatitis B surface antigen (pediatric: 10 mcg per dose; adult: 20 mcg)
- Aluminum (pediatric: 250 mcg per dose; adult: 500 mcg per dose)
- Saline solution
- Phosphate buffer
- Yeast proteins
- Sodium chloride
- Sodium phosphate dibasic dehydrate
- Sodium phosphate monobasic dehydrate

Heplisav-B[196]

- Hepatitis B surface antigen (9.0 mg/mL)
- Sodium phosphate dibasic dodecahydrate
- Sodium phosphate monobasic dehydrate
- Cytosine phosphoguanine adjuvant
- Polysorbate 80

➢ Aluminum
➢ Cytosine phosphoguanine adjuvant
➢ Formaldehyde
➢ Polysorbate 80

Package Insert Adverse Reactions

Recombivax HB: Irritability, fever, diarrhea, fatigue/weakness, diminished appetite, and rhinitis (>1% of injections in healthy infants).

Engerix-B: Injection-site soreness (22%), fatigue (14%), dizziness (1%–10%), headache (1%–10%), fever (1%–10%), injection-site redness, swelling, or hardening (1%–10%), upper respiratory tract infection (<1%), enlarged lymph nodes (<1%), anorexia (<1%), agitation (<1%), insomnia (<1%), drowsiness (<1%), tingling (<1%), flushing (<1%), low blood pressure (<1%), abdominal pain (<1%), constipation or diarrhea (<1%), nausea/vomiting (<1%), itching (<1%), rash or hives (<1%), sweating (<1%), joint, muscle, or back pain (<1%), stiffness (<1%), chills (<1%), flu-like symptoms (<1%), irritability (<1%), and weakness (<1%). Subjects reporting serious adverse events were about 2.1 percent, and potentially immune-mediated adverse events occurring within seven months of first dose were 0.7 percent.

Heplisav-B: Injection-site pain (23%–39%), fatigue (11%–17%), headache (8%–17%), general malaise (7%–9%), and fever (<1.6%). Subjects reporting serious adverse events were about 1.5 percent, and potentially immune-mediated adverse events occurring within seven months of first dose were 0.2 percent.

Parent or Healthcare Provider Adverse Events Reported through VAERS

Recombivax HB: Allergic and hypersensitivity reactions, anaphylaxis, bronchospasms, hives, joint pain or arthritis, pain in the extremities, fever, reddening of the skin, lupus, lupus-like syndrome, vasculitis, polyarteritis nodosa (inflammation of the blood vessels that damages organ systems), elevated liver enzymes, constipation, Guillain-Barré syndrome, multiple sclerosis, exacerbation of multiple sclerosis, myelitis, seizure, febrile seizure, neuropathy, Bell's palsy, radiculopathy (dysfunction of one or more nerves), Stevens-Johnson syndrome, alopecia, petechiae (brown spots on the skin as a result of bleeding), increased erythrocyte sedimentation rate, thrombocytopenia, irritability, agitation, excessive tiredness, optic neuritis, tinnitus, conjunctivitis, visual disturbances, uveitis, temporary loss of consciousness, and tachycardia.

Energix-B: Shingles, meningitis, thrombocytopenia, anaphylaxis, allergic and hypersensitivity reactions, fever, joint pain or arthritis, hives, encephalitis, encephalopathy, migraine, multiple sclerosis, neuritis, neuropathy, loss of sensation, pins-and-needles feeling, Guillain-Barré syndrome, Bell's palsy, optic neuritis, paralysis, muscle weakness, seizures, temporary loss of consciousness, transverse myelitis, conjunctivitis, tinnitus, vertigo, heart palpitations, tachycardia, vasculitis, temporary cessation of breathing, bronchospasms, asthma-like symptoms, upset stomach, alopecia, angioedema (swelling beneath the skin), eczema, erythema multiforme, Stevens-Johnson syndrome, erythema nodosum, lichen planus, purpura, abnormal-liver-function tests, and injection-site reactions.

Heplisav-B: Not reported.

Reactions Observed and Documented in Published Research

The first case studies to propose a link between the onset or worsening of multiple sclerosis (MS) and vaccination/inoculation dates back to the 1967 wherein the *British Medical Journal* describes nine cases of MS after immunization.[197] The *British Medical Journal* also states that two additional published reports in 1959 and 1965 and several German authors had previously documented a temporal relation between vaccination and the development of MS.[198,199,200] These cases of vaccine/inoculation-related MS tended to be less severe than MS that spontaneously develops. While the development of MS shortly after vaccination does not imply a causal connection, the evidence as a whole—including the clinical manifestations of the MS—supports a suspicion that vaccination has some role in an insult to health that aggravates existing MS or triggers an earlier onset of MS in a person who ultimately would have spontaneously developed the condition.

One vaccine consistently associated with MS is the HepB vaccine, especially in France where an aggressive mass HepB vaccine campaign was instituted in a short period of time during the 1990s. In 1994, French health authorities mandated that all first-year students of secondary school receive the vaccine. The very next year, the HepB vaccine was added to the routine immunization schedule for babies and preteens, and the adult population was strongly encouraged to be vaccinated. MS cases increased significantly in France the same year in which widespread vaccination happened. An upsurge in MS diagnoses among vaccinated adults triggered an investigation by the French national pharmacovigilance system (ANSM) in 1994. Ultimately, the inquiry discovered enough of an association that French health authorities abruptly discontinued school-based vaccination of preteens with HepB in 1998. That same year, adult HepB vaccination declined because of media reports of postvaccine MS.

Several studies evaluated the correlation between HepB vaccination and MS over the next decade. Most of the studies found no direct connection[201,202,203,204,205] or a statistically insignificant link between HepB vaccination and MS.[206,207,208] However, the incidence of MS after HepB vaccination is thought to be grossly underreported because it is not as severe as spontaneous MS and tends to resolve rather than become chronic. Indeed, a study found that it was underreported, and the risk of HepB vaccine-associated MS was two to two and a half times higher than the number reported by French health authorities.[209]

Based on the identified methodological limitations of the earlier studies, additional researchers set out to determine the real risk of MS after HepB vaccination not only in France but also other countries. Assessing medical records in the General Practice Research Database (GPRD) in the United Kingdom, a 2004 study found the HepB vaccine triples the risk of MS.[210] A US study published in 2005 found evidence that suggested not only did the HepB vaccine increase the risk of MS in adults fivefold, but also it increased the risk of rheumatoid arthritis, optic neuritis, alopecia, vasculitis, lupus, and thrombocytopenia.[211] A worldwide pattern of MS-like symptoms following the HepB vaccine was clearly emerging.

Later on, another neurological disorder was linked to the HepB vaccine in children. Researchers found that the risk of central nervous system inflammatory demyelination (ID) in French children dramatically increased from 1994 to 2003. The start of the significant increase in ID correlated directly with the year French authorities aggressively vaccinated children with HepB. ID is a condition that occurs when the body's immune system mistakenly attacks the protective coating around the nerves called myelin. Demyelination of the nerves causes neurological problems, including MS. Further analysis of the data determined that the HepB vaccine does not generally cause an increased risk of ID during childhood, but appears to take years to develop, increasing the risk of ID and MS later in life.[212] An evaluation of official French data and also from the national pharmacovigilance agency in 2014 revealed a significant correlation between HepB vaccination and MS. The conclusion was that MS cases increased by 65 percent in the years following the aggressive HepB vaccination campaign.[213] It should be noted that thimerosal was still used as the preservative in the HepB vaccine during this era, so it may have been the major factor contributing to increased MS and ID. Mercury is a neurotoxin that is known to damage myelin and higher mercury levels are observed in the cerebrospinal fluid and blood of people with MS. Today, HepB vaccines do not contain thimerosal.

Another central nervous system disorder, Guillain-Barré syndrome (GBS), may be associated with the HepB vaccine. GBS is a rare neurological disorder where the body's immune system attacks its own peripheral nervous system. Weakness and tingling in the extremities are usually the first symptoms, which quickly spreads, paralyzing the whole body. Certain mutated genes (e.g., CD1E and CD1A) are associated with an increased risk of GBS in humans.[214] It is possible that people who carry these mutated genes are more likely to experience GBS following receipt of the HepB vaccine. In any case, a strong association with vaccination (influenza and HepB) and the risk of GBS was observed during a fifteen-year period.[215] GBS occurred in 77.4 percent of cases within six weeks of vaccination. Researchers noted that 63.2 percent of cases were related to the influenza vaccine and 9.4 percent to HepB. The highest incidence of GBS occurred in people who received the influenza vaccine followed by the HepB vaccine, suggesting a combined toxic effect of multiple vaccines within a short period of time. Death and disability occurred 3.2 and 16.7 percent of the time in vaccine-related GBS, respectively. It can't be ruled out that a genetic predisposition is involved in the occurrence of GBS after vaccination or that mercury resulted in damaged myelin that caused the neurological conditions. Continued monitoring of neurological disorders following immunization will help uncover if this was a temporary association or continues to be a problem.

A group of studies also claim the trivalent (containing three hepatitis B virus antigens) HepB vaccine is associated with developmental delays. Developmental delays occur when a child does not reach developmental milestones at the expected times. It must be an ongoing pattern and not a temporary lag behind his peers. The odds for boys receiving special education services was approximately nine times higher in vaccinated boys compared to unvaccinated boys after adjusting for confounding variables.[216] At the time of vaccination, this vaccine still contained thimerosal, which may account for the increased risk of developmental delays. Additional studies confirm this assumption showing a significantly increased risk of developmental delays in children receiving the thimerosal-containing HepB vaccine in comparison to those receiving the thimerosal-reduced version.[217,218] However, keep in mind that most of the current vaccines contain another known neurotoxin, aluminum. It is no wonder government health agencies recommended the removal of thimerosal from vaccines.

A link between autism and HepB vaccination has also been examined in observational research. The way autism develops in the brain indicates it involves a chronic and substantial inflammatory reaction combined with brain-cell damage. Suggestive of an insult from a toxic substance rather than a developmental problem, multiple toxic substances have been implicated as a contributing factor to the development of autism, including mercury. In fact, of ninety-one studies evaluated in a review, the majority (74 percent) suggest that mercury exposure is a risk factor for autism.[219] The odds of an autism diagnosis in boys born prior to 1999 (when thimerosal was still widely used in childhood vaccines), adjusted for race, maternal education, and two-parent household, was evaluated using data from the National Health Interview Survey 1997–2002. Boys vaccinated as newborns had a threefold greater odds of being diagnosed with autism when compared to unvaccinated boys or boys vaccinated after the first month of life.[220] Non-Caucasian boys were the most likely to be diagnosed with autism. During the first year of a child's life, the brain doubles in size. Much of this growth occurs in the cerebellum—an area of the brain that coordinates voluntary movements, including speech, and is involved in social interactions. Abnormal function of the cerebellum disrupts brain circuitry that can cause neurochemical and behavioral changes related to the development of autism.[221,222,223] Introduction of mercury through thimerosal-containing vaccines during this first year of life may have contributed to cerebellar dysfunction and the development of autism.

Recognizing the concerns about the HepB vaccine and neurological disorders, the Institute of Medicine (US) Immunization Safety Review Committee assessed the risks and published its findings in 2002. They concluded that the available evidence favors denial of a causal relationship between the HepB vaccine and MS, but the evidence remains unclear whether a causal relationship exists for ID, optic

56

neuritis, GBS, and brachial neuritis.[224] Overall, this committee determined "there is weak evidence for biological mechanisms by which hepatitis B vaccination could possibly influence an individual's risk of the central or peripheral nervous system disorders."

Evidence suggests that cases of rheumatoid arthritis increase after receiving the HepB vaccine. Risk of chronic arthritis was significantly higher in adults who received the HepB vaccine when compared to adults who received the tetanus vaccine.[225] In addition, chronic arthritis has been diagnosed in children about sixteen days after HepB vaccination, which persists for at least one year. An earlier study that examined eleven cases of rheumatoid arthritis following HepB vaccination found that certain individuals may be genetically susceptible to HepB vaccine-associated rheumatoid arthritis.[226] Rheumatoid arthritis lasted for more than six months in all cases and persisted in all but two cases four years later. The subjects tested positive for a group of genes—human leucocyte antigen (HLA) class II, which have been linked to a higher risk of rheumatoid arthritis.[227,228] The researchers found that some of the proteins from the HepB vaccine bound to these genes, which may trigger the development of rheumatoid arthritis in genetically susceptible individuals. Since this study was published in 1998, thimerosal could be to blame again. Higher mercury levels have been found in people diagnosed with rheumatoid arthritis and mercury is known to provoke autoimmune and inflammatory bone and joint disorders.[229,230] It is also possible that the vaccine itself or other vaccine ingredients, like aluminum adjuvants, are provoking a sustained inflammatory response and elevated immune response that triggers autoimmunity.

Although the idea of vaccine injury is not universally accepted, emerging evidence suggests that some people may be genetically susceptible—increased likelihood of developing a particular condition because of genetic makeup—to adverse reactions or the development of conditions following vaccination. A genetic predisposition results from inherited variations (mutations) in one or more genes. However, having genetic variations doesn't guarantee a person will develop the condition associated with the gene. Instead, a trigger, usually in the form of an environmental exposure, diet, or other lifestyle factors, initiates the development of the condition. Emerging evidence suggests that further research into genetic variants and whether vaccines trigger the development of conditions in people with them is necessary.

See the *Reactions Observed and Documented in Published Research* section of chapter 9 for a discussion of immune thrombocytopenia associated with HepB vaccination.

See the *Reactions Observed and Documented in Published Research* section of chapter 4 for a discussion on sudden and unexpected deaths in children and infants in relation to vaccines containing HepB.

INFECTION RISKS	VACCINE RISKS
Chronic hepatitis B	Multiple sclerosis
Liver cirrhosis	Guillain-Barré syndrome
Liver cancer	Inflammatory demyelination
Death	Rheumatoid arthritis
	Optic neuritis
	Alopecia
	Vasculitis
	Lupus
	Thrombocytopenia
	Sudden infant death syndrome

3

Rotavirus (RV)

What Is Rotavirus Infection?

Rotavirus is a highly contagious virus that can cause severe watery diarrhea, vomiting, fever (usually greater than 102°F [39°C]), and abdominal pain. It is the most common cause of diarrhea in infants and children worldwide and reportedly caused 128,500 deaths among children in 2016, of which 95 percent occurred in sub-Saharan Africa.[231] Symptoms usually begin about two days after infection, with vomiting and diarrhea that can last from three to eight days. Additional symptoms may include dehydration and loss of appetite, which are particularly concerning in infants and young children. Parents should seek immediate medical attention if signs of dehydration like decreased urination, crying with no tears, dry mouth and throat, dizziness when standing up, or unusual sleepiness or fussiness is noticed in their children. To avoid dehydration, extra fluids should be given to children if infected.

Rotaviruses are classified into several groups depending on serotyping or genotyping of the proteins present. The most common rotavirus strains that affect humans are G1, G2, G3, G4, G9, and G12. Of these, the G1 strain accounts for the majority of infections.

Rotavirus is present in an infected person's stool several days before symptoms appear—although the incubation period is short, usually less than forty-eight hours—and remains for up to ten days after symptoms subside. Persons with a compromised immune system may have detectable levels of rotavirus for more than thirty days after infection. The virus sheds—expulsion and release of virus from the infected person—in high concentration in the stool of infected persons. Proper handwashing is very important to reduce virus spread as well as cleaning surfaces with a disinfectant. If an infected person fails to wash their hands after using the toilet, the virus can spread to anything they touch. The virus spreads easily via hand-to-mouth contact after touching a contaminated surface or the hands of an infected person. Transmission through contaminated food or water is uncommon.

Unfortunately, the clinical features and stool characteristics of rotavirus-caused infectious diarrhea are indistinguishable from other common diarrheal illnesses and may be confused with illness caused by other common pathogens, such as *Salmonella*, *Shigella*, and *Campylobacter* bacteria. Laboratory testing is required to confirm rotavirus infection (e.g., detection of rotavirus antigen in stool). Although rotavirus can be detected in the serum of infected people three to seven days after disease onset, blood tests are less commonly used to confirm diagnosis. Diarrhea that is watery, exceptionally foul smelling, and lasts more than a few days may be evidence that your child has rotavirus illness.

Mild Cases	Moderate Cases	Severe Cases
✓ A few loose stools daily	✓ Multiple loose stools daily	✓ Multiple loose stools daily
✓ Lasts several days	✓ Lasts several days	✓ Lasts several days
✓ Mild fever	✓ Mild fever	✓ Mild fever
✓ Possibly accompanied by vomiting	✓ Excessive vomiting (infants may vomit after each feeding)	✓ Excessive vomiting (infants may vomit after each feeding)
✓ Child can keep fluids down	✓ Difficult to keep fluids down (mild dehydration)	✓ Symptoms of dehydration present

Mild cases of rotavirus can usually be handled at home. Moderate cases usually require a visit to your healthcare professional. Severe cases require emergency medical attention, and infants who are severely dehydrated may require intravenous fluids. Your child can get rotavirus more than once, but subsequent infections are generally milder.

How Prevalent Is It?

In temperate climates, rotavirus infections are very common during colder months. It is so prevalent that the question is not if but when your child will get infected and how severe the illness will be. Infants who are breastfed and not taken to day care are at low risk of being infected during the first year of life (when it is riskiest). Each year, rotavirus is responsible for about 114 million cases of infectious diarrhea that require home care only, 24 million that require a visit to a healthcare professional, and 2.4 million hospitalizations in children under age five.[232] Children over age 5 tend to fare better with one in five visiting a doctor and one in fifty requiring hospitalization. Chances are that parents frequently manage a case of diarrhea at home and never even know their children were infected with rotavirus.

Nearly all children under the age of five were infected by rotavirus in the prevaccine era, causing an estimated three million infections annually in the United States alone.[233] Despite such a high infection rate, fewer than sixty deaths occurred annually during this era. Low mortality in developed countries shows that the overwhelming majority of rotavirus cases are not deadly when appropriate home or medical care is sought. It is the lack of proper medical care during serious infections, often causing severe dehydration, that makes rotavirus deadly.

What Are the Health Risks of Rotavirus Infection?

Severe diarrhea can lead to dehydration and left untreated the dehydration can become life-threatening. Globally, rotavirus infections cause thirty-three deaths per one hundred thousand population in children under age 5.[234] India and sub-Saharan Africa experience higher mortality rates. Other countries significantly affected include Nigeria, Pakistan, and the Democratic Republic of Congo. Combined, these countries account for nearly all rotavirus infection deaths. Estimates suggest the rotavirus vaccine prevented approximately twenty-eight thousand global deaths in 2016.[235] Inadequate medical care is a major reason these countries experience higher mortality rates after rotavirus infection.

Electrolyte imbalance and metabolic acidosis are also complications of rotavirus infection. Electrolytes are minerals (sodium, calcium, potassium, chloride, phosphate, and magnesium) in your body that have an electrical charge. They help regulate hydration, your body's pH level, move nutrients into and wastes out of cells, and are involved in nerve, muscle, heart, and brain function. Electrolyte imbalance occurs when you have insufficient or, less commonly, too many electrolytes in your body. This can cause irregular heartbeat, shortness of breath, confusion, fatigue, nausea, convulsions, and gastrointestinal disturbances.

Metabolic acidosis is a condition characterized by too much acid in the body fluids. This can occur from overproduction of acid by the body or when the kidneys do not remove acid from the body efficiently. It is frequently seen in critically ill individuals. Symptoms include rapid and shallow breathing, confusion, fatigue, jaundice, rapid heartbeat, and lack of appetite.

Immunocompromised children can experience prolonged rotavirus-caused infectious diarrhea or even abnormalities in multiple organs, especially the liver and kidneys. About one-third of immunocompromised individuals with rotavirus infection will require adjustments in the treatment of their preexisting condition—the condition that causes them to have a weakened immune system—during rotavirus infection.[236]

Rotavirus Vaccine

Description

The first rotavirus vaccine (RotaShield) was created by combining cow or monkey rotavirus with human rotavirus (called a combination or reassortment virus). The purpose of this combination is for the human part of the virus to provide immunity against severe illness and the monkey or cow part to weaken the vaccine virus so it doesn't cause severe vomiting or diarrhea. The rhesus-based tetravalent rotavirus vaccine (RRV-TV, RotaShield) was withdrawn from the market in 1998 because of its association with intussusception—a condition in which one part of the intestine folds into another part. The CDC estimates that this occurs in as many as one in twenty thousand infants who get the rotavirus vaccine.[237]

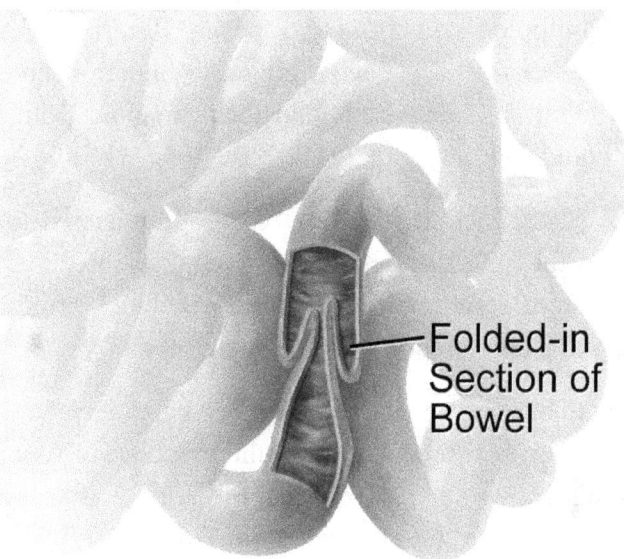

—Folded-in Section of Bowel

Intussusception of the Bowel

Currently, there are two rotavirus vaccines licensed for use in the United States: RV5 (RotaTeq) and RV1 (Rotarix). A third three-dose vaccine is under development called RV3-BB, which is intended to be given at birth (0–5 days, 8 weeks, and 14 weeks). All of these vaccines are oral solutions, rather than injections. RotaTeq is given as a three-dose series beginning at two months of age (but no later than the fifteenth week of life), then again at four and six months. Rotarix is a two-dose series given at two months (but no later than the fifteenth week of life) and four mounts of age. RVS-BB contains the single human rotavirus strain RV3 and has completed early clinical trials but is not available at the time of this writing.

Vaccine Manufacturing Process

RotaTeq uses crossbreeding of five different strains of rotavirus from infected humans and cows. These viruses are genetically engineered and grown in monkey kidney cells (VERO). The virus is then filtered out of these cells and placed in a liquid solution.

Instead of multiple strains from two species, Rotarix uses a single strain (G1p, 89-12 strain) of the most common human rotavirus. It too is grown in monkey kidney cells and then removed from the cells and added to liquid solution.

Both vaccines are whole and live when administered to humans and multiply in the intestines to produce a mild infection. The body's immune system responds to this mild infection, priming it to react effectively to a real infection if it occurs.

Something to be aware of for caregivers is that the live virus can be shed in diapers for up to fifteen days after the first dose of vaccine. Evidence suggests this occurs about 10 percent of the time after the first dose of RotaTeq but not after the second and third dose.[238] Virus shedding may be more common after Rotarix (50% average; 21%–80% range) and continues for a few weeks after the second dose.[239] People, especially children, with compromised immune systems should avoid contact with stool from an immunized child to prevent transmission and vaccine-caused illness.[240]

Ingredients

RotaTeq[241]

- Five live and whole-virus strains (cow and human)
- Sucrose
- Sodium citrate
- Sodium phosphate monobasic monohydrate
- Sodium hydroxide
- Polysorbate 80
- Cell-culture media
- Fetal bovine (cow) serum
- Porcine (pig) circoviruses PCV-1 and PCV-2 DNA (contaminant)

Rotarix[242]

- Single human rotavirus strain, live and whole
- Amino acids
- Dextran
- Dulbecco's Modified Eagle Medium (contains sodium chloride, potassium chloride, magnesium sulfate, ferric [III] nitrate, sodium phosphate, sodium pyruvate, D-glucose, concentrated vitamin solution, L-cystine, L-tyrosine, amino acids solution, L-glutamine, calcium chloride, sodium hydrogenocarbonate, and phenol red)
- Sorbitol
- Sucrose
- Liquid diluent (contains calcium carbonate, sterile water, and xanthan gum)
- Porcine (pig) circovirus PCV-1 DNA (contaminant)

Controversial Ingredients

- ➤ Monkey kidney cells
- ➤ Fetal bovine serum
- ➤ Polysorbate 80
- ➤ Porcine circoviruses DNA

RotaTeq: common—diarrhea, vomiting, irritability, ear infection, cold involving swelling of the nasal passages and back of the throat (nasopharyngitis), and constriction of respiratory passages (bronchospasms). Serious adverse events occurred in 2.4 percent of vaccine recipients and included bronchiolitis, gastroenteritis, pneumonia, fever, and urinary tract infections. Fifty-two deaths—most commonly sudden infant death syndrome—were reported across all clinical studies, of which twenty-five occurred in the RotaTeq groups. Rarely (< 0.1%), seizures were reported.

Rotarix: common—fussiness/irritability, cough, runny nose, fever, loss of appetite, and vomiting. Serious adverse events occurred in 1.7 percent of vaccine recipients within thirty-one days of vaccination. During the course of eight clinical studies, sixty-eight deaths were reported following administration of Rotarix. The most common cause of death reported was pneumonia.

Note: Children with severe combined immunodeficiency (SCIDS) should not receive the rotavirus vaccine because the live viruses in them can cause severe reactions.[243] In addition, infants with birth defects involving malformation of the gastrointestinal tract or a history of intussusception should not receive the vaccine because of a possible increased risk of intussusception.[244,245]

Parent or Healthcare Provider Adverse Events Reported through VAERS

RotaTeq: Intussusception (some fatal), Kawasaki disease, blood in stools, gastroenteritis with vaccine shedding, anaphylaxis, hives, swelling beneath the skin (angioedema), transmission of vaccine virus to others.

Rotarix: Intussusception (some fatal), recurrent intussusception (some fatal), Kawasaki disease, blood in stools, gastroenteritis with vaccine shedding, immune thrombocytopenia.

Some serious adverse events that require hospitalization, result in permanent disability, or were life-threatening are associated with rotavirus vaccines. One of these serious adverse events is intussusception mentioned earlier. Globally, intussusception is the most common cause of intestinal obstruction. Any condition, like viral enteritis and irritable bowel syndrome–diarrhea, which causes increased motility (hyperperistaltism or hypermotility) of the intestinal tract predisposes a person to intussusception. Intussusception is most likely to occur three to seven days after vaccination if it occurs. Reports in VAERS suggest intussusception and Kawasaki disease—a condition characterized by inflammation of the blood vessels throughout the body that primarily affects children under five—with intestinal involvement are significantly associated with the RotaTeq vaccine.[246,247] More recent information that included Rotarix and RotaTeq and calculated data from ten studies determined the relative risk for intussusception was 5.71 (one to seven days after the first dose), 1.69 after the second dose, and 1.14 after the third per 100,000 vaccinated children.[248] The study also found that risk of intussusception increases with the age of the infant, particularly among those receiving their first vaccination after three months of age. Based on this data, it may be best to administer the first dose of rotavirus vaccine before three months of age. It is well known that there is a small risk of intussusception associated with rotavirus infection as well. In fact, the risk of intussusception is twenty-six to ninety cases per 100,000 live births during the first three years of life (most commonly from 6–30 months of age),[249,250] suggesting it occurs spontaneously more often than could be attributable to the vaccine.

INFECTION RISKS	VACCINE RISKS
Dehydration	Intussusception
Electrolyte imbalance	Kawasaki disease
Metabolic acidosis	
Organ dysfunction	
(immunocompromised children)	
Intussusception	
Death (rare with appropriate care)	

4

Diphtheria, Tetanus, Pertussis (DTaP) & Tetanus, Diphtheria, and Pertussis (Tdap)

What Are Diphtheria, Tetanus, and Pertussis Infections?

Diphtheria is a serious bacterial infection that typically affects the mucous membranes of the nose and throat (nasopharyngeal diphtheria). If diphtheria infects the skin it is called cutaneous diphtheria. Diphtheria can be treated with intravenous antitoxin and antibiotics in a hospital. Most children recover with this treatment protocol without any lingering effects, but infection can be deadly even with treatment, especially in very young children. Delayed treatment can allow the toxin to cause excess damage to the airways. Early diagnosis by a qualified professional is important because many of the symptoms of diphtheria are similar to other common infections like strep throat and croup. The major indication of diphtheria is the white coating on the throat or inside the nose.

Diphtheria is caused by the *Corynebacterium diphtheriae* bacteria, which usually multiplies on or near the surface of the throat. Certain strains of the bacteria secrete a potent exotoxin that damages tissues in the immediate area of the infection. Whether it causes diphtheria illness depends on the ability of the bacteria to colonize the nasopharyngeal cavity or the skin, and its ability to produce this toxin. The bacteria

69

spreads by airborne droplets or secretions (when an infected person coughs or sneezes) or through direct contact with contaminated items or people. Unlike viruses, bacteria can persist on surfaces for long periods. The *Corynebacterium diphtheriae* bacterium can survive on dry inanimate surfaces for up to six months.[251] The illness spreads easily in crowded areas and among people living in unsanitary conditions.

Diphtheria can cause only mild illness (sore throat and visible coatings on the tonsils or nasal passages) or no obvious signs at all in some people. Others will experience the characteristic symptoms that usually begin two to five days after infection and may include a thick gray membrane covering the throat and tonsils, sore throat, hoarseness, nasal discharge, fever, chills, swollen lymph nodes in the neck, and difficulty or rapid breathing. Moderate cases can cause labored breathing as the throat and airway swelling. Cutaneous diphtheria causes pain, swelling, and redness of the skin, and may produce ulcers covered by a gray membrane.

Tetanus is a serious illness caused by *Clostridium tetani* bacteria that lives in the soil, saliva, dust, and manure. It can also live in the intestinal system of animals (dogs, cats, cattle, horses, sheep, rodents, and chickens). The bacteria can enter the body through a deep cut or severe burn after contact with contaminated objects. Less commonly, it enters the body through superficial wounds, crush injuries, insect bites, IV drug use, intramuscular injections, chronic sores, during surgical or dental procedures, or after a compound fracture. Once inside the body, the germ multiples and produces a potent toxin that enters the nerves and causes tightening of the muscles all over the body, frequently the jaw. Tetanus is sometimes called lockjaw because it commonly affects the jaw first. Unlike other infectious conditions, tetanus is not spread from person to person.

A tetanus immune globulin injection is given if a person suspects they may have been exposed to the bacteria or as a preventive with certain wounds—dirty wounds, puncture wounds, or trauma wounds. An injured person should have this shot within forty-eight hours of the injury. This works by providing your body with antibodies against the tetanus bacterium until your body produces its own. Derived from antibodies of donated human blood, it provides immediate, short-term protection against the bacteria. A booster tetanus vaccine is also recommended within forty-eight hours of injury if the injured person hasn't had one in the last five years.

Symptoms usually occur from three to twenty-one days after infection (average of ten days), but they can even occur several months after. The more heavily a wound is contaminated, the more quickly symptoms will occur. Generalized tetanus occurs when the toxins spread into the spinal cord and brain, affecting the entire nervous system. Symptoms of generalized tetanus include jaw cramping, painful muscle tightness all over the body, difficulty swallowing, muscle spasms (often abdominal), fever, headache, seizures, and changes in blood pressure or heart rate. If a tetanus shot and a tetanus immune globulin injection are not given in time to an unvaccinated individual after injury, the infection can progress rapidly. In this case, people can be hospitalized for many weeks and even require life support. Less commonly, tetanus will produce localized symptoms—muscle weakness and intense painful spasms—at the site of infection. Most cases of tetanus occur in children under the age of 5.

Pertussis, or whooping cough, is a highly contagious respiratory tract infection caused by the *Bordetella pertussis* bacteria. It gets the name whooping cough because people often make a "whoop" sound when they inhale after a hacking cough fit. Coughing fits are prolonged—lasting from thirty seconds to two minutes—and make it difficult to breathe during one. The bacterium attaches to the cilia (tiny, hair-like extensions) that line the upper respiratory tract and once there releases toxins and biologically active products—pertussis toxin, filamentous hemagglutinin, agglutinogens, adenylate cyclase, pertactin, and tracheal cytotoxin—that cause severe irritation and damage to the cilia. This results in swollen airways (inflammation) and reduced clearance of respiratory secretions. Community outbreaks of pertussis can even infect fully vaccinated individuals, although the illness is usually less severe.

It is spread when an infected person coughs or sneezes, releasing germ-laden airborne droplets that people nearby breathe in. Once infected, mild symptoms that resemble the common cold—severe cough, runny nose, nasal congestion, fever, and red, watery eyes—begin about seven to ten days later. Symptoms may get even worse a week or two later and include vomiting, extreme fatigue, and the characteristic "whoop" sound when you breathe in after a coughing fit. In some people, the "whoop" noise never develops. Instead, they only experience a persistent hacking cough. Pertussis affects infants differently than older children, teens, and adults. Infants may struggle to breathe, or even stop breathing temporarily, instead of coughing. Coughing fits caused by pertussis can last ten weeks or more, which gives it another nickname, the "hundred-day cough." Persistent coughs happen after pertussis infection because significant damage occurred to the airways that has not been repaired even after the infection is cleared. The majority of cases are mild in toddlers, older children, teens, and adults. Infants and young children may experience moderate-to-severe cases and require hospitalization. People are most contagious for the two weeks following the start of the cough.

How Prevalent Are They?

Diphtheria is rare in industrialized countries today. Early in the twentieth century it was common with more than 200,000 yearly cases in the United States alone. In 2017, 8,819 cases of diphtheria were reported worldwide.[252] Interestingly, a significant portion of cases is among those who have already been vaccinated. High-risk countries reported that 34 percent of pertussis cases occurred in vaccinated individuals, while 32 percent of pertussis cases were diagnosed in those already vaccinated in lower-risk countries.[253] Combining the statistics, roughly one-third of modern diphtheria cases occur in people who have been vaccinated. This suggests that vaccine efficacy is waning and some have called for additional boosters to reduce infection occurrence and a resurgence of the illness. The majority of people who are infected are under the age of 15. Diphtheria is most common in Southeast Asia, with India reporting the highest incidence.[254] Collectively, up to 99 percent of cases occur in India, Nepal, and Indonesia.

Tetanus occurs worldwide but is most common in densely populated regions with hot, damp climates and soil rich in organic matter, especially where contact with animal manure is more likely. It is estimated that at least one million cases of tetanus require medical treatment each year.[255] Neonatal tetanus (acquired through infection of the unhealed umbilical stump) accounts for about half of all cases in developing countries, whereas injury-related cases account for about 70 percent of cases in developed countries.[256] Delayed treatment of tetanus can be fatal. Tetanus is fatal in about 6 percent of mild to moderate cases and can be as high as 60 percent in severe cases.[257]

The World Health Organization reported 151,074 pertussis cases and eighty-nine thousand related deaths in 2018.[258] However, a publication modeling pertussis cases and deaths worldwide suggests more than twenty-four million cases of pertussis and 160,700 related deaths occur each year in children under age 5.[259] This is a significant discrepancy between actual reported cases and estimated cases. Africa is the hardest-hit region, accounting for 33 percent of global cases and 58 percent of total deaths. Pertussis appears to follow a five-year cycle of rises and falls in confirmed cases.

What Are the Health Risks of Diphtheria, Tetanus, and Pertussis?

One of the greatest risks of diphtheria is airway blockage. In its advanced stages the illness can damage the heart, kidneys, and nerves. The overall fatality rate for diphtheria (5–10 percent) has remained consistent for about the last fifty years, with rates higher among children younger than 5 and adults older than 40—up to 20 percent.[260] Left untreated, up to 50 percent of people can die from the illness, especially the young and old, and those with a preexisting medical condition.

Proper medical care of deep and dirty wounds—flushing of wounds with clean water and disinfectant—makes tetanus uncommon today. However, serious health problems can occur if tetanus is left untreated or if the wound is not sufficiently cleaned. They include difficulty breathing and swallowing, uncontrolled tightening of the vocal cords, pulmonary embolism (blockage of one of the arteries in the lungs caused by blood clots that have traveled from other areas of the body), broken bones, and aspiration pneumonia. Tetanus is fatal in about 11 percent of reported cases, with the elderly most likely to die from the infection.[261] In 2017, just over thirty-eight thousand deaths were attributed to tetanus worldwide, of which 30,848 were newborn children.[262,263] Infants in developing countries are obviously at the greatest risk from tetanus infection. This is primarily due to improper cord stump care (even cutting the cord with a non-sterile instrument) that delays healing and cord separation following birth.

Infants and young children are the most likely to experience serious complications of pertussis. About half of babies younger than 1 year old require hospitalization and of those treated in the hospital, many have complications, such as apnea—slowed or stopped breathing (61 percent), pneumonia (23 percent), convulsions (1.1 percent), and encephalopathy—brain disease that alters function (0.3 percent).[264] Approximately one in hundred will die (1 percent).

Older children, teens, and adults rarely experience complications from pertussis infection and may not even realize they are infected. Despite this, occasional complications do occur and include weight loss (33 percent), loss of bladder control (28 percent), pneumonia (2 percent), passing out (6 percent), and broken ribs during violent coughing fits (4 percent).[265] Other complications include dehydration, difficulty sleeping, hernias, ear infection, and epistaxis (acute hemorrhage from the nasal cavity, nostrils, or nasopharynx). More severe complications among all ages may include subdural hematomas (bleeding in the brain), refractory pulmonary hypertension (high blood pressure in the lungs and right side of the heart), pneumothorax (collapsed lung), and rectal prolapse (part of the rectum protrudes from the anus).

Diphtheria, Tetanus, and Pertussis Vaccine

Description

These three vaccines are discussed together because they are available in a combination vaccine known as DTaP (for children) or Tdap (for adolescents and adults). They can also be given individually. Combination diphtheria and tetanus (Td) vaccines are available (when pertussis vaccination is contraindicated) as well as a vaccine with tetanus only. Attempts to eradicate pertussis, tetanus, and diphtheria by the combination vaccine have proven unsuccessful partly because the vaccines only have an efficacy rate of 80–90 percent.[266] In addition, waning immunity among adults means that they are a breeding ground for pertussis and a common source of transmission to infants and others.

DTaP is given at two months, four months, and six months, with boosters given at fifteen to twenty months, and between four and six years old, and the Tdap version is given at age twelve. Tdap has a reduced dose of diphtheria and pertussis antigens and is approved for children starting at age 11 and adults age 18–64. It is also recommended for children ages 7 through 10 years who are not fully vaccinated. It is recommended that adults receive the Tdap once as well.

There are six pediatric DTaP vaccines licensed for use in the United States: Daptacel, Infanrix, Kinrix, Pediarix, Pentacel, and Quadracel. A seventh, Vaxelis, is licensed but will not be available until 2021. Two licensed Tdap vaccines are used in the United States: Adacel and Boostrix. The difference between the DTaP and Tdap vaccines is that the DTaP is meant for primary immunization in children and the Tdap is a booster given to older children, teens, and adults.

Vaccine Manufacturing Process

DTaP vaccines are each manufactured similarly by producing diphtheria and tetanus toxins grown in a medium containing *Corynebacterium diphtheriae* and *Clostridium tetani*. The acellular (contains cellular material but not complete cells) pertussis antigens—pertussis toxin

(PT), filamentous hemagglutinin (FHA), and pertactin—are isolated from *Bordetella pertussis* grown in a medium or fermentation broth. The primary difference among the vaccines is the medium used, the detoxification and filtration processes, and the preservatives and other ingredients added.

Daptacel uses a modified Mueller's growth medium (diphtheria toxin; DT) and modified Mueller-Miller casamino acid medium without beef heart 298 infusion (tetanus toxin; TT). Both toxins are purified by ammonium sulfate and detoxified with formaldehyde before being filtered. The toxoids are then individually adsorbed—the process whereby molecules from a substance adhere to the surface of another substance—onto the aluminum phosphate adjuvant. The acellular pertussis antigens are grown in a Stainer-Scholte medium modified by the addition of casamino acids and dimethyl-beta-cyclodextrin. Each of the antigens is isolated from the medium separately. Fimbriae types 2 and 3 (FIM2, FIM3)—structures on the surface of some bacteria that enable the bacteria to infect human cells and cause illness—are extracted and purified from bacterial cells. Pertussis antigens go through a multistep process of filtration and precipitation. PT is detoxified with glutaraldehyde. FHA is treated with formaldehyde and the residual aldehydes removed by ultrafiltration. The individual antigens are then adsorbed onto aluminum phosphate, and mixed with 2-phenoxyethanol and water for injection into an intermediate concentrate.

The toxins produced for Infanrix vaccines are manufactured by growing *Corynebacterium diphtheriae* in bovine extract (diphtheria toxin), and *Clostridium tetani* (tetanus toxin) in a modified Latham medium derived from bovine casein. The toxins are then detoxified with formaldehyde, concentrated by ultrafiltration, and purified through a multistep process. The acellular pertussis antigens (PT, FHA, and pertactin) are isolated from a *Bordetella pertussis* culture grown in a modified Stainer-Scholte liquid medium. Filamentous hemagglutinin and pertactin are isolated from the fermentation broth and pertactin is extracted from the cells by heat and flocculation (separation of solid particles from a liquid, forming loose flakes). All antigens are purified in a successive process. Pertactin is detoxified using glutaraldehyde and formaldehyde. Filamentous hemagglutinin and pertactin are also treated with formaldehyde. Each of these ingredients is then absorbed onto an aluminum hydroxide adjuvant.

Like other DTaP vaccines, Kinrix produces the diphtheria toxin by growing *Corynebacterium diphtheriae* on a Fenton medium containing a bovine extract. Tetanus toxin is produced by growing *Clostridium tetani* in a modified Latham medium derived from bovine casein. Both toxins are detoxified with formaldehyde. Pertussis antigens are isolated from *Bordetella pertussis* culture grown in modified Stainer-Scholte liquid medium. PT is detoxified with formaldehyde and glutaraldehyde, whereas FHA and pertactin are treated with formaldehyde. Diphtheria and tetanus toxoids and pertussis antigens are individually adsorbed onto aluminum hydroxide. Kinrix incorporates inactivated poliovirus. Three poliovirus strains are individually grown in monkey kidney cells (VERO) using calf serum and lactalbumin hydrolysate (an enzymatically hydrolyzed portion of whey protein isolate). The poliovirus strains are inactivated with formaldehyde.

Pediarix is a combination diphtheria, tetanus, pertussis, hepatitis B, and poliovirus vaccine. It produces the toxoids in a Fenton medium containing bovine extract (DT) and a Latham medium derived from bovine casein (TT), then detoxifies them with formaldehyde. The acellular pertussis antigens are isolated from a *Bordetella pertussis* culture grown in a modified Stainer-Scholte liquid medium. PT is detoxified with glutaraldehyde and formaldehyde, while FHA and pertactin are treated with formaldehyde. The hepatitis B surface antigen is obtained by culturing genetically engineered *Saccharomyces cerevisiae* cells in a synthetic medium. Inactivated poliovirus is grown in VERO cells with calf serum and lactalbumin hydrolysate and inactivated with formaldehyde. Diphtheria and tetanus toxoids and pertussis antigens are individually adsorbed onto aluminum hydroxide. HepB is adsorbed onto aluminum phosphate.

Pentacel is manufactured the same way as Daptacel but contains twice as much detoxified pertussis toxin and four times the amount of filamentous hemagglutinin. Pentacel also contains inactivated poliovirus and *Haemophilus influenzae* type b. Poliovirus type 1, type 2, and type 3 are grown in separate cultures of MRC-5 cells (diploid human cells obtained derived from a fourteen-week-old aborted Caucasian male). Diploid cells contain two complete sets of chromosomes, one from each parent. The cells are grown in a CMRL 1969 medium supplemented with calf serum. The viruses are grown in a Medium 199 without calf serum and after clarification and filtration, the viral suspensions are concentrated and purified. The individual viruses are inactivated with formaldehyde and combined to produce a poliovirus concentrate with all three types. A polymer is prepared from the *Haemophilus influenzae* type b strain grown in a semisynthetic medium. The toxoids (diphtheria and tetanus) and pertussis antigens are individually adsorbed onto aluminum phosphate and combined with aluminum phosphate, 2-phenoxyethanol, and water as an intermediate concentrate. The poliovirus is added to this intermediate concentrate.

The Quadracel vaccine used a Mueller's growth medium for diphtheria toxin and a modified Mueller-Miller casamino acid medium with beef heart infusion for the tetanus toxin. Both are purified with ammonium sulfate and individually adsorbed onto aluminum phosphate. *Bordetella pertussis* cultures are grown in a Stainer-Scholte medium modified with casamino acids and dimethyl-beta-cyclodextrin to produce the pertussis antigens. PT is detoxified with glutaraldehyde, FHA is treated with formaldehyde, and the individual antigens are adsorbed separately onto aluminum phosphate. Poliovirus type 1, type 2, and type 3 are grown in separate culture of MRC-5 cells in Connaught Medical Research Laboratories 1969 medium, supplemented with calf serum. The culture medium is replaced by Medium 199 without calf serum for viral growth. The individual polioviruses are inactivated with formaldehyde before being combined (trivalent). The toxoids (diphtheria and tetanus) and pertussis antigens are individually adsorbed onto aluminum phosphate and combined with aluminum phosphate, 2-phenoxyethanol, and water as an intermediate concentrate. The poliovirus is added to this intermediate concentrate.

The Tdap Adacel vaccine is similar to Daptacel (DTaP) but with reduced quantities of DT and PT. The pertussis antigens are produced from *Bordetella pertussis* cultures grown in Stainer-Scholte medium modified by the addition of casamino acids and dimethyl-beta-cyclodextrin. PT, FHA, and pertactin are isolated from the supernatant culture medium. PT is detoxified with glutaraldehyde and FHA is treated with formaldehyde. *Clostridium tetani* is grown in a modified Mueller-Miller casamino acid medium without beef liver heart, detoxified with formaldehyde, and purified with ammonium sulfate. DT are obtained from *Corynebacterium diphtheriae* grown in modified Mueller's growth medium, which is purified by ammonium sulfate and detoxified with formaldehyde. The toxoids (diphtheria and tetanus) and pertussis antigens are adsorbed in aluminum phosphate, 2-phenoxyethanol, and water.

TT is produced in a modified Latham medium derived from bovine casein and the DT is produced in Fenton medium containing a bovine extract to manufacture Boostrix. Both toxins are detoxified with formaldehyde. Pertussis antigens are isolated from *Bordetella pertussis* culture grown in modified Stainer-Scholte liquid medium. PT is detoxified with glutaraldehyde and formaldehyde, while FHA and pertactin are treated with formaldehyde only. Each antigen is individually adsorbed onto aluminum hydroxide.

For instances where the pertussis vaccine is contraindicated, a diphtheria and pertussis (Td) combination vaccine is available from Sanofi Pasteur. This vaccine suggests a five-dose series at 2, 4, 6, 15–18 months, and 4–6 years. DT is prepared from *Corynebacterium diphtheriae* grown with aeration in a submerged culture medium consisting of tryptic digest of casein, supplemented with cystine, maltose, uracil, inorganic salts, and vitamins. TT is converted to toxoid using formalin. The TT culture medium is the same as that used for DT. The toxins are treated with formaldehyde and adsorbed onto aluminum phosphate.

Tenivac (Td) grows *Clostridium tetani* in modified Mueller-Miller casamino acid medium without beef heart infusion. The TT is detoxified with formaldehyde and purified by ammonium sulfate. *Corynebacterium diphtheriae* is grown in modified Mueller's growth medium. DT is purified by ammonium sulfate and detoxified with formaldehyde. The toxoids are individually adsorbed onto aluminum sulfate and combined with aluminum phosphate, sodium chloride, and water for injection.

TDVAX is another tetanus diphtheria and tetanus vaccine approved for persons 7 years of age and older. Both the *Corynebacterium diphtheriae* and *Clostridium tetani* organisms are grown on a modified Mueller's medium that includes bovine extracts. They are detoxified with formaldehyde and separately purified by ammonium sulfate fractionation. The diphtheria toxoid is further purified by column chromatography. Both toxoids are individually adsorbed into aluminum phosphate.

Intended for children 7 years of age and older and adults for the prevention of tetanus, Tetanus Toxoid Adsorbed (tetanus only) is not meant for use after potential exposure to tetanus bacteria. Instead, it is given regularly to maintain sufficient antibodies to protect against tetanus infection in case of injury. The *Clostridium tetani* culture is grown in a peptone-based medium containing an extract of bovine muscle tissue and detoxified with formaldehyde. The toxin is purified by ammonium sulfate. The resulting toxoid is then adsorbed onto aluminum potassium sulfate.

Note: Some vaccine manufactures suggest careful consideration of receiving additional doses in the series if any of the following reactions have occurred after a pertussis-containing vaccine—fever of 105°F (40.5°C) within forty-eight hours, collapse or shock-like state within forty-eight hours, persistent, inconsolable crying lasting three or more hours within forty-eight hours, seizures within three days, encephalopathy within seven days, and Guillain-Barré syndrome within six weeks of prior vaccination.

Ingredients

Daptacel[267]

- Diphtheria toxoid (15 Lf)
- Tetanus toxoid (5 Lf)
- Inactivated pertussis toxin (10 mcg)
- Filamentous hemagglutinin (5 mcg)
- Fimbriae types 2 and 3 (5 mcg)
- Pertactin (3 mcg)
- 2-phenoxyethanol (3.3 mg)
- Aluminum (0.33 mg)
- Formaldehyde (≤5 mcg)
- Glutaraldehyde (≤50 ng)

Infanrix[268]

- Diphtheria toxoid (25 Lf)
- Tetanus toxoid (10 Lf)
- Inactivated pertussis toxin (25 mcg)
- Filamentous hemagglutinin (25 mcg)
- Pertactin (8 mcg)
- Sodium chloride (4.5 mg)
- Aluminum (<0.625 mg)
- Formaldehyde (≤100 mcg)
- Polysorbate 80 (≤100 mcg)

Kinrix[269]

- Diphtheria toxoid (25 Lf)
- Tetanus toxoid (10 Lf)

- Inactivated pertussis toxin (25 mcg)
- Filamentous hemagglutinin (25 mcg)
- Pertactin (8 mcg)
- Inactivated polioviruses (40 D-antigen units [DU] type 1, 8 DU type 2, 32 DU type 3)
- Aluminum ($\leq$0.6 mg)
- Formaldehyde ($\leq$100 mcg)
- Polysorbate 80 ($\leq$100 mcg)
- Neomycin sulfate ($\leq$0.05 ng; an antibiotic)
- Polymyxin B ($\leq$0.01 ng; an antibiotic)

Pediarix[270]

- Diphtheria toxoid (25 Lf)
- Tetanus toxoid (10 Lf)
- Inactivated pertussis toxin (25 mcg)
- Filamentous hemagglutinin (25 mcg)
- Pertactin (8 mcg)
- Inactivated polioviruses (40 D-antigen units [DU] type 1, 8 DU type 2, 32 DU type 3)
- Hepatitis B surface antigen (10 mcg)
- Aluminum ($\leq$0.85 mg)
- Sodium chloride (4.5 mg)
- Formaldehyde ($\leq$100 mcg)
- Polysorbate 80 ($\leq$100 mcg)
- Neomycin sulfate ($\leq$0.05 ng)
- Polymyxin B ($\leq$0.01 ng)
- Yeast protein ($\leq$5%)

Pentacel[271]

- Diphtheria toxoid (15 Lf)
- Tetanus toxoid (5 Lf)
- Inactivated pertussis toxin (20 mcg)
- Filamentous hemagglutinin (20 mcg)

- Fimbriae types 2 and 3 (5 mcg)
- Pertactin (3 mcg)
- Inactivated polioviruses (40 D-antigen units [DU] type 1, 8 DU type 2, 32 DU type 3)
- *H. influenzae* type b capsular polysaccharide (10 mcg) covalently bonded to tetanus toxoid (24 mcg)
- Aluminum (0.33 mg)
- Polysorbate 80 (10 PPM)
- Sucrose (42.5 mg)
- Formaldehyde ($\leq$5 mcg)
- Glutaraldehyde ($\leq$50 ng)
- Bovine serum albumin ($\leq$50 ng)
- 2-phenoxyethanol (3.3 mg)
- Neomycin (<4 pg)
- Polymyxin B sulfate (<4 pg)

Quadracel[272]

- Diphtheria toxoid (15 Lf)
- Tetanus toxoid (5 Lf)
- Inactivated pertussis toxin (20 mcg)
- Filamentous hemagglutinin (20 mcg)
- Pertactin (3 mcg)
- Fimbriae types 2 and 3 (5 mcg)
- Inactivated polioviruses (40 D-antigen units [DU] type 1, 8 DU type 2, 32 DU type 3)
- Aluminum (0.33 mg)
- Polysorbate 80 (10 PPM)
- Formaldehyde ($\leq$5 mcg)
- Glutaraldehyde ($\leq$50 ng)
- Bovine serum albumin ($\leq$50 ng)
- 2-phenoxyethanol (3.3 mg)
- Neomycin (<4 pg)
- Polymyxin B sulfate (<4 pg)

Adacel[273]

- Tetanus toxoid (5f)
- Diphtheria toxoid (2 Lf)
- Detoxified pertussis toxin (2.5 mcg)
- Filamentous hemagglutinin (5 mcg)
- Pertactin (3 mcg)
- Fimbriae types 2 and 3 (5 mcg)
- Aluminum (0.33 mg)
- Formaldehyde (≤5 mcg)
- Glutaraldehyde (≤50 ng)
- 2-phenoxyethanol (3.3 mg)

Boostrix[274]

- Tetanus toxoid (5f)
- Diphtheria toxoid (2.5 Lf)
- Inactivated pertussis toxin (8 mcg)
- Filamentous hemagglutinin (8 mcg)
- Pertactin (2.5 mcg)
- Aluminum (0.39 mg)
- Sodium chloride (4.4 mg)
- Formaldehyde (≤100 mcg)
- Polysorbate 80 (≤100 mcg)

Sanofi Pasteur (diphtheria and tetanus)[275]

- Diphtheria toxoid (25 Lf)
- Tetanus toxoid (5 Lf)
- Aluminum (0.33 mg)
- Free formaldehyde (<100 mcg)

Tenivac (tetanus and diphtheria)[276]

- Tetanus toxoid (5 Lf)
- Diphtheria Toxoid (2 Lf)
- Aluminum (0.33 mg)
- Formaldehyde (≤5.0 mcg)

TDVAX (tetanus and diphtheria)[277]

- Tetanus toxoid (2 Lf)
- Diphtheria toxoid (2 Lf)
- Aluminum (≤0.53 mg)
- Formaldehyde (<100 mcg)
- Thimerosal (≤0.3 mcg mercury)

Tetanus Toxoid Adsorbed, Generic (tetanus only)[278]

- Tetanus toxoid (5 Lf)
- Thimerosal, mercury derivative (≤0.3 mcg)
- Aluminum (≤0.25 mg)
- Formaldehyde (<0.2%)

Note: Lf is a measurement of potency that stands for *limits of flocculation.*

Controversial Ingredients

- Aluminum
- Formaldehyde
- Glutaraldehyde
- Polysorbate 80
- Aborted fetal cells
- Cow blood (serum)
- Monkey kidney cells (VERO)
- Mercury (tetanus only vaccine)
- Thimerosal

Package Insert Adverse Reactions

Daptacel: Fussiness/irritability (>50%), inconsolable crying (>50%), decreased activity/lethargy (>50%), muscle pain (25.8%–46.2%), injection-site reactions (>30%), fever (6%–16%), and seizure (0.3%). Approximately 4 percent of infants receiving Daptacel report at least one serious adverse reaction—bronchiolitis (1.9%), pneumonia 0.2%), meningitis (0.14%), sepsis (0.07%), pertussis (0.07%), and irritability and unresponsiveness (0.07%).

Infanrix: Injection-site reaction (pain, redness, swelling; 10%–53%), fever (20%–30%), drowsiness (15%–60%), irritability/fussiness (15%–60%), and loss of appetite (15%–60%).

Kinrix: Injection-site reaction (>50%), drowsiness (≥15%), fever (≥15%), and loss of appetite (≥15%). Only 0.1 percent of subjects experienced a serious adverse reaction in the clinical trials of the vaccine.

Pediarix: Injection-site reaction (≥25%), fever (≥25%), irritability/fussiness (≥25%), and loss of appetite (≥25%). Pediarix was also associated with higher rates of fever when compared to vaccines administered individually. About 1 percent of infants receiving Pediarix experience a serious adverse reaction, and five deaths (0.06%) were reported after vaccination.

Pentacel: Fussiness/irritability (>50%), inconsolable crying (>50%), injection-site reaction (>30%) and fever (6%–16%). Serious adverse events occurred 0.9–3.9 percent of the time and included bronchiolitis, dehydration, pneumonia, and gastroenteritis.

Quadracel: Injection-site pain (>75%), increased arm circumference (>65%), reddening of the skin (>40%), muscle pain (>50%), malaise (>35%), headache (>15%). About 0.1 percent of subjects experienced a serious adverse reaction within twenty-eight days, which increased to 0.8 percent by six months.

Adacel: Adolescents—injection-site reactions of pain (77.8%), swelling (20.9%), and redness (20.8%). Adults—injection-site reactions of pain (65.7%), redness (24.7%), and swelling (21.0%). Swollen and sore joints were reported in about 22.5 percent of subjects after vaccination. Fever is more common in adolescents than adults. Serious adverse events, including severe migraine with facial paralysis and nerve compression in the neck and left arm occurred about 1.5 percent of the time.

Boostrix: Adolescents—pain, redness, and swelling at the injection site (≥15%), increased arm circumference of injected arm (≥15%), headache

(≥15%), fatigue (≥15%), and gastrointestinal symptoms (≥15%). Adults—pain, redness, and swelling at the injection site (≥15%), headache (≥15%), fatigue (≥15%), and gastrointestinal symptoms (≥15%). Elderly, sixty-five years and older—pain at injection site (≥15%). Serious adverse events were reported in adults 1.4 percent of the time and elderly 0.7 percent (within thirty-one days) and 4.2 percent (within six months).

Sanofi Pasteur (diphtheria and tetanus): Injection-site swelling ≥51.0%), injection-site pain (≥17.0%), crying (13.0%–15.2%), injection-site redness (≥9.0%), fever (0.7%–6.6%), loss of appetite (2.9%–6.2%), and injection-site hardness (≥3.6%).

Tenivac (tetanus and diphtheria): Injection-site pain (35.3%–78.3%), headache (17.9%), injection-site redness (≥10%), injection-site swelling (≥10%), malaise (≥10%), muscle weakness, and pain in joints (≥10%). Other reported adverse events included swollen lymph nodes, rash and itching, anaphylactic reaction, dizziness, abnormal skin sensation (tingling, pricking, chilling, burning, and numbness), Guillain-Barré syndrome, temporary loss of consciousness, vomiting, and muscle pain and pain in the extremities. Serious adverse events occurred up to 1 percent of the time and were more common in individuals aged 60 or older.

TDVAX: Documented adverse reactions are mentioned in several clinical trials, but the actual reactions and their frequency of occurrence is not reported in the vaccine insert.

Tetanus Toxoid Adsorbed, Generic (tetanus only): Injection-site redness, warmth, swelling, and hardening, malaise, fever, pain, low blood pressure, nausea, joint pain, allergic or anaphylactic reaction, Guillain-Barré syndrome, nerve damage, and death.

Parent or Healthcare Provider Adverse Events Reported through VAERS

Daptacel: Swollen lymph nodes, cyanosis (bluish skin and mucous membranes), nausea, diarrhea, injection-site reactions, cellulitis, injection-site abscess, swollen limb (injected limb) involving adjacent joints, allergic reaction, hypersensitivity reaction, anaphylaxis, rash, febrile seizure, grand mal seizure, partial seizures, poor muscle tone, excessive tiredness, temporary loss of consciousness, and screaming.

Infanrix: Bronchitis, cellulitis, respiratory tract infections, swollen lymph nodes, thrombocytopenia, anaphylaxis, hypersensitivity reaction, encephalopathy, headache, poor muscle tone, temporary loss of consciousness, ear pain, cyanosis (bluish skin and mucous membranes), temporary cessation of breathing, cough, swelling beneath the skin (angioedema), reddening of the skin, itching, rash, hives, fatigue, injection-site reactions, sudden infant death syndrome (SIDS).

Kinrix: Injection-site cyst, temporary loss of consciousness, itching, hives, allergic reaction, anaphylaxis, swelling beneath the skin (angioedema), temporary cessation of breathing, collapse or shock-like state, seizures (with or without fever), swollen lymph nodes, and thrombocytopenia.

Pediarix: Cyanosis (bluish skin and mucous membranes), diarrhea, vomiting, fatigue, injection-site reactions, injection-site cyst, limb swelling (injected limb), anaphylaxis, anaphylactoid reaction, hypersensitivity reaction, upper respiratory tract infection, abnormal-liver-function test, bulging fontanelle, depressed level of consciousness, encephalitis, poor muscle tone, hypotonic-hyporesponsive episode, lethargy, temporary loss of consciousness, excessive or unusual crying, insomnia, restlessness, screaming, labored breathing, temporary cessation of breathing, reddening of the skin, rash, hives, pale appearance, and tiny purple, red, or brown spots on the skin as a result of bleeding (petechiae).

Pentacel: Cyanosis (bluish skin and mucous membranes), diarrhea, vomiting, injection-site reactions, extensive swelling of the injected limb involving adjacent joints), vaccination failure (decreased therapeutic response against Hib), anaphylaxis, anaphylactoid reaction, hypersensitivity reaction, meningitis, rhinitis, viral infection, decreased appetite, excessive tiredness, hypotonic-hyporesponsive episode, depressed level of consciousness, screaming, temporary cessation of breathing, cough, reddening of the skin, skin discoloration, and pale appearance.

Quadracel: Anaphylaxis, allergic reactions, hypersensitivity reactions, screaming, excessive tiredness, seizure, febrile seizure, hypotonic-hyporesponsive episode, poor muscle tone, cyanosis (bluish skin and mucous membranes), pale appearance, listlessness, injection-site reactions, extensive limb swelling involving adjacent joints, and injection-site cellulitis/abscess.

Adacel: Anaphylaxis, hypersensitivity reaction, pins-and-needles feeling, reduces sense of touch or sensitivity to sensory stimuli, brachial neuritis, Guillain-Barré syndrome, facial paralysis, seizure, temporary loss of consciousness, inflammation of the spinal cord (myelitis), myocarditis, itching, hives, inflammation of the muscles (myositis), muscle spasms, injection-site reactions, and extensive swelling of the injected limb involving the joints.

Boostrix: Swollen lymph nodes, allergic reactions, anaphylaxis, anaphylactoid reactions, myocarditis, extensive swelling of the injected limb, injection-site reactions, joint pain, back pain, muscle aches, seizures (with or without fever), encephalitis, facial palsy, temporary loss of consciousness, angioedema, widespread rash, hives, Henoch-Schönlein purpura, and rash.

Sanofi Pasteur (diphtheria and tetanus): Swollen lymph nodes, nausea, injection-site reactions, hypersensitivity reactions, excessive tiredness, temporary loss of consciousness, headache, rash, hives, and pale appearance.

Tenivac: Swollen lymph nodes, allergic reactions, anaphylaxis, burning or prickling sensation, dizziness, temporary loss of consciousness, Guillain-Barré syndrome, vomiting, muscle pain, pain in the extremities, injection-site reactions, fatigue, and peripheral swelling.

TDVAX: Injection-site reactions, allergic and hypersensitivity reactions, itching, peripheral swelling, general malaise, fever, dizziness, headache, seizures, muscle aches, musculoskeletal stiffness, pain or tenderness, joint pain, reddening of the skin, rash, nausea, and cellulitis.

Tetanus toxoids, adsorbed (generic): Injection-site reaction, allergic or hypersensitivity reactions, anaphylaxis (including death), general malaise, fever, pain, low blood pressure, nausea, joint pain, brachial neuritis, Guillain-Barré syndrome, nerve demyelination, neuropathy, and encephalopathy.

Reactions Observed and Documented in Published Research

Evidence suggests that the pertussis vaccine unintentionally encouraged evolutionary adaptations (genetic changes) by the *Bordetella pertussis* bacteria, allowing it to be more virulent and resistant to vaccines. Greater virulence means more people are infected, and they experience greater illness severity. An overwhelming body of evidence demonstrates unequivocally that new pertussis strains that produce more toxins have emerged from vaccinated individuals since the vaccine was introduced, and these new strains spread rapidly in global populations.[279,280,281,282,283,284,285,286,287,288,289,290,291] We are simultaneously weakening one cause of illness and bolstering several other causes.

Additionally, widespread vaccination appears to have increased the number of whooping cough cases caused by *Bordetella parapertussis*.[292,293,294,295] Bordetella parapertussis is a bacterium similar to Bordetella pertussis, which causes a pertussis-like illness without producing pertussis toxins. The data suggests that the pertussis vaccine interferes with the ability of the immune system to clear *B. parapertussis*, allowing the pathogen to more efficiently cause a whooping cough–like illness.[296] Even under-recognized species of *Bordetella*, like *Bordetella holmesii*, infections are increasing and causing whooping cough–like symptoms.[297,298] It is also possible that some people are misdiagnosed with *Bordetella pertussis* infection when they are actually infected with *Bordetella holmesii*. Vaccine manufacturers may have triggered a cascade of events by attacking one *Bordetella* species that is leading to bigger problems than the original problem they aimed to prevent. At the very least, it seems that the vaccine produces an inferior immune response when compared to natural infections.

Cases of pertussis infection in vaccinated children are on the rise, and cases of whooping cough are increasing in older age groups as well.[299] So much so that some have recommended a booster vaccine dose in adults. A study concluded that the DTaP vaccine doesn't provide sufficient protection when they observed that most pertussis cases in the United States occur in children age-appropriately vaccinated who were more than two years away from their last dose.[300,301,302] Similar ineffectiveness and waning immunity has been reported with the Tdap vaccine—vaccine effectiveness is a measly 34 percent two to four years after full vaccination.[303] The risk of a pertussis infection doubled just two years after being fully vaccinated and increased ninefold six years after completing all recommended doses of these vaccines. What the research shows is that fully vaccinated children (even after completing the entire dose series) are still at an increased risk of pertussis.

On top of this, cases of vaccinated individuals spreading pertussis bacteria to susceptible individuals have been documented. Unaware that they are infected, these individuals infected by the vaccinated population become silent carriers—infected but showing no symptoms—of the bacteria, further complicating the spread of the infection. Not only did research find that the practice of cocooning— where parents and siblings are vaccinated to protect newborns—doesn't work, but also vaccination likely exacerbated the rise in pertussis because vaccinated individuals unknowingly spread the infection.[304] Ironically, proponents of vaccine mandates claim unvaccinated individuals are a risk to them, but the evidence here suggests quite the contrary.

The ability of pertussis vaccines to cause evolutions in and resistance of pertussis bacteria may make herd immunity—protection from infection of a population due to a sufficiently high proportion of individuals within the population being immune to the disease, through natural or vaccine-induced immunity—impossible.[305] In other words, vaccinating the unvaccinated is unlikely to protect against infection. Herd immunity is very difficult to achieve because higher vaccination rates force pathogens to adapt to avoid extinction. After adaptation, the pathogen becomes more hostile in nature with the goal of maximally infecting a person without killing them. Bacterial resistance to antibiotics is a major concern and similarly applies to vaccines. The dramatic resurgence in pertussis due to bacterial adaptations is a substantial public health concern and suggests the current pertussis vaccine is inadequate to protect against pertussis infections.

Although it suffers from poor efficacy over time, the DTaP vaccine is considered very safe and well tolerated in the majority (90 percent) of individuals.[306] One of the problems with assessing vaccine safety, including DTaP and Tdap, is that many vaccines are given together making it very difficult to attribute adverse effects to a single vaccine. No vaccine is 100 percent safe, but attributing an adverse event completely to a vaccine remains complicated.

In addition to feeble long-term protection against pertussis, some vaccines are linked to febrile seizures. A febrile seizure is a full-body convulsion caused by a spike in body temperature, frequently from an infection. They occur in about 3–4 percent of children between the ages of 6 months and 5 years but are most likely to occur around 12–18 months old. Children who experience a febrile seizure before twelve months of age have about a 50 percent chance of having another, but only a small percentage progress further to develop epilepsy.

Population-based cohort studies that evaluated the health records of nearly 379,000 children found that children vaccinated according to the recommended schedule with DTaP, polio, and Hib were nearly eight times more likely to have a febrile seizure on the day of their first vaccinations.[307] This risk ratio held true even after adjusting for gestational age, birth weight, and parental history of epilepsy. The same research concluded that children who are vaccinated according to the prescribed schedule are four times more likely to experience a febrile seizure on the day of their second vaccinations, but not during the third round of vaccinations. Since the diphtheria, tetanus, pertussis, poliovirus, and Hib vaccines were given simultaneously, it was not possible to determine if only one or multiple vaccines were responsible for the increased risk of febrile seizures. Fortunately, no increased risk of epilepsy was observed in the study. Another study of nearly 680,000 children, found the DTP vaccine increased the risk of febrile seizure only on the day of vaccination, while the MMR vaccine increased risk for eight to fourteen days after vaccination.[308] The occurrence of febrile seizures following MMR and DTP vaccines caused the Italian League Against Epilepsy (LICE), in collaboration with other Italian scientific societies, to establish guidelines on vaccinations and epilepsy. They concluded that DTP and MMR vaccinations "increase significantly the risk of febrile seizures," but some cases of vaccine-induced brain damage (encephalopathy) may be "caused by an inherent genetic defect with no causal relationship with vaccination."[309]

A cohort study of 265,275 children found certain children were at an increased risk of vaccine-associated febrile seizures. Appearance, Pulse, Grimace, Activity, and Respiration (Apgar) scores are a method used to quickly summarize the health of a newborn child. Each category is scored from zero to two, depending on the observed condition, with a cumulative high score of ten. The higher the score, the better the baby is doing health wise. A score of seven or higher is a sign that the newborn is in good health. The test is performed one minute after birth to determine how well the baby tolerated the birth process and again at five minutes to assess the baby's health outside the mother's womb. The study found a significant correlation with lower Apgar scores—a score of less than or equal to three at one minute—and vaccine-associated febrile seizures, but low Apgar scores did not increase the risk of nonvaccine-associated febrile seizures.[310] In other words, lower Apgar scores alone didn't increase the risk of seizure unless the child was vaccinated. It is possible that newborns with the lowest Apgar scores are more vulnerable to vaccine injury.

Another study concluded that "vaccine administration is the second leading cause of febrile seizures."[311] The study specifically linked pertussis, measles, and influenza vaccines to febrile seizures. Three additional studies also found a link between the MMR vaccine and febrile seizures, which occurred about six to eleven days after vaccination.[312,313,314] One of these studies connected the risk of febrile seizures after vaccination to genetic and health traits: interferon-stimulated gene IFI44L and measles virus receptor CD46 for the MMR vaccine; and sodium channel genes SCN1A and SCN2A, a TMEM16 family gene (ANO3), and magnesium levels for general vaccine-associated febrile seizures.[315] More evidence that some children are predisposed to vaccine damage and a one-size-fits-all schedule is not practical or medically sound.

Further evidence gathered from the health records of 459,461 children in the CDC's Vaccine Safety Datalink suggests that the MMRV (MMR with varicella) poses a higher risk of seizure than receiving the MMR and varicella vaccines separately. This research found the MMRV vaccine increased the risk of febrile seizures eight times within seven to ten days of vaccination.[316] By contrast, the MMR and varicella vaccines separately increased seizure risk four times and the MMR vaccine alone 3.7 times. The evidence was so compelling that when presented to pediatricians and general family practitioners, almost three-quarters of which were unaware of the increased risk, only 20 percent of pediatricians and 7 percent of general family practitioners reported they would recommend the MMRV vaccine to a healthy 12–15-month-old child.[317] This points to the fact that many physicians are unaware of vaccine risks, but come to reasonable conclusions and are more willing to adapt their practice to improve patient safety when presented with sufficient evidence.

A similar increased risk of febrile seizure after MMRV and MMR and varicella vaccines given separately was noted in Canadian and German children.[318,319] Children are also four times more likely to be hospitalized with febrile seizures five to twelve days after MMRV vaccination compared to children who received only the MMR vaccine.[320] A systemic review and meta-analysis of the postmarketing data from more than 3.2 million children demonstrated that children who delay the MMRV vaccine until age 4–6 appear to be protected against vaccine-related febrile seizures, while children 10–24 months experience the highest incidence of febrile seizure after MMRV vaccination.[321] Timing of vaccination and the number of them received simultaneously can be the difference between an adverse reaction or not.

A family history of seizures, including siblings, or a personal history of seizures may predispose children to vaccine-associated seizures. A 2004 study evaluating data from over 537,000 children associated a family or personal history of seizures to MMR vaccine-related seizures.[322] Children with siblings that had a history of seizures were twice as likely to experience febrile seizures after receiving the MMR vaccine, while those with a personal history were twelve times more likely to experience febrile seizures during the two weeks following MMR vaccination than at other times. These findings are not surprising because research has consistently identified an increased risk of seizures when a family history of seizures among a first-degree relative—sibling, parent, or offspring—is known.

Contrary to the above studies' findings, Chinese researchers concluded that there is no causal relationship between vaccines and febrile seizures.[323] Instead, they propose that febrile seizures are due to a set of complex factors, including age, genetics (genetic epilepsy syndrome), vaccine type, how many vaccines are received at one, and timing of vaccination. It's interesting that they mention vaccines three times after concluding there is no causal association. The study authors stated that "parents should be informed that some vaccines could be associated with an increased risk of FS [febrile seizure], particularly, in children with personal and family history of FS." A meta-analysis and systemic review of thirty-one published studies and unpublished clinical trials involving about 40,000 children also found no direct link between MMRV or MMR and febrile seizures.[324] It is true that it is very difficult to identify vaccines as the definitive cause of seizures after vaccination, but a strong correlation appears to exist, and emerging evidence suggests that vaccines can be a trigger in predisposed children.

Nonfebrile seizures, also called afebrile seizures, are convulsions that occur without a high fever. They can occur in children of all ages and may be a sign of epilepsy. Some research has also linked vaccines with nonfebrile seizures. A large German database of adverse events following immunization was searched for reports of seizures or epilepsy. Of the adverse seizure events included, 49 percent were febrile seizures and 15.4 percent were nonfebrile seizures.[325] Severe childhood epilepsies (Dravet syndrome, West syndrome, Lennox-Gastaut syndrome, or Doose syndrome) were diagnosed in 11.7 percent of the children, with the vaccine-associated event being the first documented seizure in more than half of the children. On average, seizures occurred twenty-four hours after receipt of an inactivated vaccine and 7.5 days after attenuated vaccines, suggesting the inactivated vaccines may have a higher risk of vaccine-associated seizures.

The DTaP, Tdap, and tetanus vaccines may also increase the risk of allergies and asthma. Children who received these vaccines are twice to five times as likely as their unvaccinated peers to be diagnosed with asthma and 63 percent more likely to be diagnosed with an allergy-related respiratory symptom.[326,327,328] Researchers in New Zealand found that 23 percent of children who received the DTP (diphtheria-tetanus-pertussis) and polio vaccines had asthma and 30 percent sought medical treatment for other allergies.[329] Children who received the DPT vaccine later than recommended were also significantly less likely to develop asthma.[330,331] Looking at the pertussis vaccine alone, vaccinated children were more than twice as likely to have asthma, hay fever, or food allergies when compared to unvaccinated children.[332] Conflicting research found little to no evidence of vaccine-related allergies.[333,334] However, given the consistency of estimates relating to vaccine-related allergies and their dramatic rise over the last decade, the control of confounding known risk factors for asthma and allergies, and a growing amount of observed cases, a vaccine-related cause of allergies is still plausible.

Surprisingly, few studies examine the introduction of vaccines in low-income countries and their impact on child survival. However, evidence suggests that the introduction of the DTP vaccine in the West African country of Guinea-Bissau appeared to have a negative effect on infants receiving it. The DTP and oral polio (OP) vaccines were introduced in Guinea-Bissau in June 1981, roughly three years after a three-month nutritional weighing schedule was initiated among children in the country. Infants were vaccinated during these weighing visits between the ages of three and five months. Comparison of deaths among vaccinated and unvaccinated children aged 3–5 months showed that vaccinated children were five times more likely to die than unvaccinated children.[335] Interestingly, the risk of mortality was even higher among children who received the DTP vaccine and not the OP vaccine. These children were ten times more likely to die. Another study found that children vaccinated at 3–5 months in Guinea-Bissau had a better nutritional status and less diphtheria, pertussis, and tetanus infections between the ages of 6 and 35 months, suggesting the vaccine did its job to protect against the three infections.[336] However, the research also noted that vaccinated children were more than twice as likely to die of any cause when compared to unvaccinated children. Girls fared worse than boys. A systemic review found that while the measles and tuberculosis (Bacillus Calmette-Guérin) vaccines reduced mortality in children, receiving the DTP vaccine was associated with increased mortality.[337] This research highlights how all causes of infant mortality increased after the introduction of DTP and not necessarily other vaccines.

The United States just recently (2018) and other countries have used a hexavalent vaccine that contains diphtheria toxoids, tetanus toxoids, acellular pertussis, inactivated poliovirus, Hib conjugate (meningococcal protein conjugate), and hepatitis B (recombinant) antigens all in a single syringe. It is administered as a three-dose series between the ages of 6 weeks through 4 years, typically at 2, 4, and 6 months of age. The package insert for one of the vaccines lists that six deaths (0.2 of participants) occurred in the two US studies, none of which were deemed as vaccine caused.[338] The causes of death were asphyxia (when the body is deprived of oxygen), hydrocephalus (accumulation of cerebrospinal fluid within the brain), sepsis, two cases of sudden infant death syndrome (SIDS), and one of unknown cause. In addition, irritability (61.8 percent), excessive sleepiness (56.3 percent), abnormal crying (52.0 percent), decreased appetite (28.9 percent), fever (19.2 percent), and vomiting (13.1 percent) were common adverse effects. Emerging evidence indicates that while more convenient for families because the child and parent endure fewer shots, the hexavalent vaccine may not be safer.

SIDS involves the sudden and unexpected death of a seemingly healthy baby under age 1—usually while sleeping—in which the immediate cause of death is unknown. Sudden unexplained death in childhood (SUDC) is the death of a seemingly healthy child over age 1 of which the cause remains unexplained after thorough investigation. Dysfunction of central nervous system leading to poor control of the respiratory system during sleep, cardiac activity, and arousal may play a central role in these unexpected deaths.[339] The clinical safety studies conducted by the manufacturer of one hexavalent vaccine may underestimate the risk of SIDS and SUDC according to published data evaluating the use of hexavalent vaccines in countries that have used them for more than a decade. A study evaluating the risk of SUDC within twenty-eight days after receipt of a hexavalent vaccine found that children in their second year of life were significantly more likely to die within one or two days following hexavalent vaccination.[340] The researchers conducted multiple sensitivity analyses to gage any limitations in data sources and ruled out the deaths as coincidental. The findings do not prove a causal relationship, but do emphasize the need to intensify surveillance of unexpected deaths following hexavalent vaccination and more closely scrutinize vaccines as a contributing factor.

Another group of researchers assessed health data from three million infants vaccinated in Italy between 1999 and 2004, of which 1.5 million received hexavalent vaccines. They found 604 sudden unexpected deaths occurred in infants during this time period. Data analysis showed a statistically significant twofold increased risk of SIDS within fourteen days after the first dose of a hexavalent vaccine.[341] Similarly, another group of researchers identified a twofold increased risk in SIDS in German children within three days of receiving a second dose of a pentavalent (five antigens in one vaccine) vaccine.[342] Even data from one of the European manufacturers of a hexavalent vaccine show 97 percent of the reported cases of SIDS following hexavalent vaccination occur within ten days after receipt.[343] Commentary on these confidential periodic safety update reports (PSURs) submitted by the manufacturer, researchers noted that the manufacturer deleted deaths acknowledged in PSUR 16 when they submitted PSUR 19.[344] Deletion of these deaths from the 2016 report gave the vaccine a more favorable safety profile in the 2019 report. Furthermore, the researchers challenged the European Medicines Agency's due diligence in reviewing these reports because they accepted the manufacturer's report with the deleted data, stating "as a result of which numerous children were unnecessarily exposed to the risk of death." In the end, the researchers concluded that "the number of observed deaths soon after vaccination among children older than 1 year was significantly higher than that expected by chance once the deleted deaths were restored and included in the analysis."

Autopsies performed on six children ranging from 4 to 17 months old whose death was attributed to SIDS or SUDC following vaccination revealed a possible explanation for the deaths that occur within days after hexavalent vaccination. The forensic postmortem examination found neuropathological (nervous system tissue) and histological (tissue studied under a microscope) abnormalities in the brain and

99

extraordinary brain swelling and inflammation, which made them dissimilar to typical SIDS and SUDC cases.[345] The cases were reported as possible, but not definitive, serious vaccine side effects. In addition, the scientists felt it important to "inform vaccinating physicians and pediatricians as well as parents about such possibly fatal complications after application of hexavalent vaccines." Would informing physicians of these risk result in a similar agreeance to discontinue hexavalent vaccines as was seen with MMRV?

Another case study involving the death of a 2-month-old female infant within twenty-four hours after hexavalent vaccination concluded the death was vaccine related. Postmortem examination found significant fluid buildup in the lungs, damaged and enlarged air sacs in the lungs, degranulating mast cells (this increases inflammation and can trigger anaphylaxis), and a high level of beta-tryptase (a marker for anaphylaxis seen in SIDS and SUDC cases).[346] Based on the findings, the pathologists concluded that the sudden respiratory failure and cause of the death was "likely due to post hexavalent immunization-related shock."

Further evidence of vaccine involvement in SIDS was documented in a case of a 3-month-old female that died suddenly and unexpectedly after receiving a hexavalent vaccine. Pathologists performed an autopsy and found an inadequate number of brain cells (hypoplasia) in the arcuate nucleus of the hypothalamus.[347] The arcuate nucleus is a group of neurons involved in breathing control and responses to chemical stimuli. This hypoplasia can lead to death by disrupting synchronization between the brain's coordination of breathing and autonomic nervous system function, responses to chemical stimuli, and the ability to integrate sensations in order to maintain optimal performance levels during sleep. A disruption of cardiac function was also noted. Additional data from thirteen cases of unexpected deaths within seven days after hexavalent vaccination also found hypoplasia of the arcuate nucleus in five of the thirteen cases.[348] Although the study doesn't prove a causal relationship between hexavalent vaccines and unexpected deaths in infants and children, birth defects involving primary nervous system structures that regulate vital functions were ruled out in all thirteen cases. In other words, they could not find a preexisting condition that explained the unexpected and untimely deaths. Based on this, the pathologists concluded "that vaccine components could have a direct role in sparking off a lethal outcome in vulnerable babies."

Notwithstanding, multiple independent studies claiming a relationship between hexavalent vaccines and SIDS or SDUC, some researchers consider the vaccines to have a good safety record extending over a decade of use.[349,350] This "clinically acceptable safety" profile extends to premature and low-birth-weight infants according to a summary of ten clinical studies and fifteen years of postmarketing safety surveillance.[351] Instead, it is proposed that placing children on their stomachs to sleep is the greatest risk of SIDS.

Evaluation of sudden and unexpected deaths after all vaccinations reported that the most common vaccine received immediately prior to death was the Hib vaccine.[352] In their conclusion, they state that at least some of the deaths are suspected as vaccine related, but causation can't be conclusively determined.

As with hexavalent vaccines, a number of studies come to contrasting conclusions about vaccines and whether they cause SIDS. Several studies have found no direct link to SIDS and the DTaP, hepatitis B, or other vaccines.[353,354,355,356,357] It cannot be stated with certainty that SIDS and SDUC are caused by vaccination, but there does appear to be a suspicious correlation.

Damage to the protective covering of nerves (myelin) in the peripheral nervous system has long been known to follow certain viral (cytomegalovirus, Epstein-Barr virus, vaccinia virus, HIV, rubeola virus, paramyxovirus, rubella virus) and bacterial infections (*Campylobacter jejuni, Mycoplasma pneumoniae*). Guillain-Barré syndrome (GBS) is a rare disorder in which the immune system mistakenly attacks the nerves and damages their myelin (called demyelination). GBS is occasionally reported in people who receive a tetanus vaccine or tetanus immune globulin.[358] Enough of a correlation was established that the Institute of Medicine concluded "there is biologic plausibility for a causal relation between vaccines [tetanus, tetanus and diphtheria, and tetanus immune globulin] and demyelinating disorders" and the "evidence favors a causal relationship between tetanus toxoid [and tetanus/diphtheria and tetanus immune globulin] and GBS." Over half of all people who developed GBS following a tetanus vaccine or immune globulin had a history of a respiratory or gastrointestinal infection one to four weeks prior to vaccination. This provides a clue as to why some people may be prone to nervous system disorders after vaccination. If a person receives a vaccine while they are sick with a viral illness—and possibly some bacterial illnesses—the pathogen could enter the central nervous system as the immune system is further challenged by vaccine antigens. Based on this, it is best to postpone some vaccines until at least four weeks (possibly six) after your child recovers from other illnesses.

See the *Reactions Observed and Documented in Published Research* section of chapter 9 for a discussion of immune thrombocytopenia associated with pertussis, DTaP, and Tdap vaccinations.

See the *Reactions Observed and Documented in Published Research* section of chapter 9 for a discussion about how certain childhood infections may protect against cancer development later in life.

INFECTION RISKS	VACCINE RISKS
Tetanus	Allergies (food, seasonal)
Lockjaw	Asthma
Difficulty breathing/swallowing	Febrile seizure
Pulmonary embolism	Nonfebrile seizure
Aspiration pneumonia	Thrombocytopenia
Broken bones	Cancer risk later in life
Death (11%)	Sudden infant death syndrome

Diphtheria
Airway blockage
Organ damage
Death (5%–10%)

Pertussis
Pneumonia
Convulsions
Encephalopathy
Death (1%; infants)
Subdural hematoma
Pulmonary hypertension
Collapsed lung
Rectal prolapse

Sudden unexplained death of a
child
Guillain-Barré syndrome

5

Haemophilus Influenzae Type B (Hib)

What Is Haemophilus Influenzae Type B Infection?

Haemophilus influenzae type b (Hib) is a bacterium responsible for multiple types of infections, including meningitis, severe pneumonia, pericarditis (infections of the covering of the heart), and serious infections of the blood, throat (epiglottitis), joints, and bones. Hib can also cause mild throat, respiratory, and ear infections. If Hib is limited to the bloodstream it is called bacteremia, which can lead to sepsis—a dangerous whole-body infection that can damage organs and even cause death if not treated quickly—or other illnesses. Children younger than 5 most often experience Hib infections, but they can also affect older children, adolescents, teens, and adults.

Hib is transmitted from one person to others through respiratory droplets expelled when an infected person sneezes or coughs. A person does not need to be exhibit symptoms to spread the bacteria. People who are not sick but infected are the most common cause of Hib transmission. People who have close contact with an infected person or have certain medical conditions (HIV, sickle cell disease, cancer requiring chemotherapy, radiation therapy, or bone marrow transplant) are also at a greater risk of infection.

Hib symptoms mimic the common cold at first. It is possible for a child to experience a mild case where a sinus infection or bronchitis is diagnosed, be treated with antibiotics, and no one is the wiser that the child had Hib. Moderate cases involve lethargy, general malaise, and possibly labored breathing. Labored breathing usually provokes physicians to perform a chest X-ray and blood test. While blood tests results are awaited, antibiotics are administered. Hospitalization and several days of intravenous antibiotics are ordered if Hib infection is confirmed by blood test. Severe cases involving meningitis, pneumonia, or epiglottitis are more readily detected by physicians.

Symptoms of Hib infection vary depending on the part of the body infected but frequently begin within seven days after exposure. Symptoms of bacteremia include fever, chills, fatigue, diarrhea, abdominal pain, nausea with or without vomiting, difficulty breathing, mental confusion, and anxiety. Hib pneumonia usually presents as cough, shortness of breath, chest pain, fever, chills, sweating, headache, fatigue, and muscle aches. Symptoms of Hib meningitis—infection of the tissue covering the brain and spinal cord—include stiff neck, fever, headache, light sensitivity, nausea with or without vomiting, and mental confusion. Severe sore throat is the characteristic symptom of Hib-related epiglottitis, but it may also be accompanied by fever, abnormal high-pitched sound when breathing (stridor), difficulty breathing or swallowing, drooling, and improvement of symptoms when leaning forward. Hib-related pericarditis is characterized by a sharp, piercing chest pain (center of left side of chest) that is worse when breathing in, shortness of breath, heart palpitations, general malaise, cough, and abdominal or leg swelling. Pericarditis can mimic other conditions, especially a heart attack. Confirmation of Hib infection is determined by one or more laboratory tests. The most common methods to detect the infection use body fluid (blood or spinal fluid) samples.

Breastfeeding is protective against Hib infection and the incidence of Hib caused meningitis in children younger than six months old because breast milk contains Hib antibodies.[359,360,361] Small amounts of Hib antibodies transferred from mother to child provide some level of protection against infection. Despite this fact, breastfed infants are encouraged to receive Hib vaccinations according to the routine recommended schedules.

How Prevalent Is It?

The global burden caused by Hib infections is substantial. The World Health Organization estimates that Hib causes three million serious illnesses and 386,000 deaths each year.[362] A more recent report estimated that Hib caused 8.13 million serious illnesses and 371,000 deaths in children under age 5 worldwide during the year 2000.[363] The majority of cases occur in economically developing countries. Just ten countries (all in Asia and Africa) account for 61 percent of childhood Hib deaths. Without vaccination, scientists estimate that between 1.2 and 2.1 percent of children under age 5 would contract Hib pneumonia each year.[364] Children between the ages of six months and two years of age are at greatest risk of Hib infection.

What Are the Health Risks of Haemophilus Influenzae Type B Infection?

Even with proper treatment, some Hib infections result in long-term problems—blindness, deafness, mental retardation, and learning disabilities—or even death. Brain damage or hearing loss may occur if Hib causes meningitis. Cerebrospinal fluid gets trapped between the surface of the brain and the outer lining of the brain (subdural effusion) in about a third of meningitis cases caused by Hib.[365] Bacteremia can result in the loss of limbs. Globally, Hib causes about 199,000 deaths in children each year, mainly from meningitis and pneumonia.[366] Fatalities usually only occur if the illness is very aggressive from the beginning or if Hib infection is not diagnosed soon enough or treatment delayed. Hib-related deaths rarely occur in developed countries with adequate medical care, like the United States—0.23 deaths per 100,000 population.[367] The greatest number of fatalities occur in the elderly and infants under age 1.[368] Complications can develop quickly, and left untreated, can result in lifelong effects and death, stressing the need for proper medical care if Hib is suspected.

107

Haemophilus Influenzae Type B Vaccine

Description

There are three conjugate Hib vaccines currently in use: ActHIB, Hiberix, and PedvaxHIB. They require three or four doses, depending on the vaccine chosen. ActHIB and Hiberix are given at 2 months, 4 months, 6 months, and 15 months. The first two doses of PedvaxHIB work faster than the other brands so the six-month dose is skipped. ActHIB and Hiberix are combined with tetanus toxoid, but PedvaxHIB is combined with meningococcal proteins. These vaccines are called conjugated because they combine a weak antigen with a strong antigen as a carrier to trigger a stronger immune system response to the weak antigen. Without using a stronger antigen to get the immune system to respond to the weak antigen, T cell activation and more rapid and long-lasting immunologic memory would not be possible.

In addition, Comvax, Pentacel, and TriHIBit are combination shots that contain the Hib vaccine. Comvax combines Hib and HepB, Pentacel (see chapter 4) contains Hib, DTaP, and poliovirus, and TriHIBit was a Hib and DTaP combination that is no longer being manufactured.

Vaccine Manufacturing Process

Each manufacturer makes the Hib vaccine by the same process to start. Hib bacteria is grown in a culture medium, and batches of bacteria are removed from the medium, broken up, sugars (polysaccharides) on the outer coating of the bacteria removed, and purified. The remaining parts of the bacteria are discarded, and the sugars are inserted into the vaccine.

ActHIB grows Hib bacteria in a semisynthetic medium, molecularly (covalently: chemical bonding involving the sharing of an electron between atoms) bound to tetanus toxoid. The tetanus toxoid is prepared by extraction, ammonium sulfate purification, and formaldehyde inactivation of *Clostridium tetani* grown in a modified Mueller-Miller medium with casein derivatives. ActHIB is reconstituted with sodium chloride.

Hib is grown in a synthetic medium during production of the Hiberix vaccine. The tetanus toxin is prepared from *Clostridium tetani* grown in a semisynthetic medium and detoxified with formaldehyde. Hib sugars are covalently bound to the tetanus toxoid and lyophilized (freeze-dried in high vacuum to remove the water and preserve perishable materials) in the presence of lactose. The conjugate is added to a saline solution.

PedvaxHIB uses a complex fermentation medium to grow both Hib and *Neisseria meningitidis* serogroup B. The Hib sugars are purified from the culture broth using ethanol, enzyme digestion, phenol, and diafiltration. The meningococcal proteins are purified by detergent, ultracentrifugation, diafiltration, and sterile filtration. Hib is covalently bonded to the outer membrane of the meningococcal proteins and added to a saline solution.

The Hib and meningococcal part of the Comvax vaccine is produced the same way as PedvaxHIB but adds hepatitis B antigens produced in the same way as Recombivax HB (see chapter 2). They are combined to produce Comvax.

Ingredients

ActHIB[369]

- Hib sugars (10 mcg)
- Tetanus toxoid (24 mcg)
- Formaldehyde (<0.5 mcg)
- Sucrose (8.5%)
- Saline

Hiberix[370]

- Hib sugars (10 mcg)
- Tetanus toxoid (25 mcg)
- Lactose (12.6 mg)
- Formaldehyde (≤0.5 mcg)
- Saline

PedvaxHIB[371]

- Hib sugars (7.5 mcg)
- *Neisseria meningitidis* serogroup B11 proteins (125 mcg)
- Aluminum (225 mcg)
- Saline

Comvax[372]

- Hib sugars (7.5 mcg)
- *Neisseria meningitidis* serogroup B11 proteins (125 mcg)
- Hepatitis B surface antigen (5 mcg)
- Aluminum (225 mcg)
- Saline
- Sodium borate (35 mcg)
- Yeast proteins
- Formaldehyde (0.0004% [w/v])

Controversial Ingredients

- ➢ Formaldehyde
- ➢ Aluminum

Package Insert Adverse Reactions

ActHIB: Children 2–20 months—Fussiness/irritability (75.8%), inconsolable crying (58.5%), decreased activity/lethargy (51.1%), and fever (9.3%). Children 15–20 months—Drowsiness (36.4%), irritability/fussiness (27.3%), tenderness (20%), loss of appetite (12.7%), and firmness at the injection site (5.5%). On average, 3.4 percent of children experienced a serious adverse event within thirty days of vaccination in one study, but they received other injections simultaneously.

Hiberix: First three doses—Irritability (67%–70%), drowsiness (49%–60%), injection-site pain (43%–49%), redness (19%–29%), loss of appetite (28%–29%), and swelling (13%–19%). Fourth dose—Irritability (58%), pain (41%), drowsiness (39%), redness (30%), loss of appetite (28%), swelling (18%), and fever (15%). Serious adverse reactions were reported just 0.6 percent of the time.

PedvaxHIB: Fever (18.1%), swelling (2.5%), and skin reddening (2.2%). No serious vaccine-related adverse reactions were reported during the clinical trial.

Comvax: Irritability (57.0%), drowsiness (49.5%), injection pain, soreness, reddening (34.5%), unusual crying (10.6%), loss of appetite (3.9%), vomiting (2.1%), and diarrhea (1.7%).

Parent or Healthcare Provider Adverse Events Reported through VAERS

ActHIB: Anaphylaxis, hypersensitivity or allergic reactions, hives, itching, rash, seizures, extensive limb swelling, and peripheral swelling.

Hiberix: Extensive swelling of vaccinated limb, injection-site reactions, allergic reactions, anaphylaxis, anaphylactoid reactions, rash, hives, angioedema, seizures (with or without fever), hypotonic-hyporesponsive episode, cyanosis, pale appearance, excessive tiredness, vasovagal responses, and temporary cessation of breathing (premature infants).

PedvacHIB: Swollen lymph nodes, hypersensitivity reactions, febrile seizure, and injection-site abscess.

Comvax: Anaphylaxis, angioedema, hives, erythema multiforme, thrombocytopenia, seizure, febrile seizure, injection-site reactions, abscess at injection site, swollen lymph nodes, extensive swelling of injected limb, allergic reactions (including anaphylaxis), seizures, shock, hives, rash, fainting, and apnea.

Reactions Observed and Documented in Published Research

Like the pertussis vaccine, the Hib vaccine targets some strains but not all, leading to the emergence of other, often more virulent strains (called strain replacement), including nontypeable strains.[373,374,375] The *Haemophilus influenzae* type A (Hia) strain has become a major cause of invasive bacterial illness in some areas of the world since the introduction of the Hib vaccine.[376] An increase in deadly infections by Hia and non-b strains are especially severe in the elderly—frequently requiring intensive care and with a high mortality rate—and young children (under 2 years of age).[377,378,379,380] Cases of non-b strains (a, c, d, e, f, and nontypeable infections) and the related meningitis cases they cause significantly increased in adults following the widespread use of Hib vaccines.[381,382] Mainly occurring in children under age 2, Hia infection–related complications have significantly increased: meningitis (increased eightfold within one year after implementation of the Hib vaccination program), hospitalization (84 percent), and death (9 percent).[383,384] This is another case of waging a war on a single strain of bacterial species that creates a favorable environment for other strains of the same species to thrive and become more active in infecting humans. Continuance of this practice against multiple pathogens may cause us to win small battles but lose the war on infectious disease as we awaken previously inactive pathogens. However, the increase in Hia meningitis is considered small in relation to the significant reduction of Hib meningitis due to vaccination.

Type 1 diabetes (insulin-dependent diabetes mellitus: IDDM) is a chronic autoimmune condition characterized by little or no insulin production by the pancreas. A significant number of viral infections have been linked to type 1 diabetes, including rotavirus, mumps virus, cytomegalovirus, rubella, coxsackievirus B, and enteroviruses.[385] Emerging evidence indicates that a common virus family, enteroviruses, are the most likely to increase a child's risk for developing IDDM.[386] Enteroviruses are a group of viruses that usually cause mild illnesses (like the common cold) to more severe illnesses (like polio and hand, foot, and mouth disease). Poliovirus, coxsackievirus, and enterovirus-D68 are all examples of enteroviruses. Cases of IDDM in susceptible children seem to parallel the seasonal pattern of enterovirus infections, and enterovirus infections often precede the production of islet autoantibodies.[387,388] Islet autoantibodies are proteins produced by the immune system that appear when insulin-producing beta cells in the pancreas are damaged. It is believed that these enteroviruses disrupt the immune system and provoke an autoimmune attack on islet cells in the pancreas. Islet cells (beta cells) perform the very important job of producing insulin in response to elevated blood sugar levels. Increased production of islet autoantibodies has been verified in children with type 1 diabetes.[389] The data also shows that children usually experienced an enterovirus infection more than a year before they tested positive for the islet autoantibodies. Pancreas islet cells express specific receptors that enteroviruses can use to sustain a productive and persistent viral infection that eventually damages or destroys the islet cells. More research is necessary, but the evidence thus far suggests that enteroviruses may contribute to the onset of IDDM?

Similarly, islet autoantibodies have been documented in children a few years after receiving a Hib vaccine. Evaluation of eleven years of health data supports a causal relationship between the Hib vaccine, and other vaccines, and the development of IDDM.[390,391,392,393] The mechanisms by which the Hib vaccine may trigger IDDM three to four years after vaccination imply that all vaccines have the potential to induce diabetes in genetically susceptible individuals. Vaccines contain antigens that interact (cross-react) with pancreatic islet cell proteins, which may produce an autoimmune response that destroys insulin-producing cells and causes IDDM.[394,395] For example, the whole-cell pertussis vaccine contains heat-shock proteins that mimic antigens produced by the body. These heat-shock proteins are capable of initiating an interaction that damages islet cells. Islet cells in the pancreas are responsible for producing hormones, including glucagon and insulin that are important for the control of glucose levels. Islet autoantibodies act as markers of an autoimmune response that is damaging islet cells. They can be detected long before the cells are completely destroyed and help estimate a person's risk for developing IDDM.[396]

Several independent studies show that autoantibodies to islet cells correspond with Hib vaccine timing.[397,398,399,400] On average, diabetes is diagnosed three years after detection of islet autoantibodies in children.[401] There are multiple types of autoantibodies. Islet cell cytoplasmic autoantibodies (ICA), glutamic acid decarboxylase autoantibodies (GADA), insulinoma-associated-2 autoantibodies (IA-2A), insulin autoantibodies (IAA), and zinc transporter-8 autoantibodies (ZnT8A) are the five most commonly associated with diabetes. German researchers evaluated how closely the presence of islet autoantibodies match the risk of developing IDDM by studying children who are at a greater risk of IDDM due to a family history. What they found was that children who had two of the above antibodies by age two had a 50 percent risk of developing IDDM by age 5.[402] Likewise, the delay between a Hib vaccine and onset of IDDM is about two to four years, hinting that autoantibody development could have occurred on or around the time of vaccination. Since the timing of autoantibody presence to IDDM development is comparable for children at a higher risk of diabetes and children who receive a vaccine, the researchers believe there is a strong correlation between vaccination and the development of IDDM.

In addition to mimicking antigens in the body, vaccines may trigger an inflammatory response or overstimulate the immune system to increase the risk of diabetes. Vaccines can activate a systemic inflammatory response, increasing the risk of IDDM.[403] Vaccines also stimulate a potent immune response that activates macrophages. Macrophages play a crucial role in the initiation, maintenance, and resolution of inflammation and are key immune cells involved in metabolism. They produce cytokines like IL-1, TNF-alpha, and IL-6, and enzymes such as 12-LOX, and 15-LOX that increase inflammation. Unchecked and prolonged secretion of these cytokines and enzymes can destroy insulin-secreting islet cells and elevate cortisol levels, contributing to the development of both type 1 and type 2 diabetes and metabolic syndrome.[404,405] Simply put, the macrophages can travel to the pancreas and take up residence in islet cells where they will continue to release cytokines that increase inflammation and subsequently damage their ability to produce insulin. Poor regulation of macrophage activity produces a state of chronic inflammation and metabolic syndrome, which increases the risk of diabetes. Type 1 diabetics have increased macrophage activity and it is believed that this increased activity contributes to the development of IDDM. Once activated, macrophages also release alpha interferon, which impedes the replication of viruses, but a sustained release of alpha interferon is linked to causing IDDM.[406,407] Alpha interferon binds to islet cells and provokes secretion of chemicals that attract immune cells, like macrophages and natural killer cells, to the pancreas and sparks an autoimmune reaction in susceptible individuals. In addition, alpha interferon impairs insulin production further reducing blood sugar control. Macrophage activation and increased alpha interferon production after vaccination represent potential novel mechanisms whereby vaccines could contribute to the onset of IDDM.

While diet and exercise are typically the major cause of obesity and metabolic syndrome, they cannot explain the onset of these conditions in 6-month-old infants. In this case, the cause is more likely a sustained inflammatory response triggered by a foreign substance that challenges the immune system.[408,409,410] It is plausible that this immune challenge that makes the immune system overactive is a vaccine antigen or ingredient. What the research shows is that Hib vaccination significantly increases the risk of diabetes and this risk is exponentially increased if the child receiving these vaccines has a family history of IDDM.[411,412,413,414,415] Children who have a family history of diabetes may be at an increased risk of diabetes following Hib vaccination. Both a disruption of inflammatory control and the ability of vaccinations to trigger autoimmune attacks on islet cells suggest they may increase the risk of metabolic syndrome and diabetes.

Mumps infection can also affect the pancreas and is linked to the development of diabetes. Indeed, some evidence suggests that introduction of the MMR vaccine in Finland in 1982 reduced the risk of type 1 diabetes.[416] This may be because fewer people experienced mumps infections, so the virus had less opportunity to infect and damage the pancreas. Strong immune and inflammatory responses following vaccination, recruit natural killer (NK) cells to the pancreas. Once there, NK cells can destroy islet cells, potentially contributing to autoimmune reactions and the development of IDDM. Whether vaccine virus antigens similarly provoke immune and inflammatory responses linked to diabetes is up for debate. The available evidence is weaker for an association with MMR vaccination and IDDM. Nevertheless, documented cases of IDDM after the mumps vaccine suggest there is a relationship.[417,418] The theory of molecular mimicry states that if foreign peptides and peptides produced naturally by the body (self-antigens) are sufficiently similar, the foreign antigens cause autoreactive T and B cells to attack healthy cells.

Despite molecular similarities between self-antigens and foreign antigens that can differ by as little as one amino acid, the body typically does a good job of recognizing and destroying autoreactive T cells that could damage healthy cells. However, sometimes they escape detection and are activated by a foreign antigen that is molecularly similar. Such may be the case with glutamic acid decarboxylase (GAD65) antibodies. GAD65 is an enzyme present in high concentrations in the brain and pancreatic beta cells. The presence of GAD65 antibodies is used to detect predispositions to IDDM. Protein sequencing allowed scientists to identify similarities between chicken embryo proteins used in some viral vaccines and human GAD65. Given their similarity, chicken embryo proteins can cross-react with human GAD65 proteins to create islet cell autoantibodies and initiate an autoimmune process that causes IDDM.[419] This provides yet another mechanism by which vaccines may play a role in autoimmune diseases and IDDM.

A review that evaluated an association between IDDM and multiple different vaccines (Hib, diphtheria, pertussis, tetanus, MMR, and poliovirus) found that there was no causal relationship between any childhood vaccination and IDDM.[420] Two additional studies also found no association between vaccines and IDDM.[421,422] But the latter two studies were considered methodologically flawed and show a nearly identical risk to studies that do show a relationship between diabetes and vaccination, and therefore may actually support a mild association. Right now, scientists have not pinpointed the definite cause for the dramatic rise in IDDM diagnoses across the world. The answer likely lies in a host of lifestyle, environmental, nutrition, and genetic factors.

See the *Reactions Observed and Documented in Published Research* section of chapter 4 for a discussion on vaccine-associated seizures and the Hib vaccine.

See the *Reactions Observed and Documented in Published Research* section of chapter 4 for a discussion on sudden and unexpected deaths in children and infants in relation to vaccines containing HepB.

INFECTION RISKS	VACCINE RISKS
Impaired vision/hearing	Type 1 diabetes
Mental retardation	Type 2 diabetes
Learning disabilities	Metabolic syndrome
Meningitis	Seizures
Pneumonia	Sudden infant death syndrome
Loss of limbs	Sudden unexplained death of a
Death (very rare)	child

6

Pneumococcus

What Is Pneumococcal Infection?

Pneumococcal infection is caused by *Streptococcus pneumoniae* bacteria, which can cause serious infections like pneumonia, meningitis, and bloodstream infections (septicemia). It is also responsible for milder common infections, such as sinusitis and ear infections (otitis media). The bacteria are primarily transmitted through exposure to respiratory droplets expelled—through coughing or sneezing—by an infected person. It colonizes the back of the nose (nasopharynx) once it enters the body. Infection of other body parts involves direct contact with infected blood or body fluids or invasion of the bloodstream. How long a person is contagious after infection isn't known, but it is presumed that a person can spread the infection as long as the bacteria is present in respiratory secretions. Confirmation of infection is determined via blood test.

Approximately ninety distinct pneumococcal serotypes (distinct strains of a microorganism distinguished by the antigens on their surfaces) have been identified but only a fraction of these cause illness.[423] Infection and colonization (presence of the bacteria on a body surface, like the skin, mouth, or airways) by multiple serotypes at once occurs fairly frequently.[424] It is very virulent—frequently causes illness and harmful effects—because it is shielded from the immune system by a

119

polysaccharide capsule. Imagine the virus with a force field around it as it travels through your body. This force field barrier prevents the surface of the bacteria from coming into contact with cells that can identify its presence. In some ways, it's like the force field gives the virus a level of invisibility to travel through the body undetected.

Of note, introduction of vaccines has changed the serotypes infecting young children. Before the introduction of the vaccine, serotypes 19F, 6A, 6B, and 23F were common in children under age 5 while serotypes 3 and 23F were rather common in adolescents and adults. Serotypes 19A (resistant to antibiotics), 6C, 11A, 15A, and 15B/C became more common after the vaccine was introduced.[425,426] This is troubling because serotypes that used to be rare are now common and bacterial resistance to antibiotics is happening. More and more new serotypes not covered by vaccines are responsible for severe infections, suggesting we have started a war on *Streptococcus pneumoniae* in which it is making regular adjustments to win. The benefits of protection against strains included in the vaccine may come at the cost of an increased prevalence of and susceptibility to other strains.

The severity of pneumococcal illness is dependent on the serotype a person is infected with. Serotype 1 rarely colonizes the nasopharynx, and serotypes 4, 5, and 7F also poorly colonize the nasopharynx. Other serotypes, like 15C and 6B, colonize the nasopharynx more readily and can last in the body for up to twenty weeks.[427] Many people are infected with the bacteria and carry it without any noticeable symptoms.

Symptoms of pneumococcal infection depend on the part of the body infected. Pneumococcal pneumonia, which is an infection of the lungs, is the most common serious form of pneumococcal infection. Symptoms involve fever, chills, cough, chest pain, and rapid or difficult breathing in children. These symptoms can also be observed in adults who are infected, but they may experience confusion and decreased alertness as well. Pneumococcal meningitis is an infection of the tissue covering the brain and spinal cord. This type of pneumococcal infection is characterized by a stiff neck, headache, fever, light sensitivity, and confusion. Infants with meningitis may experience loss of appetite, vomiting, or poor alertness. An infection of the blood, pneumococcal bacteremia can cause symptoms that include fever, chills, and decreased alertness. Sepsis is a complication caused by the body's response to infections—the body releases too many chemicals into the body in response to an infection, triggering changes that can damage multiple organs. Symptoms, such as disorientation, high heart rate, fever, extreme pain, shortness of breath, and clammy or sweaty skin, may be noticed if sepsis occurs. Infection of the middle ear or sinuses can cause mild illnesses. About half of middle ear infections are caused by *pneumococcus* bacteria.[428] Symptoms include ear pain, fever, red and swollen eardrum, and sleepiness. An infection of the sinuses, called sinusitis, results in pain, swelling, and tenderness around the cheeks, eyes, and forehead. Because ear and sinus infections are also caused by other bacteria, they may be simply treated by antibiotics, and the child will likely recover without the provider or parents even realizing she had *Streptococcus pneumoniae*.

How Prevalent Is It?

Pneumococcal infections are quite common, causing nearly nine million cases of pneumonia worldwide—of which 3.5 million were severe—in 2015.[429] The same review found that *Streptococcus pneumoniae* caused about thirteen cases of meningitis per 100,000 children under age 5. Pneumococcal infections most commonly affect the very young and very old (infants and the elderly). About 30–60 percent of infants and 1–10 percent of adults contract the infection.[430,431] In 2014, European countries reported 4.8 cases per 100,000 people, which were higher in those aged 65 or older (13.8 cases per one hundred thousand) and infants (11.3 cases per one hundred thousand).[432] Importantly, 68 percent of cases in children under age 5 were caused by serotypes not covered by any pneumococcal vaccine. A Swedish study reported that any pneumococcal infection occurred at a rate of 15.5 per 100,000 people—again with the elderly and children under 2 being the most affected—

121

and 1.1 case of meningitis per 100,000 people.[433] Sub-Saharan Africa, followed by South Asia, has the highest incidence of pneumococcal illness, which can reach 416 cases per 100,000 population.[434]

What Are the Health Risks of Pneumococcal Infection?

Respiratory infections are a leading cause of childhood mortality worldwide. Pneumonia caused by *Streptococcus pneumoniae* is the leading cause of childhood mortality, accounting for more deaths than all the other causes combined.[435] The World Health Organization estimates that pneumococcal infections are responsible for nearly five hundred thousand deaths in children under age 5 every year.[436] The mortality rate in Sweden averaged 10 percent, varying from 3 percent in children under 18 years of age and peaking at 22 percent in individuals aged 80 or older.[437] Another study concluded that around 11 percent of all deaths in children under age 5 are caused by pneumococcal infections.[438] Most of these deaths occur in developing countries in sub-Saharan Africa and Asia. In developed countries, up to 20 percent of people infected with *Pneumococci* die, while this number spikes to closer to 50 percent in the developing world.[439] Many of the people who die after infection have a preexisting condition, such as a chronic respiratory disease, cancer, cardiovascular disease, or an autoimmune condition. These individuals may have weakened immune systems that predispose them to bacterial infections.

Infants that contract pneumococcal meningitis have severe, lasting effects—hearing loss, eyesight loss, learning or language disabilities, and seizures—about 25 percent of the time.[440] Around 15 percent of children with pneumococcal meningitis die. More than twelve thousand cases of bacteremia are caused by pneumococcal infection each year. These severe infections have about a 20 percent fatality rate overall, but this rate is even higher for the elderly and may be as high as 60 percent.[441] Breastfed infants that are not taken to daycare or exposed to large groups (including church, grocery stores, schools, etc.) are less likely to be infected.

Moderate infections require hospitalization and intravenous antibiotics for one to two weeks. Severe infections will require hospitalization and an aggressive antibiotic regimen, possibly combined with respiratory therapy. Infants, toddlers (especially up to age 2), the elderly, and people with a compromised immune system are more likely to experience severe illness.

Pneumococcal Vaccine

Description

Pneumococcal vaccines are conjugates of multiple serotypes: Synflorix (pneumococcal polysaccharide conjugate vaccine, PCV10) contains ten serotypes—1, 4, 5, 6B, 7F, 9V, 14, 18C, 19F, and 23F; Prevnar 13 (pneumococcal conjugate vaccine, PCV13) contains thirteen serotypes— 1, 3, 4, 5, 6A, 6B, 7F, 9V, 14, 18C, 19A, 19F, and 23F; while Pneumovax 23 (pneumococcal polysaccharide vaccine, PPSV23) contains twenty-three serotypes—1, 2, 3, 4, 5, 6B, 7F, 8, 9 N, 9 V, 10A, 11A, 12F, 14, 15B, 17F, 18C, 19F, 19A, 20, 22F, 23F, and 33F. The original vaccine only covered seven strains and is no longer being manufactured. These vaccines will likely require regular adjustment to add serotypes that are being identified as responsible for severe infections currently.

Prevnar 13 vaccine is given during a child's most vulnerable years at two months, four months, six months, and between 12 and 15 months. It can also be given to older children and adults. Synflorix is administered in three doses (2 months, with additional doses occurring with at least one month between doses, with or without a booster—the booster can be given from 9 months onward—preferably between 12 and 15 months), or a two-dose schedule with a booster dose (first dose as early as six weeks old, second dose two months later, and the booster dose at least six months after the second dose, preferable between 12 and 15 months). Pneumovax 23 is not approved for use in children 2 and younger but is primarily used in adults and people with certain immune disorders or chronic illnesses. When the vaccine is given depends on if and when an individual received previous pneumococcal vaccines.

Vaccine Manufacturing Process

Prevnar 13 is a suspension of sugars (saccharides) of the capsular antigens of thirteen *Streptococcus pneumoniae* serotypes, individually linked to nontoxic diphtheria protein. Pneumococcal serotypes are kept alive in a soy culture, and then the bacteria are broken up to obtain sugars from the outer covering of the germs. The nontoxic diphtheria toxin is isolated from cultures of *Corynebacterium diphtheriae* grown in a casamino acids and yeast-extract-based medium or in a chemically defined medium. It is purified with ammonium sulfate. The pneumococcal sugars and diphtheria protein are combined with aluminum.

Conjugated with Hib, and diphtheria and tetanus toxoids, Synflorix is adsorbed onto aluminum sulfate. Beyond this, not much is known about the actual manufacturing process, although it is assumed the sugars are isolated similarly to Prevnar 13 and the diphtheria and tetanus toxoids are obtained by a similar process used for DTaP and Tdap vaccines.

Pneumovax is not conjugated to other antigens like the previous two vaccines, which may be why it is ineffective in children—it lacks an adjuvant to provoke a sufficient immune response. The pneumococcal sugars are likely obtained the same way as explained for Prevnar 13.

Ingredients

Prevnar 13[442]

- Pneumococcal sugar serotypes 1, 3, 4, 5, 6A, 7F, 9V, 14, 18C, 19A, 19F, 23F (2.2 mcg each)
- Pneumococcal sugar serotype 6B (4.4 mcg)
- Diphtheria protein (34 mcg)
- Polysorbate 80 (100 mcg)
- Succinate buffer (295 mcg)
- Aluminum (125 mcg)

Synflorix[443]

- Pneumococcal sugar serotypes 1, 5, 6B, 7F, 9V, 14, 23F (1 mcg each)
- Pneumococcal sugar serotypes 4, 18C, 19F (3 mcg each)
- Hib protein D (9–16 mcg)
- Tetanus toxoid protein (5–10 mcg)
- Diphtheria toxoid protein (3–6 mcg)
- Sodium chloride (4.3 mg)
- Aluminum

Pneumovax 23[444]

- Pneumococcal sugar serotypes 1, 2, 3, 4, 5, 6B, 7F, 8, 9N, 9V, 10A, 11A, 12F, 14, 15B, 17F, 18C, 19F, 19A, 20, 22F, 23F, and 33F (25 mcg each)
- Saline solution with 0.25 percent phenol

Controversial Ingredients

- ➢ Aluminum
- ➢ Polysorbate 80

Package Insert Adverse Reactions

Prevnar 13: Infants/toddlers—Irritability (>70%), injection-site tenderness (>50%), decreased appetite (>40%), decreased sleep (>40%), fever (>20%), injection-site redness (>20%), and injection-site swelling (>20%). Children 5–17—injection-site tenderness (>80%), injection-site redness (>30%), injection-site swelling (>30%), limitation of arm movement (>10%), vomiting (>5%), fever/chills (>5%), and rash (>5%). Adults—injection-site pain (>50%), fatigue (>30%), headache (>20%), muscle pain (>20%), joint pain (>10%), decreased appetite (>10%), injection-site redness (>10%), vomiting (>5%), fever/chills (>5%), and rash (>5%). Serious adverse events occurred in 8.2 percent of infants and toddlers, with bronchiolitis, gastroenteritis, and pneumonia being the most common reported. Three deaths, as a result of sudden infant death syndrome, also occurred. Up to 1.4 percent of adults reported a serious adverse event within one month of vaccination.

Synflorix: Infants and children—Irritability (55%) and injection-site pain (39%–58%). Appetite loss, drowsiness, and fever were also very commonly observed.

Pneumovax 23: Injection-site soreness/pain/tenderness (60.0%–77.2%), injection-site swelling (20.3%–39.8%), injection-site redness (16.4%–34.5%), headache (17.6%–18.1%), fatigue (13.2%–17.9%), and general muscle aches (11.9%–17.9%). Adverse reactions were worse in those receiving their second dose of Pneumovax 23 approximately three to five years after their first dose.

Parent or Healthcare Provider Adverse Events Reported through VAERS

Prevnar 13—Injection-site dermatitis, hives, or itching, enlarged lymph nodes near injection, cyanosis (bluish skin and mucous membranes), hypersensitivity reactions, anaphylactic reaction including shock, decreased muscle tone, angioneurotic edema (swelling and massive intracellular protein loss and plasma expulsion in the subcutaneous tissue), apnea, and pale appearance.

Synflorix—Anaphylaxis and hypotonic-hyporesponsive episode (sudden onset of poor muscle tone, poor responsiveness, pale appearance, and cyanosis after immunization).

Pneumovax 23—Cellulitis or cellulitis-like reactions, general malaise, fever, warmth at injection site, decreased limb mobility, swelling in the injected area, nausea and vomiting, enlarged lymph nodes, thrombocytopenia (low blood platelet count) in people with previously stabilized thrombocytopenia, hemolytic anemia (red blood cells are destroyed faster than they can be created) in people with hematologic disorders, high white blood cell count, anaphylactic reactions, serum sickness (an immune response to proteins in medicines that is similar to an allergy), angioneurotic edema, arthritis, joint pain, Guillain-Barré syndrome, pins or pricking sensation, febrile seizure, neuropathy that affects the nerve roots, rash, and hives.

Reactions Observed and Documented in Published Research

The sheer number of *Streptococcus pneumoniae* serotypes (about ninety) means that not all strains are covered by the vaccines. Strains not covered by vaccines are likely to rapidly replace strains targeted by the vaccine as causes of infections in humans. Evidence shows that this is already happening. The introduction of the PCV7 vaccine in 2000 significantly reduced the incidence of serious pneumococcal disease initially, but it was a two-edged sword. While strains covered by the vaccine were diminishing, serious infections from strains not covered in the vaccine significantly increased.[445] In effect, the overall rates of pneumococcal infection have not changed substantially since the first introduction of the PCV7 vaccine because of strain replacement.[446,447] Even worse, the introduction of PCV7 promoted the rapid replacement of strains covered by this vaccine with strains that are resistant to antibiotics.[448,449] Unfortunately, a rebound in pneumococcal-related meningitis cases also occurred.[450]

Another study found that introduction of PCV7 shifted the illnesses from children to adults, particularly elderly persons.[451,452] During their lifetimes, adults built up a natural immunity to pneumococcal strains that were common and that they were exposed to. However, when the vaccine was introduced, it targeted the common strains that adults had a natural immunity against. Aided by the vaccine, previously nonvirulent strains emerged that adults and the elderly had no natural immunity to and that became more active and virulent. The result was that adults and the elderly experienced higher rates of infection and illness.

Further research found that strains of *Streptococcus pneumoniae* strongly compete against each other, which explains why new strains emerge when a limited number of strains are targeted by the vaccine.[453] To some degree, the dozens of *Streptococcus pneumoniae* strains naturally kept one another in check as they competed for hosts to infect. By introducing a vaccine that only targets a limited number of strains, we are essentially aiding strains not covered in vaccines by eliminating some of their competition.

The PCV13 that covered more strains was introduced in 2010 hoping to crush some of the emerging strains. Nevertheless, the same outcome of decreased vaccine strains—the thirteen included in PCV13—and increased infections by nonvaccine strains were observed.[454] Even more troubling, an increase in sepsis caused by nonvaccine strains of *S. pneumoniae* has been documented.[455] About 69 percent of sepsis cases were caused by nonvaccine strains following the introduction of PCV-13 and 8 percent of these cases are fatal. Vaccines seem to be shifting the balance of power among *S. pneumoniae* strains rather than eradicating the illness. As happened with the introduction of the PCV7 vaccine, adults over age 65 experienced a significant increase in pneumococcal illness shortly after the introduction of PCV13.[456,457,458] The pneumococcal vaccine is creating a moral dilemma where vaccine policy makers must decide if the lives of infants are more important than the lives of the elderly. This book won't get embroiled in that debate, but the intent is to point out a serious shortcoming and flaw in some vaccines. As the great Albert Einstein said, "The definition of insanity is doing the same thing over and over again and expecting different results." Unless a vaccine with all ninety *S. pneumoniae* strains is introduced, a pneumococcal vaccine will do little to eradicate illness caused by the bacteria.

INFECTION RISKS	VACCINE RISKS
Meningitis	Strain replacement
Pneumonia	Illness burden shifted to adults
Death (15%–20% of severe	and the elderly
cases)	
Learning disabilities	
Hearing or eyesight impairment	
Seizures	

7

Poliovirus

What Is Poliovirus Infection?

Polio, also called poliomyelitis, is caused by a contagious human enterovirus (viruses that typically live in the gastrointestinal tract and sometimes spread to other areas of the body) called the poliovirus. There are three wild types of poliovirus: type 1, type 2, and type 3. Two types are believed to be eradicated: type 2 since 1999 and type 3 in 2019. Type 1 remains active and causes illness. Vaccine-derived polio can be caused by the oral poliovirus vaccine, which contains an attenuated (weakened) vaccine virus.

The virus can cause one of two illnesses: (1) illness that does not involve the central nervous system and causes mild symptoms (nonparalytic polio) and (2) illness involving the central nervous system, which causes paralysis (paralytic polio) in less than 1 percent of poliovirus infections.[459] The majority of people infected with poliovirus—90–95 percent—don't show any symptoms and aren't even aware they are infected.[460]

Poliovirus is highly contagious and spreads from person-to-person contact. It only enters the body through the mouth via contact with infected feces, or less commonly by ingesting respiratory droplets (cough or sneeze) of an infected person. Good hygiene is critical to prevent infection. The virus can live in an infected person's feces for weeks, making it easy to contaminate food and water in unsanitary conditions. Touching the mouth after contact with infected feces can cause infection. An infected person—even those who display no symptoms—can spread the virus to others.

People with nonparalytic polio can experience flu-like symptoms for two to several days, which may include fever, headache, sore throat, neck pain and stiffness, back pain and stiffness, vomiting, muscle weakness or tenderness, or pain and stiffness of the limbs. If the poliovirus affects the brain and spinal cord (central nervous system) more serious symptoms may occur, such as paresthesia (feelings of pins and needles) and meningitis. The most severe form of polio, paralytic polio, is characterized by progressive muscle or joint weakness and pain, muscle wasting, fatigue, abnormal reflexes, difficulty breathing or swallowing, and decreased tolerance to cold temperatures. Diagnosis of poliovirus infection is confirmed with a sample of throat secretions, stool, or cerebrospinal fluid.

A polio infection can lead to lifelong symptoms decades after recovering from the initial infection, something known as post-polio syndrome. When this occurs, polio survivors usually begin to experience gradual muscle weakness of muscles previously affected by the polio infection. Occasionally, pain from joint degeneration and skeletal deformities like scoliosis may precede the muscle weakness. Progressive muscle weakness, generalized fatigue, and loss of muscle mass may also be experienced. The symptoms of post-polio syndrome range from mild to moderate. It is rarely life-threatening, but the condition may reduce quality of life.

How Prevalent Is It?

Wild poliovirus cases have substantially decreased by about 99 percent since 1988 and polio is virtually unheard of in the Western hemisphere. Most cases of wild poliovirus are reported in Africa and Asia. Today, there are more vaccine-caused (by the oral poliovirus vaccine) polio cases than those caused by the wild virus.[461] When a person receives the oral polio vaccine, the weakened vaccine virus replicates in the intestine for a limited period. The vaccine virus is excreted in the person's feces and can spread to the immediate community if there is inadequate sanitation and poor vaccine coverage. Indeed, some of the most vulnerable countries to wild-type virus infections had zero cases of wild virus reported compared to one to 103 vaccine-caused cases in 2019.[462] Children who receive oral polio vaccine can also spread it to others they come in contact with so parents and siblings should be aware. More than 90 percent of vaccine-caused polio infections were due to the type 2 component in the oral polio vaccine, instigating a change in the vaccine that removed type 2 poliovirus from the vaccine. Unfortunately, vaccine-caused polio can still cause paralysis (although less commonly than wild virus), making it a somewhat risky vaccine.

Comparison of Wild and Vaccine-Caused Polio Cases[463,464,465]

Year	Vaccine-Caused Cases	Wild Virus Caused Cases
2018	104	33
2019	302	168

What Are the Health Risks of Poliovirus Infection?

Beyond the rare case of paralytic polio, from 2 to 10 percent of people with paralytic polio die from the infection because it paralyzes the muscles that help them breathe.[466] High blood pressure is a common complication of polio and may progress to hypertensive encephalopathy (general brain dysfunction due to high blood pressure). Gastric bleeding is also a risk. Rarely myocarditis (inflammation of the heart muscle) will occur.

Polio Vaccine

Description

There are two types of poliovirus vaccine, oral polio vaccine (OPV) and inactivated poliovirus vaccine (IPVC). The United States has exclusively used the IPVC since 2000, but OPV is still the predominant vaccine used in other countries because it is cheaper and easier to use. The four-dose IPVC is given at 2 months, 4 months, between 6 and 18 months, and again between 4 and 6 years old. The OPV is given as at least three doses at minimum intervals of four weeks (suggested at birth, 6, 10, and 14 weeks). Polio vaccine is also included in some combination shots (Pentacel, Pediarix, and Kinrix).

Vaccine Manufacturing Process

The IPVC grows each of the three types of poliovirus in monkey kidney cells (VERO) in Eagle MEM modified medium, supplemented with newborn calf bovine serum. For viral growth, the culture medium is replaced by M-199, without calf bovine serum. The viruses are inactivated with formalin—an aqueous (water) solution of formaldehyde—after purification.

There are three types of OPV: monovalent (contain one strain), bivalent (contain types 1 and 3 poliovirus), and trivalent (contain all three types of poliovirus; withdrawn in 2016). OPV is made by weakening the included strains of poliovirus (two or three) by passing them through monkey kidney cells (VERO) at specific temperatures. The weakened viruses produce an immune response—production of antibodies in the intestines—after swallowing. They act as a first line of defense against poliovirus because the virus enters the body through the gastrointestinal tract. The risk with this vaccine is its ability to replicate itself effectively in the intestines, which can cause vaccine-caused polio and, in rare cases, (one case per million doses) cause paralytic polio.[467]

Ingredients

Inactivated poliovirus vaccine (IPVC)[468]

- Type 1 inactivated poliovirus (40 D-antigen units)
- Type 2 inactivated poliovirus (8 D-antigen units)
- Type 3 inactivated poliovirus (32 D-antigen units)
- 2-phenoxyethanol (0.5%)

- Formaldehyde (≤0.02%, roughly 100 mcg)
- Neomycin (<5 ng)
- Streptomycin (<200 ng)
- Polymyxin B (<50 ng)
- Cow blood (<50 ng)

Oral polio vaccine (OPV)[469,470]

- Type 1 inactivated poliovirus ($10^{5.9}$ + 0.5 $TCID_{50}$)
- Type 2 inactivated poliovirus ($10^{5.0}$ + 0.5 $TCID_{50}$)
- Type 3 inactivated poliovirus ($10^{5.7}$ + 0.5 $TCID_{50}$)
- Neomycin (<25 mcg)
- Streptomycin (<25 mcg)
- Magnesium chloride

Controversial Ingredients

- ➢ Monkey kidney cells (VERO)
- ➢ Cow blood
- ➢ Formaldehyde
- ➢ 2-phenoxyethanol

Package Insert Adverse Reactions

IPVC: Fever (38%), injection-site pain (13.0%), injection-site redness (3.2%), and injection-site hardening of tissues (1.0%). Other reactions included irritability, sleepiness, fussiness, and crying.

OPV: OPV is generally well tolerated, but there is a small risk of nonparalytic polio and very rarely paralytic polio, particularly among infants receiving their first dose and people they come in contact with.

Parent or Healthcare Provider Adverse Events Reported through VAERS

IPVC—Swollen lymph nodes, agitation, rash or mass at injection site, allergic reaction (including anaphylaxis), general joint or muscle aches, seizure (including febrile), headache, pins-and-needles feelings, excessive tiredness, rash, and hives.

OPV—Not reported largely because OPV was almost always given at the same time as DTaP, DT, or Td vaccines, and the adverse reactions seemed more likely associated with these three vaccines.

Reactions Observed and Documented in Published Research

Nonpolio acute flaccid paralysis (NPAFP) is characterized by the sudden onset of paralysis or weakness in any part of the body of a child young than 15 years old. Polio immunization activities intensified in India in 1999 as part of a campaign to eradicate polio from India and the world. However, Indian doctors began to question the practice of widespread administration of the OPV a few years later when a surge in polio cases was observed. Virtually all of the polio cases were among children who received four doses of OPV and many in children who received ten doses of OPV.[471] The findings suggest that the OPV vaccine was not effective in preventing polio infections.

In addition, to the vaccine failures observed, the OPV significantly increased cases of NPAFP. In 2011, India experienced 47,500 new cases of NPAFP, which is clinically indistinguishable from polio paralysis but twice as deadly. During this outbreak, more than 43 percent of children diagnosed with NPAFP had residual paralysis after sixty days or died.[472] That year the rate of NPAFP was 13.35 cases per one hundred thousand people compared to the expected rate of 1–2/100,000 and strongly correlated with the number of oral poliovirus vaccines administered.[473] Cases of NPAFP directly increased in correspondence with the number of oral polio vaccines doses administered, and was the only correlation that showed a positive relationship.[474] Some Indian states experienced higher rates of 25-35/100,000. In total, more than 640,000 children developed NPAFP in the years 2000–2017, suggesting that OPV may have contributed to an additional 491,704 paralyzed children. The incidence of NPAFP is up to thirty-five times higher than international norms in regions of India where children were vaccinated multiple times as recommended (the oral polio vaccine is recommended as a four- or five-dose series). Based on this, India made a switch from a trivalent

OPV to a bivalent OPV and also incorporated the injectable polio vaccine to reduce the significant rise in NPAFP experienced in the country due to the aggressive OPV vaccination campaign.

Scientists and health professionals endeavored to identify what was causing an increase in NPAFP. Recent research suggests that other nonpolio enteroviruses—like echoviruses and coxsackievirus—may contribute to the development of NPAFP.[475,476,477] It is possible that this represents an emergence of opportunistic viruses after extensive eradication of poliovirus by vaccination. Decades of aggressive vaccination worldwide has driven poliovirus to the brink of extinction, but potentially allowed viruses in the same family to thrive. Here again, aggressive vaccination campaigns against one infectious illness may have cause the emergence of others. The axiom of Hydra "cut off one head and two will take their place" may become the mantra of vaccines if they continue to be associated with the rise of emerging infectious illnesses. Recognizing nonpolioviruses may be the replacement for polio infections, health officials are scrambling to find answers to these emerging viruses that represent a global health concern.

See the *Reactions Observed and Documented in Published Research* section of chapter 4 for a discussion on vaccine-associated seizures and the poliovirus vaccine.

See the *Reactions Observed and Documented in Published Research* section of chapter 4 for a discussion on sudden and unexpected deaths in children and infants in relation to vaccines containing HepB.

INFECTION RISKS	VACCINE RISKS
Paralysis (1%)	Paralysis (1/1,000,000)
Death (2%–10% of paralysis cases)	Death
High blood pressure	Seizures
Hypertensive encephalopathy	Sudden infant death syndrome
Myocarditis	Sudden unexpected death of a child
Gastric bleeding	

8

Influenza

What Is Influenza Infection?

Influenza, or the flu, is a contagious respiratory system—nose, throat, and lungs—infection caused by a group of viruses known as influenza. There are actually four types of influenza viruses: A, B, C, and D. Types A and B are responsible for the increased human cases (called an epidemic) observed during colder months. Influenza A viruses may cause epidemics (affecting a greater number of people than usual for the locality) or global pandemics (affects worldwide populations) of flu. Influenza C is not believed to cause flu epidemics and only results in mild illness. The last type, influenza D, primarily affects cattle and is not known to be a cause of infection in humans. A different strain of the virus carrying different mutations usually predominates each year.

In addition to the types of influenza virus, influenza A viruses are subdivided according to proteins (hemagglutinin and neuraminidase) found on the surface of the virus. The two protein subtypes mean there are potentially 198 different influenza A subtypes, but only about 131 have been detected in nature so far. At a deeper level, influenza subtypes are further divided into clades (groups) and subclades (subgroups). Clades and subclades basically group the viruses according to similar genetics and common ancestors. Mutations of these viruses have also been observed—for instance, the 2009 H1N1 pandemic virus was a mutated strain that combined human, swine, and bird flu viruses.

Unlike influenza A viruses, type B viruses are not divided into subtypes. Instead, they are classified according to lineage and the antigenic properties of the surface glycoprotein hemagglutinin: Yamagata (B/Yamagata/16/88) and Victoria (B/Victoria/2/87). Influenza B viruses are also further classified into clades and subclades. All told, this means that thousands of influenza viruses are out there, of which a smaller group causes human infections each year.

Flu is considered seasonal in that it occurs more frequently during specific seasons. The northern hemisphere typically experiences increased cases of flu in early fall, peaking in mid-February. Temperate regions in the southern hemisphere experience peak influenza activity during May through August. Tropical areas can experience flu throughout the year.

For the majority of people, influenza resolves on its own without any medical intervention. Plenty of rest, lots of fluids, and some of grandma's chicken soup is all that is needed. However, children under age 5 (especially those under 12 months), the elderly (over age 65), people with chronic illnesses or a weakened immune system, women who are pregnant or recently delivered (two weeks postpartum), and individuals who are severely obese are at a greater risk of complications from the flu.

The initial symptoms—runny nose, sore throat, sneezing—imitate a common cold but come on more suddenly and tend to be more severe. Characteristic signs of the flu are fever, chills, sweats, muscle aches, headache, general fatigue, nasal congestion, and a dry, persistent cough. The majority of flu cases resolve without consequence, but moderate cases involving complications require medical attention. Severe cases with complications frequently place the individual in the hospital. Antiviral medications intended to help resolve the flu more quickly if given within the first forty-eight hours of the first symptoms also exist. The flu is typically diagnosed by symptom presentation and nasal swab.

Like other infectious illnesses, the flu is easily spread by respiratory droplets expelled when an infected person coughs or sneezes. Droplets can remain in the air for hours—a cubic meter of air can contain fifteen thousand flu viruses in very high-traffic areas.[478] These infection-spreading droplets can even be released when talking, singing, or exhaling.[479] Research shows that airborne flu particles are in sufficient levels in public places (day care centers, public transportation centers, etc.) to infect others frequently.[480] Less commonly, people may get the flu by touching an infected surface or object and then touching their noses or mouths. With so much flu virus hanging out in the air of crowded places, it's no wonder that so many people get the flu during the most active months.

How Prevalent Is It?

Worldwide, influenza is estimated to cause three to five million severe illnesses each year, and about 290,000–650,000 flu-related deaths. Most of these deaths occur in high-risk populations, like among people over age 65.[481] Many of the deaths attributed to the flu are from flu-related complications—the person develops a secondary infection (bacterial pneumonia) or the flu aggravates an existing chronic illness (congestive heart failure, or chronic obstructive pulmonary disease)—rather than the flu itself. For example, a person with diabetes (many of whom have poor immune function) and mild kidney failure. If they get the flu and become dehydrated—making kidney function worse—they may not be able to fight the flu because of an already lowered immune response and spiral out of control. The flu acts as the tipping point toward death in vulnerable individuals.

Experts suggest that influenza begins in the west and spreads to the east across the globe because the virus dies out across the world during the year everywhere but in the west. Despite this fact, more cases of flu are reported in the east than the west, particularly in Southeast Asia. This is likely due to dense populations in many Asian countries.

What Are the Health Risks of Influenza?

The vast majority of people with the flu have only mild illness and require no medical care. However, some people develop complications as a result of the flu, a portion of which are life-threatening or result in death. Moderate complications of the flu include ear infections and sinus infections. More serious complications include pneumonia (from the flu virus itself or an opportunistic bacteria that infects the person while or immediately after having the flu), myocarditis (heart inflammation), encephalitis (brain inflammation), myositis (muscle inflammation), sepsis, and multi-organ failure. Flu can also exacerbate existing chronic conditions, such as heart disease or asthma.

It is not surprising that older people bear the greatest burden of severe flu cases. Statistically, the elderly account for up to 70 percent of flu-related hospitalizations and 90 percent of flu-related deaths each year.[482] About 1,500 total flu-related deaths are reported every year. However, 36,000 deaths per year is often reported by the press and many medical organizations because they include both pneumonia and flu deaths that are reported in the same group in the *Morbidity and Mortality Weekly Report* database. The older a person is, the more likely they will experience flu-related complications. Individuals aged 85 or older are 2.2–6.4 times more likely to be hospitalized than adults aged 65–74. Those aged 75–84 are 1.4–3.0 times more likely to be hospitalized. The H3N2 flu virus is particularly dangerous for the elderly. H3N2 flu infections cause more severe illness and result in more hospitalization in the elderly. Older adults tend to have a weaker immune system making it hard for them to fight flu infection.

The flu can be serious for children younger than 5 years old as well. Children younger than 2 are at a high risk of developing flu-related complications. Like elderly adults, young children who get the flu are at a greater risk of developing pneumonia. In addition, they can quickly become dehydrated, experience secondary infections (sinus or ear infections), exacerbation of existing medical conditions, and, in rare cases, encephalopathy or death. Since 2004–2005, flu-related deaths in children reported to the CDC have ranged from 37–187 per "flu season," with an average of about a hundred.[483] Even in the worst years of the flu, the number of childhood deaths doesn't come anywhere near the grossly inflated thousands reported by media and some medical organizations.

Influenza Vaccine

Description

Two types of influenza vaccine are widely available: injectable influenza vaccine (IIV) and live inactivated influenza vaccine (LAIV). Of the thousands of influenza viruses a person might be exposed to, both of these vaccines typically protect against three of four influenza viruses—H3N2, pandemic A (H1N1), and one or both of the two influenza B lineage viruses. Common brand names of the IIV include quadrivalent (four strains)—Afluria, Fluarix, FluLaval, and Flucelvax; trivalent (three strains)—Fluad, Fluvirin, and Fluzone. Flublok is a quadrivalent recombinant (produced by inserting the DNA encoding of an antigen to stimulate an immune response) vaccine for persons aged 18 or older. FluMist and Fluenz Tetra are common LAIV vaccines. Immunization against the flu is recommended at or near the start of "flu season" in your locale for most people six months of age or older.

The IIV is given as an injection and is approved for a wider range of ages and individuals. Research suggests that IIV may be more effective than LAIV for certain influenza types (pandemic H1N1).[484] People who are allergic to eggs should not receive vaccines manufactured in egg cells. LAIV is a live-virus nasal spray approved for use in people aged 2–49 with limitations. Pregnant women, children taking aspirin or salicylate-containing medications, people with a weakened immune system, children with asthma (aged 2–4) or a history of wheezing in the last twelve months, people who have taken influenza antiviral drugs, and people who care for severely immunocompromised individuals should not get LAIV. In addition, children aged 5 and older with asthma, certain underlying medical conditions (lung disease, heart disease, kidney disease, diabetes, liver disorders, neurological or neuromuscular disorders, or metabolic disorders), moderate-to-severe acute illness with fever, and Guillain-Barré syndrome (within six weeks following a previous dose of influenza vaccine) should be cautioned against using LAIV.

It should be noted that a high number of people who receive flu vaccines experience flu-like symptoms—fever, headache, and body aches—for a few days after vaccination. This can occur for a few reasons. Flu-like symptoms can be due to a reaction to the vaccine as your body produces antibodies. It takes about two weeks for the flu shot to take effect, so it is also possible that you could contract the actual flu during this time. In addition, the viruses in the vaccine you received may not match the strain you were exposed to. So people can have flu-like symptoms as the body creates antibodies to the vaccine virus or get the actual flu because antibodies weren't created yet or the vaccine didn't protect against the flu you were exposed to.

Vaccine Manufacturing Process

The influenza vaccine takes about six months to produce and is based on viral propagation in embryonated eggs or cell cultures. Egg-based flu vaccines are the most common. In this method, laboratories grow influenza viruses in fertilized hen's eggs for incubation. After several days to allow for viral replication, the fluid containing virus is harvested from the eggs. The virus is inactivated (killed) for IIVs and the virus antigen purified. The virus is weakened in LAIVs. Following inspection and approval from a regulatory body, the vaccine is then released for shipment and administered to the public.

As the name suggests, cell-based flu vaccines grow flu viruses in animal cells. Next, the viruses are inoculated into cultured mammalian cells and allowed to replicate for a few days. The virus-containing fluid is removed from the cells and purified. Following inspection and approval from a regulatory body, the vaccine is then released for shipment.

Recombinant vaccines are the third way to make flu vaccines. These vaccines are created synthetically by taking DNA (genetic instructions) for making hemagglutinin found in flu viruses and combining it with a baculovirus (a virus that infects invertebrates). The baculovirus helps transport the DNA instructions for making flu virus hemagglutinin antigen into a host cell—insect cell line (*Spodoptera frugiperda*). Next, the recombinant hemagglutinin antigen grows rapidly in the host cell line. The antigen is collected, purified, and packaged as a vaccine. Following inspection and approval from a regulatory body, the vaccine is then released for shipment.

Vaccine	Age Rec.	Type	Culture	Thimerosal
Afluria	6 mos.–64 yrs.	IIV	Egg	24.5mcg/0.5mL*
Fluad	≥65 yrs.	IIV	Egg	No
Fluarix	≥6 mos.	IIV	Egg	No
Flublok	≥18 yrs.	IIV	N/A	No
Flucelvax	≥4 yrs.	IIV	Cell	<25mcg/0.5mL*
Fluenz Tetra	2–17 yrs.	LAIV	Egg	No
FluLaval	≥6 mos.	IIV	Egg	<25mcg/0.5mL*
FluMist	2–49 yrs.	LAIV	Egg	No
Fluvirin	≥4 yrs.	IIV	Egg	≤1mcg/0.5mL 25mcg/5mL
Fluzone	≥6 mos.	IIV	Egg	<25mcg/0.5mL[+]
Fluzone (HD)	≥65 yrs.	IIV	Egg	No

* 5.0mL dose only; 0.25mL and 0.5 mL doses don't use thimerosal.
[+] Multidose units only.

Ingredients

Note: Ingredients listed are those on the vaccine package insert at the time of this writing. Ingredients, especially the influenza virus strains used in each vaccine, are subject to change according to the predicted most active strains of the season.

Afluria[485]

- Inactivated influenza virus
  - A/Singapore/GP1908/2015 IVR 180A (H1N1)
  - A/Singapore/INFIMH-16-0019/2016 IVR-186 (H3N2)
  - B/Maryland/15/2016
  - B/Phuket/3073/2013 BVR-1B
- Hemagglutinin (60 mcg; 15 mcg from each virus)
- Sodium chloride (4.1 mg)
- Monobasic sodium phosphate (80 mcg)
- Dibasic sodium phosphate (300 mcg)
- Monobasic potassium phosphate (20 mcg)
- Potassium chloride (20 mcg)
- Calcium chloride (0.5 mcg)
- Egg protein, ovalbumin (<1 mcg)
- Sucrose (<10 mcg)
- Neomycin sulfate (≤ 81.8 ng)
- Polymyxin B (≤14 ng)
- Beta-propiolactone (≤1.5 ng)
- Sodium taurodeoxycholate (≤ 10 ppm)

Fluad[486]

- Inactivated influenza virus
  - A/Brisbane/02/2018 IVR-190 (H1N1)
  - A/Kansas/14/2017 X-327 (H3N2)
  - B/Maryland/15/2016
- Hemagglutinin (60 mcg; 15 mcg from each virus)
- Squalene based oil-in-water emulsion adjuvant, MF59 (9.5 mg squalene)
- Polysorbate 80 (1.175 mg)
- Sorbitan trioleate (1.175 mg)
- Sodium citrate dehydrate (0.66 mg)

- Citric acid monohydrate (0.04 mg)
- Cetyltrimethylammonium bromide (≤12 mcg)
- Formaldehyde (≤10 mcg)
- Egg protein, ovalbumin (< 0.4 mcg)
- Neomycin (≤0.02 mcg)
- Kanamycin (≤0.03 mcg)
- Barium (<0.5 mcg)
- Hydrocortisone (≤0.0025 ng)

Fluarix[487]

- Inactivated influenza virus
  - A/Brisbane/02/2018 (H1N1)
  - A/Kansas/14/2017 X-327 (H3N2)
  - B/Maryland/15/2016
  - B/Phuket/3073/2013 BVR-1B
- Hemagglutinin (60 mcg; 15 mcg from each virus)
- Octoxynol-10 (≤0.115 mg)
- Alpha-tocopheryl hydrogen succinate (≤0.135 mg)
- Sodium deoxycholate (≤65 mcg)
- Polysorbate 80 (≤0.55 mg)
- Formaldehyde (≤5 mcg)
- Gentamicin sulfate (≤0.15 mcg)
- Egg protein, ovalbumin (≤0.05 mcg)
- Hydrocortisone (≤ 0.0015 mcg)

Flublok[488]

- Inactivated influenza virus
  - A/Brisbane/02/2018 (H1N1)
  - A/Kansas/14/2017 X-327 (H3N2)
  - B/Maryland/15/2016
  - B/Phuket/3073/2013 BVR-1B
- Hemagglutinin (180 mcg; 45 mcg from each virus)
- Sodium chloride (4.4 mg)
- Monobasic sodium phosphate (0.195 mg)

- Dibasic sodium phosphate (1.3 mg)
- Polysorbate 20 (27.5 mcg)
- *Spodoptera frugiperda* cell proteins (≤19 mcg)
- Baculovirus and cellular DNA (≤10 ng)
- Triton X-100 (≤100 mcg)

Flucelvax[489]

- Inactivated influenza virus
  - A/Idaho/07/2018 (H1N1)
  - A/Indiana/08/2018 (H3N2)
  - B/Iowa/06/2017
  - B/Singapore/INFTT-16-0610/2016
- Hemagglutinin (60 mcg; 15 mcg from each virus)
- Dog kidney cell proteins—MDCK (≤25.2 mcg)
- Protein other than hemagglutinin (≤240 mcg)
- Dog kidney cell DNA (≤10 ng)
- Polysorbate 80 (≤1500 mcg)
- Mercury (25 mcg)
- Cetyltrimethylammonium bromide (≤18 mcg)
- Beta-propiolactone (<0.5 mcg)

Fluenz Tetra[490]

- Reassortant influenza virus, live attenuated
  - A/Brisbane/02/2018 (H1N1)pdm09–like strain ($10^{7.0\pm0.5}$ FFU)
  - A/Kansas/14/2017 X-327 (H3N2)–like strain ($10^{7.0\pm0.5}$ FFU)
  - B/Colorado/06/2017–like strain ($10^{7.0\pm0.5}$ FFU)
  - B/Phuket/3073/2013–like strain ($10^{7.0\pm0.5}$ FFU)
- Sucrose
- Dipotassium phosphate
- Potassium dihydrogen phosphate
- Gelatin (porcine, Type A)
- Arginine hydrochloride
- Monosodium glutamate monohydrate
- Egg protein, ovalbumin (<0.024 mcg)

- Gentamicin
- Water

Note: Processed in monkey kidney cells (VERO)

FluLaval[491]

- Inactivated influenza virus
  - A/Brisbane/02/2018 (H1N1)
  - A/Kansas/14/2017 X-327 (H3N2)
  - B/Maryland/15/2016
  - B/Phuket/3073/2013 BVR-1B
- Hemagglutinin (60 mcg; 15 mcg from each virus)
- Mercury (<25 mcg)
- Egg proteins, ovalbumin (≤0.3 mcg)
- Formaldehyde (≤25 mcg)
- Sodium deoxycholate (≤50 mcg)
- Alpha-tocopheryl hydrogen succinate (≤320 mcg)
- Polysorbate 80 (≤887 mcg)

FluMist[492]

- Weakened influenza virus strains
  - A/Switzerland/3330/2017 (H1N1), ($10^{6.5-7.5}$ FFU)
  - A/Kansas/14/2017 X-327 (H3N2), ($10^{6.5-7.5}$ FFU)
  - B/Phuket/3073/2013, B Yamagata lineage ($10^{6.5-7.5}$ FFU)
  - B/Colorado/06/2017, B Victoria lineage ($10^{6.5-7.5}$ FFU)
- Monosodium glutamate (0.188 mg)
- Gelatin, porcine (2 mg)
- Arginine (2.42 mg)
- Sucrose (13.68 mg)
- Dibasic potassium phosphate (2.26 mg)
- Monobasic potassium phosphate (0.96 mg)
- Egg protein, ovalbumin (<0.024 mcg)
- Gentamicin (<0.015 mcg)

Fluvirin[493]

- Inactivated influenza virus
  - A/Singapore/GP1908/2015 (H1N1)
  - A/Hong Kong/4801/2014 (H3N2)
  - B/Brisbane/60/2008, wild type
- Hemagglutinin (45 mcg; 15 mcg from each virus)
- Mercury (0.5 mL dose: ≤1 mcg; 5 mL dose: 25 mcg)
- Egg proteins, ovalbumin (≤1 mcg)
- Polymyxin (≤3.75 mcg)
- Neomycin (≤2.5 mcg)
- Beta-propiolactone (≤0.5 mcg)
- Nonylphenol ethoxylate (≤0.015% w/v)

Fluzone (0.25 mL dose)[494]

- Inactivated influenza virus
  - A/Brisbane/02/2018 (H1N1)
  - A/Kansas/14/2017 (H3N2)
  - B/Phuket/3073/2013 BVR-1B (Victoria lineage)
  - B/Maryland/15/2016 (Yamagata lineage)
- Hemagglutinin (30 mcg; 7.5 mcg from each virus)
- Mercury (12.5 mcg, multidose only)
- Sodium phosphate–buffered isotonic sodium chloride solution
- Formaldehyde (≤50 mcg)
- Octylphenol ethoxylate (≤125 mcg)

Fluzone (0.5 mL dose)[495]

- Inactivated influenza virus
  - A/Brisbane/02/2018 (H1N1)
  - A/Kansas/14/2017 X-327 (H3N2)
  - B/Phuket/3073/2013 BVR-1B (Victoria lineage)
  - B/Maryland/15/2016 (Yamagata lineage)
- Hemagglutinin (180 mcg; 60 mcg from each virus)
- Mercury (25 mcg, multidose only)

- Sodium phosphate–buffered isotonic sodium chloride solution
- Formaldehyde (≤100 mcg)
- Octylphenol ethoxylate (≤250 mcg)

Fluzone (high dose)[496]

- Inactivated influenza virus
  - A/Brisbane/02/2018 (H1N1)
  - A/Kansas/14/2017 X-327 (H3N2)
  - B/Maryland/15/2016 (Yamagata lineage)
- Hemagglutinin (60 mcg; 15 mcg from each virus)
- Sodium phosphate–buffered isotonic sodium chloride solution
- Formaldehyde (≤100 mcg)
- Octylphenol ethoxylate (≤250 mcg)

Controversial Ingredients

- Mercury
- Monkey kidney cells
- Insect cell proteins
- Baculovirus and cellular DNA
- Gelatin (pig)
- Chick embryo protein
- Monosodium glutamate
- Formaldehyde
- Cetyltrimethylammonium bromide
- Squalene based oil-in-water emulsion adjuvant
- Polysorbate 80
- Polysorbate 20
- Sodium deoxycholate
- Sodium taurodeoxycholate
- Octoxynol-10
- Nonylphenol ethoxylate
- Octylphenol ethoxylate

Afluria: Injection-site pain (≥50%), redness and swelling (≥10%), headache (≥10%), muscle pain (≥10%), fatigue (≥10%), general malaise (≥10%), nausea (≥7.0%), diarrhea (≥5.0%), fever (2.1%–4.5%), and vomiting (1.8%–2.4%).

Fluad: Injection-site pain (25.0%) and tenderness (21.1%), muscle pain (14.7%), fatigue (13.3%), headache (13.2%), joint pain (8.5%), chills (6.7%), diarrhea (4.8%), and fever (3.6%). Serious adverse events were reported 1.1–4.3 percent—within thirty days and six months, respectively—of the time during fourteen randomized trials. Neuroinflammatory and immune conditions were reported 0.9 percent of the time after vaccination.

Fluarix: Injection-site pain (17.2%–56.2%), muscle aches (17.5%–28.8%), injection-site redness (13.1%–23.0%), irritability (16.2%–20.9%), fatigue (18.8%–19.9%), injection-site swelling (7.9%–18.5%), drowsiness (12.5%–17.2%), headache (15.1%–16.4%), loss of appetite (13.4%–15.5%), joint pain (5.6%–9.8%), gastrointestinal symptoms (9.8%), fever (4.2%–8.9%), and shivering (3.1%–6.4%).

Flublok: Injection-site tenderness (34%–48%), injections site pain (19%–37%), headache (13%–20%), fatigue (12%–17%), muscle aches (13%), joint pain (8%–13%), nausea (5%–9%), and chills/shivering (5%–7%).

Flucelvax: Injection-site tenderness (46%–58%), injection-site swelling (18%–22%), headache (19%–22%), sleepiness (19%), fatigue (13%–18%), muscle aches (12%–16%), irritability (16%), injection-site hardening (13%–16%), loss of appetite (9%–10%), injection-site bruising (4%–9%), chills (4%–7%), nausea (8%–9%), joint pain (4%–6%), vomiting (2%4%), diarrhea (3%–4%), and fever (1%–4%).

Fluenz Tetra: Very common—decreased appetite, headache, nasal congestion, general malaise. Common—muscle pain, fever. Uncommon—hypersensitivity reactions (including facial swelling, hives, and very rare anaphylactic reactions), nosebleed. The clinical trial of the vaccine found that 6.1 percent of infants (6–11 months of age) were hospitalized within 180 days after vaccination compared to 2.6 percent of those receiving IIV.

FluLaval: Injection-site pain (39.4%–65.4%), irritability (8.1%–49.4%), drowsiness (7.7%–36.7%), loss of appetite (9.0%–28.9%), muscle aches (12.0%–28.5%), fatigue (8.4%–22.1%), headache (10.5%–22.0%), joint pain (6.3%–12.9%), gastrointestinal symptoms (5.5%–9.6%), shivering (3.0%–7.0%), fever (1.9%–5.6%), injection-site swelling (1.0%–6.2%), and injection-site redness (0.4%–5.3%).

FluMist: Runny nose or nasal congestion (51%–58%), reduced appetite (13%–21%), irritability (12%–21%), fever (4%–16%), lethargy (7%–14%), sore throat (5%–11%), headache (3%–9%), muscle aches (2%–6%), chills (2%–4%), and hospitalization due to wheezing requiring bronchodilator therapy or accompanied by respiratory distress occurred 2.1–5.9 percent of the time within forty-two or 180 days of vaccination.

Fluvirin (adult reports only): Injection-site pain (≤55%), headache (≤30%), muscle pain (≤21%), general malaise (≤19%), fatigue (≤18%), injection-site redness (≤16%), injection-site hardening (≤14%), injection-site swelling (≤11%), injection-site mass (≤8%), sore throat (≤8%), injection-site inflammation (≤7%), chills (≤7%), nausea (≤7%), painful joints (≤7%), cough (≤6%), wheezing (≤4%), chest tightness (≤4%), injection site bruising (≤4%), and injection-site reaction (≤4%).

Fluzone (0.25 mL or 0.5 mL dose): Injection-site pain (57.0%–66%), irritability (47.4%–54.0%), injection-site tenderness (47.3%–54.1%), abnormal crying (33.3%–41.2%), muscle pain (26.7%–38.6%), drowsiness (31.9%–37.7%), injection-site bruising (34.1%–37.3%), general malaise (31.9%–38.1%), appetite loss (27.3%–32.3%), injection-site swelling (12.9%–24.8%), headache (8.9%–23.1%), vomiting (10.0%–14.8%), and fever (7.0%–14.3%).

Fluzone (high dose): injection-site pain (35.6%), muscle aches (21.4%), general malaise (18.0%), headache (16.8%), injection-site bruising (14.9%), injection-site swelling (8.9%), and fever (3.6%).

Afluria—low blood platelet count (thrombocytopenia), allergic or immediate hypersensitivity reactions (including anaphylaxis and serum sickness), neuralgia, pins-and-needles sensation, seizures (including febrile), encephalomyelitis, encephalopathy, neuritis or neuropathy, transverse myelitis, Guillain-Barré syndrome, vasculitis, rash, hives, itching, cellulitis, and flu-like illness.

Fluad—thrombocytopenia, enlarged lymph nodes, allergic reactions (including anaphylactic shock, anaphylaxis, and angioedema), muscle weakness, encephalomyelitis, Guillain-Barré syndrome, seizure, neuritis or neuralgia, pins-and-needles feeling, temporary loss of consciousness, sensation of passing out, vasculitis, renal vasculitis, hives, itching, rash, and erythema multiforme.

Fluarix—enlarged lymph nodes, tachycardia, vertigo, conjunctivitis, eye irritation, pain, redness, or swelling, eyelid swelling, abdominal pain, swelling of the mouth, throat, or tongue, lack of energy, chest pain, flu-like illness, feeling hot, injection-site mass, abscess, cellulitis, warmth, injection site reaction, body aches, anaphylactic reactions, hypersensitivity, pharyngitis, rhinitis, tonsillitis, seizure, encephalomyelitis, Guillain-Barré syndrome, erythema multiforme, facial swelling, itching, seating, hives, Stevens-Johnson syndrome, Henoch-Schönlein purpura, and vasculitis.

Flublok—Not reported.

Flucelvax—Allergic or immediate hypersensitivity reactions (including anaphylaxis), temporary loss of consciousness, sensation of passing out, pins or needles feeling, itching, hives, rash, extensive swelling of injected limb.

Fluenz Tetra—Guillain-Barré syndrome and exacerbation of Leigh syndrome.

FluLaval—Eye pain, light sensitivity, difficulty swallowing, vomiting, chest pain, injection-site inflammation, physical weakness/lack of energy, injection-site rash, flu-like symptoms, abnormal gait, injection-site bruising, injection-site abscess, allergic reactions (including anaphylaxis and angioedema), rhinitis, laryngitis, cellulitis. Muscle weakness, arthritis, dizziness, decreased sense of touch or sensation, feelings of pins or needles, increased sensitivity to pain, excessive tiredness, temporary loss of consciousness, sensation of passing out, Guillain-Barré syndrome, seizure, facial or cranial nerve paralysis, encephalopathy, limb paralysis, insomnia, vocal cord spasms (dysphonia), labored breathing, bronchospasm, throat tightness, hives, localized or generalized rash, itching, sweating, flushing, and pale appearance.

FluMist—Pericarditis, exacerbation of Leigh syndrome, nausea, vomiting, diarrhea, hypersensitivity reactions (including facial swelling, hives, and anaphylactic reactions), Guillain-Barré syndrome, Bell's palsy, meningitis, eosinophilic meningitis, vaccine-associated encephalitis, nose bleed, and rash.

Fluvirin—Local injection-site reactions, hot flashes, chills/shivering, fever, general malaise, fatigue, physical weakness or lack of energy, facial swelling, hypersensitivity reactions (including throat/mouth welling), anaphylactic shock and death (rare), vasculitis, loss of consciousness, feeling of passing out, diarrhea, nausea, vomiting, abdominal pain, enlarged lymph nodes, thrombocytopenia, loss of appetite, joint pain, muscle pain, muscle weakness, headache, dizziness, neuralgia, confusion, febrile seizure, Guillain-Barré syndrome, myelitis, neuropathy, paralysis (including Bell's palsy), labored breathing, chest pain, cough, pharyngitis, rhinitis, Stevens-Johnson syndrome, sweating, itching, hives, rash, and injection-site cellulitis.

Fluzone (0.25 mL or 0.5 mL dose)—Thrombocytopenia, enlarged lymph nodes, anaphylaxis, allergic/hypersensitivity reactions, eye redness, Guillain-Barré syndrome, seizure (including febrile), myelitis,

Bell's palsy, eye neuritis/neuropathy, brachial neuritis, temporary loss of consciousness, dizziness, feelings of pins and needles, vasculitis, flushing, difficulty breathing, cough, wheezing, throat tightness, oropharyngeal pain, rhinorrhea, rash, itching, Stevens-Johnson syndrome, physical weakness or lack of energy, pain in extremities, chest pain, and vomiting.

Fluzone (high dose)—Thrombocytopenia, enlarged lymph nodes, anaphylaxis, allergic/hypersensitivity reactions, eye redness, Guillain-Barré syndrome, seizure (including febrile), myelitis, Bell's palsy, eye neuritis/neuropathy, brachial neuritis, temporary loss of consciousness, dizziness, feelings of pins and needles, vasculitis, flushing, difficulty breathing, pharyngitis, rhinitis, cough, wheezing, throat tightness, itching, Stevens-Johnson syndrome, physical weakness or lack of energy, pain in extremities, chest pain, chills, vomiting, nausea, diarrhea, and joint pain.

Reactions Observed and Documented in Published Research

The biggest flaw of flu vaccines is their failure to cover more than a few strains among the dozens that may infect humans each year. Throughout the year, national influenza centers in more than a hundred countries collect data on which flu viruses are making people sick across the world. Data from these centers is pooled at five main centers to select which strains of the flu to include in the next vaccine. While founded in data, the efforts represent a major guessing game that frequently fails. This fact alone means that flu vaccines are not likely to be very effective.

Evidence demonstrates that this is particularly true in children under age 2. A review of seventy-five studies concluded that scant evidence exists that vaccinating children under age 2 protects them against the flu.[497] Even more alarming, the authors concluded that "extensive reporting bias of safety outcomes from trials" of flu vaccines prevented meaningful analysis to determine the true safety of the vaccines in this age group. A follow-up review of forty-one clinical trials six years later determined that flu vaccines probably reduce flu in children aged 3–16 years old from 18 percent (without vaccination) to 4 percent (with vaccination), but again no compelling evidence was documented for children under age 2.[498] In spite of convincing evidence that there is little benefit for children under 2, health organizations adamantly advocate that children 6 months and older receive an annual flu shot. This practice is potentially and unnecessarily exposing very young children to mercury and other controversial ingredients.

Even when the vaccine strains chosen closely match the most virulent strains of the year, effectiveness of the flu vaccine is surprisingly low.[499] A review of six European studies from October 2018 to January 2019 concluded that the flu vaccine was effective in preventing influenza A between 32 and 43 percent of the time, more effective against H1N1, and less effective against H3N2.[500] Similarly, during the 2018–2019 season, the US CDC reported effectiveness ranging from 7 percent (children aged 9 to 17) to 48 percent (children 6 months to 8 years) against influenza A, better effectiveness against H1N1, and significantly lower effectiveness for H3N2.[501] In fact, the effectiveness was negative for 20 percent of people aged 50–64 against H3N2, meaning elderly individuals who were vaccinated had a higher rate of H3N2 flu illness than those who never got the shot. On average, the efficacy of the flu vaccine ranges between 10 percent and 60 percent each year. But evidence that it frequently misses the mark can be found in dismal numbers like the 2004–2005 season when flu shots protected against the flu only 10 percent of the time, or the 2012–2013 season, where it was only 9 percent effective in seniors.[502] Mounting evidence indicates that getting an annual flu shot is not only not protective but may be detrimental to long-term health.

Elderly individuals are particularly vulnerable to flu complications. As reported earlier, the majority of deaths caused by flu complications occur in people of 65 years or older. The preponderance of hospitalizations occurs in the same age group. But data from 1968 to 2001 showed that despite a fourfold increase in vaccination rates from 1980 to 2001, flu-related mortality rates remained constant.[503]

Importantly, the authors also identified a decline in mortality in the decade following the pandemic flu of 1968. This idea was strengthened by a later study that found people exposed to pandemic flus of the twentieth century were relatively immune to emergent seasonal strains because the emergent viruses resembled those that had previously circulated.[504] This suggests that exposure to pandemic flu confers natural immunity against nonpandemic influenza viruses and reduces the risk of flu-related deaths.

The purpose of the flu shot is not just to prevent illness, but also to minimize hospitalization and death. Some research assessed data from 1996 to 2005 and found that the flu vaccine reduced all causes of mortality by 4.6 percent.[505] Other research suggests that flu shots reduce mortality in people with heart failure,[506] while yet another study concluded that "influenza vaccination is still associated with substantial reduction in mortality risk."[507] The reality is that the evidence as to whether the flu vaccine decreases mortality rates is conflicting.

Scientific papers indicate that receiving influenza vaccines reduces a person's protective immunity against the more virulent pandemic strains. In other words, receiving a regular flu shot may increase your risk of infection with pandemic flu. On the contrary, unvaccinated individuals naturally exposed to circulating flu viruses are likely to acquire cross protection against other flu strains. Cross protection (called heterosubtypic immunity) means that exposure to influenza viruses can provide some protection from other similar but unrelated subtypes. Cross protection does not fully protect against the flu, but it can limit virus replication and reduce the severity of the illness. Infants are immunologically naïve to influenza viruses and researchers hypothesize that an annual flu vaccine in infants may prevent cross protection from occurring against pandemic strains.[508] This is hardly ideal considering pandemic flus are typically more severe and lethal. Currently, the evidence suggests that natural immunity conferred from wild viruses—both pandemic and seasonal—helps the immune system more effectively eliminate seasonal and pandemic strains of the flu. If you get a pandemic flu, it will likely confer some protection against seasonal flus, and if you get a seasonal flu, you will probably have a less severe case of a pandemic flu. Research indicates that vaccines might interfere with this cross protection.

Some evidence suggests that this hypothesis is true. Analysis of four epidemiological studies in Canada showed that receipt of the 2008–09 trivalent inactivated influenza vaccine increased the risk of pandemic H1N1 (swine flu) illness that required medical intervention during the spring and summer of 2019.[509] Similar results were observed in active duty members of the military. Members of the military that received a seasonal influenza shot were significantly more likely to get infected with H1N1 pandemic flu.[510] From this data, it appears the seasonal flu shot not only increased the risk of pandemic flu infection but also its severity. It seems logical to allow protection against more lethal and severe pandemic flus instead of seasonal flu outbreaks by allowing the public to be exposed to seasonal strains.

Type A viruses are responsible for flu pandemics, and the circulating strains constantly change. Exposure to one type A virus can help reduce the severity of other type A strains according to the available research. Experimental research in animals suggests that an annual flu vaccine reduces cross protection against influenza A viruses caused by new subtypes.[511] It also shows that prior infection with influenza viruses confers protection against more virulent strains and allows animals to clear the infection more quickly.[512,513] Another study found that animals vaccinated with a specific influenza A (A/California/7/2009) were protected against influenza A/H1N1 subtype viruses circulating during 2009 and 2010, but the protection was ineffective against the 2015 strain.[514] Remarkably, mice vaccinated against seasonal influenza and then infected with influenza A/H5N1 (bird or avian flu) virus had drastically more severe influenza and frequently died more often than mice who did not receive vaccination prior to exposure to H5N1 influenza.[515] Comparable results were observed in ferrets.[516] The experimental research suggests that vaccines interfere with cross protection and may increase the incidence and severity of pandemic flus. Since animal models of human influenza are considered predictive of vaccine effectiveness, the results of these studies can't be ignored and are concerning for those receiving annual flu shots.

Research conducted among members of the US Air Force indicates that the influenza vaccine may interfere with immunity against certain other respiratory viruses as well. Called virus interference, the research showed that receiving an influenza vaccination increases the risk of human coronavirus and human metapneumovirus (hMPV) infections.[517] hMPV is a leading cause of acute respiratory infection and particularly affects children, the elderly, and those with a compromised immune system. Coronaviruses are a large family of viruses that usually cause mild to moderate—sometimes no symptoms at all—upper respiratory infections. Still, coronaviruses have caused serious epidemics and pandemics, including severe respiratory illness and death, multiple times during the twenty-first century. However, the same research showed that the influenza vaccine significantly decreased influenza, parainfluenza, RSV (respiratory syncytial virus), and noninfluenza coinfections. The basic assumption that vaccines do not change the risk of infections with other respiratory pathogens appears to be flawed and not based in facts.

On the contrary, experimental research shows that vaccines may provide some cross protection against influenza B type viruses.[518] The scientists observed that the trivalent live attenuated influenza vaccine provided some cross protection against wild B strains that were not included in the vaccine. Further research found that inactivated virus vaccines did not control virus growth in the lungs of mice, but consistent immunization with an inactivated virus reduced the severity of infection caused by pandemic flu.[519] Cross protection may be somewhat strain dependent. Both type A and type B flu viruses cause human illness, but type A viruses cause more severe and long-lasting illness.[520] Therefore, cross protection against influenza A may be more important than cross protection against type B viruses.

Evidence suggests that receiving repeated flu vaccines each year as recommended may reduce long-term immunity to the flu. Interestingly, when 1,441 people were followed for an entire flu season, infection rates were similar in both the vaccinated and unvaccinated.[521] You heard that right, the vaccine provided no significant protection. Even more remarkably, the researchers reported that people who were vaccinated during two consecutive years were not protected against the flu and in fact had an increased risk of flu illness. Another meta-analysis found that the flu vaccine was less effective against H3N2 and B in people vaccinated in consecutive years.[522] Puzzlingly, the article was retracted because of "a few erroneous inclusions and an omission of estimates which impacted the conclusion for the influenza A (H3N2) and influenza B analyses." Contrary to these findings, a study conducted by scientists associated with a flu vaccine manufacturer reported that vaccination in consecutive years "was not associated with reduced vaccine effectiveness in children."[523] However, something to keep in mind when relying on studies initiated by vaccine manufacturers or policy makers is the fact that it is estimated that 70 percent of studies overestimate vaccine effectiveness, and more than half have a high risk of bias.[524] Compounding this is the fear marketing approach adopted by the CDC and other health organizations.[525] The conclusion was that flu vaccine studies that report favorable outcomes are riddled with methodological flaws and are unduly influenced by industry funding.

The flu is known to exacerbate asthma and frequently lands people with asthma in the emergency room. When people with asthma get the flu, it can cause inflammation and narrowing of the airways to the point that it literally takes their breath away. Based on this, it is important that people with asthma protect themselves against the flu. The question is whether the flu vaccine provides sufficient protection. A study encompassing eight years of data found that it did not, and on the contrary, children who received their annual flu vaccine were three times more likely to be hospitalized compared to children with asthma who did not get vaccinated.[526]

Contradicting evidence reported that getting a flu shot reduced asthma attacks that required an emergency room visit or hospitalization by 59–78 percent.[527] The intranasal flu vaccine carries a warning that children younger than 5 with asthma or recurrent wheezing may be at an increased risk of wheezing following administration. However, two separate studies concluded that neither the LAIV nor IIV vaccines exacerbate asthma or increase respiratory events requiring medical attention in young children.[528,529] On the other hand, the last two studies were funded and sponsored by organizations involved in vaccine policy, and reports to VAERS (representing real world experience) do show that labored breathing or airway tightening can occur after flu vaccines.

Interestingly, some research indicates that receiving the annual flu shot puts children at a greater risk of other respiratory infections. Researchers in Hong Kong conducted a randomized and placebo-controlled trial in 115 children to determine the incidence of respiratory infections with and without vaccination. Although the children who received the flu vaccine experienced fewer cases of flu based on blood tests, the actual reduction in flu cases was not statistically significant when compared to unvaccinated children. However, vaccinated children were four times more likely to develop a nonflu acute respiratory illness when compared to children who received a placebo.[530] Most of the nonflu infections were caused by rhinoviruses and coxsackieviruses/echoviruses. The vaccine may be disrupting nonspecific immune system function—the innate immune system each person is born with—in a previously unknown way. By vaccinating children against the flu, we may be preventing nonspecific immunity against other respiratory infections.

Another concern is the recommendation by health organizations that all pregnant women receive the flu vaccine regardless of their trimester. While the available evidence suggests that infection with influenza during pregnancy is rarely a threat to a healthy pregnancy, the injection of mercury (via thimerosal) present in most flu vaccines is implicated in neurodevelopmental disorders, toxicity, and fetal death. A critical assessment of the recommendations by the CDC's Advisory Committee on Immunization Practice (ACIP) concluded that ACIP's policy of "routinely administering influenza vaccine during pregnancy is ill-advised and unsupported by current scientific literature, and it should be withdrawn."[531] Why did the two medical doctors who wrote the commentary come to this conclusion? Several reasons were mentioned: (1) inadequate evidence that the flu is more dangerous during pregnancy, (2) no noteworthy differences in illness rates among vaccinated and unvaccinated individuals, (3) vaccinated pregnant women are four times more likely to be hospitalized for flu-like symptoms than unvaccinated pregnant women, and (4) the presence of mercury above limits considered safe by the EPA.

A significant increase—more than a tenfold increase—in spontaneous abortions (miscarriage) was noted in pregnant women who received both the pandemic (A-H1N1) and seasonal influenza vaccines during the 2009–2010 season.[532] In efforts to protect the mother and her unborn child against two types of flu, these vaccines may have contributed to the loss of fetal lives. The conclusion was that "a synergistic fetal toxicity" likely occurred from receiving both thimerosal-containing (50 mcg of mercury total) vaccines too close together. These results highlight the potential risk of fetal exposure to even low levels of mercury.

Many healthcare workers (physicians, nurses, etc.) receive compulsory flu vaccinations each year. Numerous healthcare organizations have mandatory flu vaccine policies where employees who opt out are terminated. The publicized reason behind this forced vaccination is to protect the welfare and lives of patients and employees. However, there is a substantial lack of scientific evidence for these forced vaccination policies and their alleged protection of patients.[533,534,535] The same is likely true for coworkers. Indeed, forced vaccination of healthcare workers doesn't appear to be beneficial for their patients. Healthcare workers should have the same right to an informed choice to accept or reject flu vaccines that the public enjoys without being subject to legal, institutional, or peer coercion.

While flu vaccines, in general, are considered safe and well tolerated, they are not used without risks of side effects. Some of these adverse effects are more common in children, while others are more common in adults. At a minimum, flu vaccines need to meet a higher safety standard and be subject to independent analysis of efficacy with high methodological standards and an absence of bias.

As a final note, physical interventions—teaching children good handwashing and avoiding touching your eyes, nose, or mouth— and staying home when sick are highly effective against the spread of respiratory viruses like the flu. A systemic review of fifty-eight studies that evaluated the effectiveness of public health measures to reduce the spread of respiratory infections, concluded that handwashing and wearing masks (when sick) significantly reduces the spread of respiratory viruses.[536] A follow-up study by the same authors that included sixty-seven studies confirmed their previous results that handwashing and wearing masks (particularly an N95 respirator) protected against respiratory viruses.[537] In other words, significant evidence proves handwashing as a simple but effective way to reduce flu illness, while wearing a mask when sick and symptomatic may also be helpful.

See the *Reactions Observed and Documented in Published Research* section of chapter 4 for a discussion on vaccine-associated seizures and the flu vaccine.

See the *Reactions Observed and Documented in Published Research* section of chapter 9 for a discussion of immune thrombocytopenia associated with influenza vaccination.

See the *Reactions Observed and Documented in Published Research* section of chapter 9 for a discussion about how certain childhood infections may protect against cancer development later in life.

INFECTION RISKS	VACCINE RISKS
Secondary infections: pneumonia, myocarditis, encephalitis, myositis, sepsis	Reduced protection against pandemic or seasonal flu
Multi-organ failure	Nonflu respiratory infections
Dehydration	Seizure
Death	Immune thrombocytopenia
	Increased cancer risk later in life
	Miscarriage

9

Measles, Mumps, and Rubella (MMR)

What Are Measles, Mumps, and Rubella Infections?

Measles, also called rubeola, is a highly contagious infectious illness caused by the rubeola virus. Being infected with wild rubeola virus confers lifelong immunity. Prior to 1963—when a vaccine was first introduced—virtually all children got measles by age 15, which granted them this lifelong immunity. Despite being declared eradicated in the United States, measles cases are on the rise. In 2014, 667 cases were reported in twenty-seven states. Outbreaks were also reported in 2013 and 2015. And a measles outbreak (1,282 cases) occurred in thirty-one states in 2019 in both unvaccinated and vaccinated children, suggesting possible vaccine failure.

Rubeola virus lives in the nose and throat mucus of infected people and spreads when they cough or sneeze. Droplets expelled by infected persons can remain in the air where they coughed or sneezed for up to two hours. People contract the virus when they breathe in enough contaminated air or touch a contaminated surface and then touch their mouths, noses, or eyes. Rubeola virus is one of the world's most contagious illnesses. So contagious that up to 90 percent of people in close contact to an infected person that are not immune also become infected. Spread of the virus can occur about four days before and after the characteristic rash appears.

Early symptoms of measles include high fever, cough, runny nose, and red, watery eyes. Symptoms appear about seven to fourteen days after infection. Within three days of initial symptoms, white spots (Koplik spots) appear on the inside of the mouth. The tell-tale rash—small, raised bumps on top of flat, red spots—breaks out three to five days after the initial symptoms (about seven to eighteen days after infection). This rash usually starts on the face at the hairline and spreads downward to the upper neck, trunk, arms, legs, and feet. A fever over 104°F may accompany the appearance of the rash. The rash lasts for about five to six days and the fever can last up to twelve days.

Atypical measles is an unusual form of measles that occurs in adults who received the measles vaccine before 1968. The vaccine used prior to 1968 did not confer long-term immunity to measles. Instead, it only provided partial immunity. The main symptom of atypical measles is a rash that begins on the extremities and progresses toward the trunk. The rash may itch and be fluid filled. Atypical measles can be confirmed by very high antibody levels in the blood (titers).

Mumps—also called parotitis—is a viral infection characterized by swelling of one or both sides of the salivary glands (usually parotid) causing the cheeks to appear puffy. The jaw is swollen and tender. It most often affects children between the ages of 5 and 9, but can also affect adults. One to two days prior to the swollen salivary glands a person usually experiences fever, headache, general malaise, and loss of appetite. Symptoms tend to decrease after seven days and completely resolve in about ten days. Mumps is often so mild in children that the child may only have a mild fever and sore throat. About one-third of small children infected with mumps exhibit no symptoms.[538] Mumps infections with no symptoms are also observed in people who have received two doses of the MMR vaccine—two-thirds of mumps cases during an epidemic occurred in vaccinated children.[539] Waning immunity despite vaccination suggests that vaccination does not confer lifelong immunity like infection with wild virus.

Caused by the paramyxovirus, mumps is spread from person to person via direct contact with airborne droplets of respiratory secretions. The average incubation period for the virus is from twelve to twenty-five days, with an average of sixteen to eighteen days. An infected person is most contagious one to two days after parotid swelling appears. Infection is confirmed by physical exam (parotid swelling on one or both sides) and laboratory test of body fluids (throat, saliva, or spinal fluid). Treatment of mumps usually involves hydration and avoidance of acidic foods.

Rubella, or German measles, is a viral infection that causes a rash on the body. The rash typically begins on the face and spreads from the center of the body to the rest of the body over the course of twenty-four hours. It is usually mild and accompanied by a mild fever, swollen lymph nodes, headache, muscle or joint pain, inflamed or red eyes, and runny or stuffy nose. Up to half of people who are infected with rubella virus don't show any symptoms.[540] The rash is characterized by a flat, red area on the skin that is covered with small bumps. German measles appears similar to other rashes and so it is confirmed through a blood test that checks for the presence of rubella antibodies. Because rubella is generally mild in older children and adults, it can be treated at home.

Young children frequently exhibit no symptoms until the rash appears, but with only a mild fever and generic rash it may go unrecognized. In adolescents and adults, eye pain (primarily while looking sideways and upward), sore throat, headache, swollen lymph nodes, fever, chills, body aches, and nausea often precede the rash.

Rubella is most devastating when the virus is acquired during fetal development in early pregnancy. Rubella can be transmitted from a pregnant woman to her developing baby through the bloodstream. In this case, the virus can cause congenital rubella syndrome, which can cause miscarriages, stillbirths, and a combination of birth defects—cataracts, hearing impairment, developmental delay, multiple organ dysfunction, congenital heart disease, and others. This risk is greatest during the first twelve weeks of gestation and gradually decreases until the risk of complications is rare after the twentieth week.[541] Pregnant women may be treated with antibodies (hyperimmune globulin) to help fight the virus, but this may not prevent congenital rubella syndrome in her baby.

Rubella is spread via breathing in tiny droplets of respiratory secretions from an infected person. Once inside the body, the virus replicates in the lymph nodes, nose, and throat. It spreads to other areas of the body over the next five to seven days (this is also when the fetus is infected in pregnant women). People are most contagious when the rash is erupting, but they can shed the virus from seven days prior to and fourteen days after the rash appears, meaning they may spread the virus without even knowing they have it.

How Prevalent Are They?

The World Health Organization estimates that there were 7,585,900 and 9,769,400 cases of measles in 2017 and 2018, respectively, suggesting a sharp increase in measles activity. Countries highly impacted by measles include the Democratic Republic of the Congo (DRC), Liberia, Madagascar, Somalia, and Ukraine, which account for nearly half of all global cases.[542] Estimates peg the odds of getting measles at less than a fraction of a percent, but infections are rising globally.

Before a mumps vaccine was available, less than 1 percent of the population was infected by mumps annually, with peaks every two to five years.[543] The World Health Organization estimated the global incidence of mumps cases at 311,599 in 2015 but that number has risen to 499,512 in 2018.[544] China reports the most cases (accounting for nearly half of all global cases), followed by Japan, Nepal, Iraq, and Ghana. Despite rising mumps cases, chances of getting the mumps remain low today.

Actual cases of rubella are believed to be underreported worldwide. Rubella outbreaks typically occur in the spring and large epidemics occur every three to nine years. Rubella cases are reported far less frequently than measles—measles cases outnumber rubella cases more than ten to one. Globally, from 2014 to 2018, an average of about 24,618 reported rubella cases and 415 reported congenital rubella syndrome cases were reported each year.[545] Rubella is still considered a public health problem because of the risk of maternal infection and congenital rubella syndrome.

What Are the Health Risks of Measles, Mumps, and Rubella Infections?

Although usually self-limiting, rarely measles can be serious, and complications do occur. Young children under age five and adults over age 20 are at a higher risk of complications that range from mild—ear infections (one in ten children) and diarrhea (fewer than one in ten children)—to serious, like pneumonia and encephalitis. In addition, pregnant women and people with compromised immune systems are more likely to suffer measles complications. Measles complications, range in occurrence from pneumonia (5 percent of cases) to encephalitis (0.05–0.1 percent of cases).[546] Those who survive measles encephalitis often have chronic neurological problems.

Pneumonia and ear infections that accompany measles may be caused by opportunistic viruses or bacteria. Rubeola virus suppresses cell-mediated immune responses, which makes a secondary bacterial infection—called bacterial superinfections—more likely. Bacterial superinfections of the respiratory tract are fairly common complications of measles because of the weakened state of the immune system. Pneumonia is the primary cause of measles-related death in young children, but encephalitis is more likely to cause measles-related mortality in teens. An estimated one to three children for every one thousand who are infected with measles will die from respiratory or neurological complications.

Persons with compromised immune systems may experience severe complications of measles, such as giant cell (primary) pneumonia and measles encephalitis. Measles encephalitis can occur in immunocompromised persons up to six months after measles infection. Other rare complications of measles include inflammation of the heart (myocarditis or pericarditis) and thrombocytopenic purpura—an immune disorder in which the blood clots abnormally.

Complications of atypical measles include nodular pneumonia (pneumonia accompanied by abnormally swollen clumps of cells in the lungs), swelling of both the liver and spleen, and neurological disorders like muscle weakness and tingling, pricking, or numbness with no apparent cause.

Rarely, the measles virus can disrupt the immune system's memory abilities. Normally, your immune system has the ability to remember and quickly recognize antigens that the body has previously encountered. This allows for a more rapid immune response against a subsequent infection by the same pathogen. In the case of "immune amnesia" caused by measles, the immune system doesn't maintain this memory, making the person more susceptible to previous infections.

Another possible long-term complication is subacute sclerosing panencephalitis (SSPE), which is a very rare, but fatal condition of the central nervous system. The condition is believed to be caused by a persistent measles-related viral infection in the brain. It develops about seven to ten years after a person has recovered from measles earlier in life. Risk of SSPE is greater in people who had measles before the age of 2. Symptoms of SSPE presents as gradual behavioral and intellectual decline and seizures that eventually progresses to coma and death.

Worldwide about 140,000 people died from measles complications in 2018.[547] Most of these deaths occurred in children under 5 years of age.

Mumps generally resolves without any complications or lasting effects. The most common complication in postpubertal males—occurring in 3.3–10 percent of males infected—is testicular inflammation (orchitis), which usually only affects one testicle.[548] Abrupt swelling of one or both testicles is typically accompanied by tenderness, fever, nausea, and vomiting. Orchitis commonly occurs after mumps but may precede it or occur alone.

Postpubertal females may experience ovarian inflammation—1 percent or less—called oophoritis.[549] Inflammation can occur in one or both ovaries. The inflammation may go unnoticed until sudden and severe pelvic or abdominal pain prompts the individual to seek medical attention. Fever, chills, vomiting, burning sensation or pain while urinating, and heavy vaginal discharge that may be foul smelling are additional signs of oophoritis.

The mumps virus has an affinity to infect the central nervous system, but it rarely results in clinical manifestations, such as encephalitis and meningitis. Cerebrospinal fluid pleocytosis—increased cell count, particularly white blood cells, in cerebrospinal fluid—occurs frequently, perhaps greater than 65 percent of the time in mumps cases, but may only manifest as a headache or migraine.[550] Mumps encephalitis is a more serious complication of mumps and affects men more than women. Estimates suggest that it occurs between 0.02 percent and 0.3 percent of the time.[551] Mumps meningitis occurs less than 1 percent of the time if the virus spreads into the outer protective layer of the brain (the meninges).[552] Unlike bacterial meningitis, which can be life-threatening, viral meningitis symptoms are milder, resembling the flu, and the risk of serious complications is low.

Congenital rubella syndrome is virtually nonexistent in the Americas and much of Europe but still occurs in Asia and Africa. Risk of congenital defects is 90 percent if the infection occurs in the first eleven weeks of gestation, 33 percent in weeks eleven to twelve, 17.5 percent in weeks thirteen to sixteen, and virtually nonexistent after week sixteen.[553] Besides congenital rubella syndrome, other complications of rubella may occur. Arthritis or pain in multiple joints is commonly reported in adolescents and adults with confirmed rubella. Less commonly, thrombocytopenia and encephalitis, which can be fatal, occur in about one out of every six thousand rubella cases.[554] Global initiatives are still ongoing to reduce the incidence of maternal rubella infection and the incidence of congenital rubella syndrome.

Measles, Mumps, and Rubella Infections Vaccine

Description

During a measles outbreak in Boston, Massachusetts in 1954, John F. Enders and Dr. Thomas C. Peebles successfully isolated the rubeola virus from a 13-year-old named David Edmonston. Almost ten years later, they transformed the Edmonston-B strain of measles virus into a vaccine and licensed it in the United States. The vaccine was improved by Maurice Hillerman and colleagues in 1968 (called the Edmonston-Enders strain) to make the virus weaker. Hillerman also created the mumps vaccine from the virus that infected his 5-year-old daughter in 1967. It was recommended for routine use in the United States in 1977. Hillerman was instrumental in creating the combination measles, mumps, and rubella (MMR) vaccine in 1971.

The MMR (M-M-R II) vaccine is given in two doses between 12 and 15 months and again between ages 4 and 6. It is given later than other vaccines because some antibodies against the infections are transferred from mother to baby, which makes the MMR vaccine less effective though the first 12 months of life. A vaccine with MMR and varicella (chickenpox)—MMRV (Proquad or Priorix-Tetra)—also exists. The following would contraindicate receiving the MMR vaccine: currently pregnant, a weakened immune system, parent or sibling with a history of immune problems, severe, life-threatening allergies, hemophilia, a recent blood transfusion, tuberculosis diagnosis, currently experiencing a mild illness, and receipt of other vaccinations in the last four weeks.

Vaccine Manufacturing Process

Live measles and mumps viruses are produced in chick embryo culture. M-M-R II uses a weakened measles virus derived from Enders' attenuated Edmonston and the Jeryl Lynn strain of mumps virus. An attenuated rubella virus (Wistar RA 27/3 strain) is grown in lung cells from an aborted female of three months' gestation (WI-38 human diploid lung fibroblasts). Measles and mumps viruses are grown in Medium 199 (a buffered salt solution containing vitamins and amino acids and supplemented with fetal bovine serum) containing SPGA (sucrose, phosphate, glutamate, and recombinant human albumin) and neomycin. The growth medium for rubella virus is minimum essential medium (MEM)—a buffered salt solution containing vitamins and amino acids and supplemented with fetal bovine serum; and containing recombinant human albumin (synthetically produced human blood protein), neomycin, sorbitol, and hydrolyzed gelatin.

The process of growing the measles, mumps, and rubella viruses is the same as for the M-M-R II vaccine. The Oka/Merck strain varicella-zoster virus is propagated in cells (MRC-5) derived from the lung tissue of a 14-week-old male fetus. Bovine serum and human albumin (the major protein found in human blood) are also used in the manufacturing process. The MMRV vaccine called Priorix-Tetra grows the viruses (measles—Schwarz strain; mumps—Jeryl Lynn strain) separately in chick embryo cells or MRC-5 cells (rubella—Wistar RA 27/3 strain; varicella-zoster—OKA strain).

Ingredients

M-M-R II[555]

- Measles virus, live attenuated ($\geq$1,000 $TCID_{50}$)
- Mumps virus, live attenuated ($\geq$12,500 $TCID_{50}$)
- Rubella virus, live attenuated ($\geq$1,000 $TCID_{50}$)
- Sorbitol (14.5 mg)
- Sodium phosphate
- Sucrose (1.9 mg)
- Sodium chloride
- Hydrolyzed gelatin (14.5 mg)
- Recombinant human albumin ($\leq$0.3 mg)
- Fetal bovine serum (<1 PPM)

- Buffer and media ingredients
- Neomycin (25 mcg)
- Residual human cells (DNA and protein fragments)

Proquad[556]

- Measles virus, live attenuated ($\geq$3.00 $\log_{10}$ TCID$_{50}$)
- Mumps virus, live attenuated ($\geq$4.30 $\log_{10}$ TCID$_{50}$)
- Rubella virus, live attenuated ($\geq$3.00 $\log_{10}$ TCID$_{50}$)
- Varicella virus, live attenuated ($\geq$3.99 $\log_{10}$ TCID$_{50}$)
- Sucrose ($\leq$21 mg)
- Hydrolyzed gelatin (11 mg)
- Sodium chloride (2.4 mg)
- Sorbitol (1.8 mg)
- Monosodium L-glutamate (0.40 mg)
- Sodium phosphate dibasic (0.34 mg)
- Human albumin (0.31 mg)
- Sodium bicarbonate (0.17 mg)
- Potassium phosphate monobasic (72 mcg)
- Potassium chloride (60 mcg)
- Potassium phosphate dibasic (36 mcg)
- Residual human cells (DNA and protein fragments)
- Neomycin (<16 mcg)
- Bovine calf serum (0.5 mcg)
- Egg protein, ovalbumin
- Other buffer and media ingredients

Priorix-Tetra[557]

- Measles virus, live attenuated ($\geq$10$^{3.0}$ CCID$_{50}$)
- Mumps virus, live attenuated ($\geq$10$^{4.4}$ CCID$_{50}$)
- Rubella virus, live attenuated ($\geq$10$^{3.0}$ CCID$_{50}$)
- Varicella virus, live attenuated ($\geq$10$^{3.3}$ CCID$_{50}$)
- Lactose
- Amino acids
- Sorbitol

- Mannitol
- Neomycin
- Residual human cells (DNA and protein fragments)
- Egg protein, ovalbumin

TID=tissue culture infectious doses; CCID=cell-culture infected dose

Controversial Ingredients

- ➤ Aborted fetal cells
- ➤ Human albumin
- ➤ Cow blood
- ➤ Recombinant human albumin
- ➤ Monosodium glutamate
- ➤ Chick embryo protein
- ➤ Egg protein, ovalbumin

Package Insert Adverse Reactions

M-M-R II: Panniculitis (painful bumps, or nodules, formed under the skin), atypical measles, fever, temporary loss of consciousness, headache, dizziness, general malaise, irritability, vasculitis, pancreatitis, diarrhea, nausea, vomiting, mumps, diabetes, thrombocytopenia, enlarged lymph nodes, leukocytosis (increased white blood cells), anaphylaxis, arthritis, painful joints, muscle aches, encephalitis, encephalopathy, measles encephalitis, pneumonia, pneumonitis, cough, sore throat, rhinitis, Stevens-Johnson syndrome, hives, erythema multiforme, rash, measles-like rash, itching, injection-site reactions, nerve deafness, ear infection, retina inflammation, optic neuritis, conjunctivitis, epididymitis, orchitis, and death. A review by Merck—the manufacturer of the vaccine—scientists concluded that adverse experiences occur at an overall rate of 30.5 per million doses.[558]

Proquad: Injection-site pain, tenderness, or soreness (15.9%–22.0%), fever (8.3%–21.5%), injection-site redness (8.4%–12.4%), injection-site swelling (8.0%–14.4%), irritability (2.4%–6.7%), measles-like rash (0.9%–4.3%), rash (0.6%–2.3%), and varicella-like rash (0.1%–2.1%).

Priorix-Tetra: Fever (29.3%–61.2%), injection-site redness (27.0%–31.0%), rash (11.5%–20.3%), injection-site swelling (8.4%–12.3%), injection-site pain (9.5%–10.2%), and irritability.

Parent or Healthcare Provider Adverse Events Reported through VAERS

M-M-R II—Death (136 through September 30, 2010), subacute sclerosing panencephalitis (a progressive neurological disorder), aseptic meningitis, encephalopathy, autism, febrile seizure, deafness, hypersensitivity reaction, anaphylaxis, thrombocytopenia, measles, mumps, rubella, injection-site reactions, arthritis, spontaneous abortion, stillbirth, and congenital rubella syndrome.[559]

Proquad—Subacute sclerosing panencephalitis, encephalitis, aseptic meningitis, measles, atypical measles, pneumonia, respiratory infection, infection, chickenpox-related influenza, shingles, orchitis, epididymitis, cellulitis, skin infection, retinitis, bronchitis, parotitis, sinusitis, impetigo, herpes simplex, candidiasis, rhinitis, aplastic anemia, thrombocytopenia, enlarged lymph nodes, anaphylaxis, facial swelling, measles encephalitis, myelitis, cerebrovascular accident, Guillain-Barré syndrome, optic neuritis, ocular palsies, eyelid or eye irritation, Bell's palsy, polyneuropathy, lack of voluntary coordination of muscles (ataxia), headache, seizures (including febrile), daytime sleepiness, dizziness, temporary loss of consciousness, tremors, feelings of pins and needles, necrotizing retinitis (in immunocompromised persons), nerve deafness, ear pain, extravasation blood (leakage of blood from a vessel into surrounding tissues), pneumonitis, pulmonary congestion, wheezing, bronchial spasm, sore throat, nose bleed, mouth ulcers, abdominal pain, passage of fresh blood through the anus (hematochezia), Stevens-Johnson syndrome, Henoch-Schönlein purpura, erythema multiforme, acute hemorrhagic edema of infancy, itching, thickening of the skin, panniculitis, arthritis, joint pain, muscle aches, and injection-site complaints.

Priorix-Tetra—meningitis, encephalitis, cerebrovascular accident, cerebellitis, Guillain-Barré syndrome, myelitis, neuritis, shingles, measles-like syndrome, mumps-like syndrome (including orchitis, epididymitis, and parotitis), thrombocytopenia, allergic reactions (including anaphylaxis), vasculitis, erythema multiforme, chickenpox-like rash, joint pain, arthritis, and febrile seizures.

Reactions Observed and Documented in Published Research

Childhood infections serve a valuable function and are important for the normal development of the immune system. The immune system is literally built and fine-tuned by exposures to germs and pathogens on a day-to-day basis. Indeed, a healthy immune system cannot be developed without regular exposure to germs and pathogens. Each exposure to an infectious agent "trains" the immune system to behave in a specific protective way. The immune system learns to distinguish between harmful pathogens, healthy cells and tissues, and microbes that live in harmony or synergy with the human body. Children are exposed to thousands of pathogens every day through the air they breathe, the food they eat, items that they touch, and the things they put in their mouths. In reality, pathogen exposure during childhood establishes a stronger immune system and less illness in their later years.

Interestingly, a measles or mumps infection during childhood appears to afford long-term cardiovascular benefits. Men who contracted the measles during childhood were significantly less likely to die from cardiovascular disease compared to men who were never infected.[560] In addition, a mumps infection in childhood resulted in a significantly reduced risk of dying from a stroke. The researchers also observed that women who had the measles or mumps as a child were significantly less likely to die from cardiovascular disease or a stroke. Over the last few decades, the role the immune system has in cardiac development and function has been documented and recognized. Discoveries show that immune cells infiltrate the heart during gestation and remain there to perform important housekeeping functions throughout life.[561] Immune cells also play a crucial role after a heart attack by heading to the heart to remove dying tissue, kill pathogens, and promote healing.

Conversely, abnormal immune system function can play a part in cardiovascular disease like stroke, atherosclerosis, and heart failure. It is possible that early childhood infections train the immune system to perform essential housekeeping duties and terminate the initial inflammatory response once repair is complete without contributing to a sustained and overwhelming inflammatory response that results in tissue damage.

Other data indicates that a measles infection during childhood decreases the risk of food and airborne allergies and eczema.[562,563,564,565] Infants are born with the capacity to mount an immune response due to their exposure to environmental allergens, through their mother, while in the womb.[566] Once born, these responses are changed by infections, nutrition, additional allergens, and the balance of healthy to unhealthy bacteria in the gut. It has also been documented that a heightened inflammatory response at birth predisposes children to food allergies.[567] Perhaps, avoiding a benign measles infection prevents required training for the immune system and predisposes some children to allergies. Further research is necessary to evaluate vaccines and their relationship with allergies.

Children who delayed receiving the MMR vaccine until later in life had a significantly reduced risk of developing hay fever.[568] Interestingly, children with eczema associated with food sensitivities experienced notable improvements in their symptoms after they contracted measles.[569] This suggests a natural infection with the measles provokes an immune response that protects against disease later in life and may improve current conditions related to improper immune responses. Comparison of unvaccinated children—from Steiner schools that practiced the anthroposophic lifestyle—to vaccinated children identified that children who never received the MMR vaccine had a lower prevalence of allergies.[570,571] However, this can't rule out that other lifestyle or environmental factors protected children against allergies, particularly since people who follow an anthroposophic lifestyle limit doctor's visits (limits opportunities to be diagnosed with allergic diseases), antibiotics, and medicines used for fevers. What is clear is that exposure to pathogens, particularly viruses, has and will continue to shape human biology and reducing those exposures may alter favorable human adaptations.

Immune system irregularities involving immunoglobulin E (IgE) production, helper T cells, cytokines (IL-4, IFN-gamma), and possibly other immune cells are involved in the development of allergy during childhood.[572] The immune system comprises a complex and vital network of cells and organs, each of which performs a unique role while maintaining communication with other immune cells and organs to perform their collective protective functions. Disruption of any of these cells or organs or their regular communication can cause immune system irregularities and dysfunction.

Vaccines contain ingredients (organisms, parts of organisms, inactivated toxins, adjuvants, and other ingredients) that generate protective immune responses against these components. They also can trigger abnormal immune responses and irregularities. Gelatin components in the DTaP vaccine increase IgE production.[573] Production of IgE antibodies in response to influenza vaccine components, especially 2-phenoxyethanol, causing anaphylaxis has also been documented.[574] Two types of T cells are involved in immune responses to pathogens: killer T cells (also called CD8 cells) and helper T cells (also called CD4 cells). Killer T cells are the primary cells that eliminate cells infected by viruses, whereas helper T cells bolster the responses of killer T cells and antibody-producing B cells. Animal models demonstrate that some viral vaccines can trigger robust helper-T-cell responses but poor or no killer-T-cell or B-cell response, leading to a devastating inflammatory response.[575] If this occurs, the helper T cells are sounding the alarm for other immune cells to fight the infection, but the other cells are not properly responding to the call to action. Elevated inflammatory cytokines, like IFN-gamma, IL-4, and IP-10, in the blood are commonly reported following vaccination.[576,577,578] Since most immune responses to vaccines are regulated by helper T cells,[579] it is plausible that vaccines are promoting an inflammatory response that increases the risk of allergies. Elevated levels of cytokines associated with allergies add to the evidence that vaccines, or vaccine ingredients, may trigger abnormal immune and inflammatory responses that could promote allergies.

Another connection between childhood infections and risk of disease later in life is cancer. More than a century of evidence shows that certain infections can either contribute to or reduce the risk of cancer. In a process called immunosurveillance, cells in the immune system look for and recognize foreign pathogens, and precancerous and cancerous cells throughout the body. Maintaining a delicate balance between immunosurveillance and inflammation is key to protection against cancer. Cancer can occur in an inflammatory dominant body environment.[580] An impressive amount of data suggests that infections early in life protect against various cancers.[581] Contrarily, vaccination may prevent this natural anticancer protection from developing.

The theory is that events—like childhood infections—help train the immunosurveillance system to better discriminate pathogens and precancerous/cancerous cells from healthy cells. Ordinarily, the immune system detects problematic cells in infected, injured, or inflamed tissues because they express excessive amounts of certain cell proteins. Regular exposure to these cells with high levels of cell proteins teaches the immune system to better detect and eliminate them. Since cancer cells also express abnormal levels of cell proteins, previous exposure to cells expressing these same levels of proteins allows the immune system to more readily identify cancer cells. For example, mucin 1 (MUC1) is one of many proteins that produce mucus to protect and lubricate the airways, digestive system, reproductive system, and other organs and tissues. Increased expression of MUC1 plays a dynamic role in protection against infection by a variety of pathogens and helps to regulate inflammatory responses to these infections. Let's say you are exposed to a respiratory pathogen. Cells that express MUC1 in the lungs engage in a defensive strategy to reduce infection by the pathogen.[582] In addition, MUC1 levels increase during inflammatory responses to airway infections, which helps resolve airway inflammation during the later stages of the infection. MUC1 expression is also increased in intestinal cells during infections to limit pathogen access to the surface of the digestive tract.[583] Altered expression of MUC1 during infections stimulates immune responses, including natural antibodies, to cells that display higher MUC1 levels. Years of exposure to infections and increased expression of MUC1 means that anti-MUC1 antibodies are present in the bloodstream of healthy individuals. These circulating antibodies provide protection against infectious pathogens and malignant cells that overexpress MUC1.

MUC1 is often overexpressed in colon, ovarian, breast, lung, melanoma, and pancreatic cancers.[584] Because the immune system was programmed—called immune memory—by a previous event to recognize the overexpression of MUC1, cancer cells that overexpress MUC1 are targeted for destruction by the immune system.[585] Essentially, the immune system already contains anti-MUC1 antibodies that target cancer cells expressing MUC1, which might prevent cancer from occurring in the first place. Indeed, overexpression of MUC1 is associated with aggressive, metastatic cancer that evades therapy and reduces survivability, and people without anti-MUC1 antibodies have an increased risk of cancer.[586] In this way, childhood infections that involve increased MUC1 expression prime the immune system to efficiently deal with cancer cells with high levels of MUC1.

Some viruses, like measles, mumps, and chickenpox, have even been known to cause spontaneous cancer remission and kill cancer cells.[587,588,589,590,591,592] These viruses have an affinity to infect and kill cancer cells. As the infected cell breaks down, it releases virus particles into other cancerous cells in the tumor, shrinking tumor size. Unfortunately, mumps vaccination only triggers the immune system to develop anti-mumps antibodies and not anticancer antibodies so the vaccine does not afford the same cancer protection.[593] In fact, some evidence suggests that certain vaccines—MMR, DPT, and hepatitis B—

181

increase the risk of leukemia.[594,595,596] It is plausible that avoidance of these childhood infections limits the immune system's training to identify and kill cancer cells proficiently. Conflicting research disputes the findings that vaccines increase childhood leukemia risk, but confirm that exposure to pathogens at an early age reduces leukemia risk.[597,598] A large amount of evidence suggests that childhood infections promote the development and maturity of the immune system so it can function more efficiently without overreacting.

Other experts suggest a general hygiene hypothesis, which says that exposure to pathogens during childhood allows the immune system to develop resistance to chronic diseases. In essence, exposure to viruses, bacteria, and parasites teaches the immune system to differentiate harmless substances from harmful pathogens. At the heart of this theory is immune system balance—teaching the immune system not to overreact, which in turn decreases the likelihood of autoimmune conditions. An oversimplified analogy for this important immune system training is learning to identify trees. When you were very young you identified all trees at trees, but as you grew older and saw more trees you learned to distinguish a spruce tree from a maple tree and so forth. In a similar manner, exposure to various types of infected cells allows your immune system to distinguish them as healthy or harmful. Below is a list of febrile (fever) infections that may provide protection against cancers later in life.

- Mumps infection may confer protection against ovarian cancer.[599,600,601]
- Mumps, measles, rubella, or chickenpox infections may confer protection against ovarian cancer (measles infection provided the greatest protection—53%).[602]
- Measles, rubella, and chickenpox infections may confer protection against genital, prostate, skin, lung, gastrointestinal, ear-nose-throat cancers, and cancers listed as "others."[603]

- Chickenpox or shingles infections and other infectious illnesses (e.g., cold and flu) may confer protection against brain tumors—glioma and meningioma.[604,605,606,607,608]
- Measles infection may confer protection against non-Hodgkin's lymphoma, and rubella, pertussis, measles, mumps, chickenpox, and influenza infections may confer protection against Hodgkin's lymphoma.[609,610,611,612,613,614,615]
- Measles and pertussis infections may confer protection against chronic lymphoid leukemia, and pertussis may decrease the risk of acute myeloid leukemia; other infections may protect against childhood leukemia, particularly acute lymphoblastic leukemia (the more serious the childhood infection, the lower the risk for leukemia).[616,617,618,619,620,621,622,623,624]
- Influenza, chickenpox, measles, and mumps infections may confer protection against malignant melanoma.[625,626]

The golden question is, are we decreasing mostly benign childhood infections for an increased incidence of cancer and an amplified risk of death from cancer? Cancer mortality has simultaneously increased as the number of deaths due to infectious illnesses have reduced because of the introduction of vaccines. Certainly other environmental, nutritional, and lifestyle factors are contributing to the observed increase in cancer mortality, but the influence of vaccines cannot be ruled out. One study found that for every 2 percent reduction in mortality from infectious illnesses a 2 percent increase in cancer mortality was witnessed ten years later.[627] We may simply be shifting the cause of death from infections to cancer since this is a one-to-one tradeoff. In some ways, acute childhood infections seem to counter chronic conditions and mortality later in life.

The diverse ecosystem of microorganisms—viruses and bacteria—in and on our bodies is vital for health and the development of a competent and capable immune system.[628,629] As part of a symbiotic relationship, certain pathogens receive a place to live (in or on us) and eat, and in return, they help support our immune defenses against other pathogens and provide a long list of other benefits. This is particularly true of exposure to beneficial bacteria as early in childhood as possible, which benefits a developing infant's immune system. Essentially, good bacteria help "program" the immune system of infants to respond better to pathogens without overreacting to substances in food and the environment. It is possible that artificial stimulation of the immune system through vaccination, as opposed to through natural immunity gained by childhood infections, disrupts normal immune system development in favor of abnormal immune responses.

Surprisingly, recent evidence suggests that natural infection with measles also disrupts immune memory. Immune memory is the ability of the immune system to rapidly recognize a threat that the body was previously exposed to and initiate a corresponding immune response. After an infection, antibodies created in response to an earlier infection remain in the body and serve as an important defensive mechanism in subsequent infections. The immune system also creates memory B and T cells that contain information about each threat the body has previously encountered. Scientists discovered that the measles virus erases part of immune memory making it less effective in protecting against threats it has already handled. In fact, measles can erase from 11 to 73 percent of antibodies circulating in the blood against other viruses and bacteria.[630] Severe measles illness tended to cause greater immune amnesia than mild illnesses. To make it simple, if you had 100 antibodies against the flu, a measles infection could reduce those antibody levels to somewhere between 27 and 89. This is like providing only 27–89 percent of a wanted poster to a bounty hunter. Obviously, the bounty hunter with 27 percent of the poster is going to struggle to find the criminal. Similarly, the immune system has a diminished ability to respond to infections with fewer antibodies. Fortunately, the immune system regains its memory of previous threats slowly as it is exposed to these threats again. Clearly, measles significantly affects immunity and overall well-being beyond our current understanding.

Ample evidence exists that fully vaccinated individuals can transmit measles to other fully vaccinated individuals. Called secondary vaccine failure—when vaccine's efficacy diminishes to nonprotective levels and a vaccinated person contracts the infection—measles is making a comeback despite being declared eliminated in the United States in 2000. Primary vaccine failure refers to when a person fails to create sufficient antibodies to protect against an infection after receiving a vaccine. A case in 2011 where a 22-year-old woman transmitted measles to four other people (two that were fully vaccinated and two that were considered immune to measles based on the presence of IgG antibodies) documents that fully vaccinated individuals spread measles to other fully vaccinated individuals.[631] The presence of IgG antibodies indicates prior exposure to measles virus either through natural infection or vaccination. Too few antibodies means that you are not immune to the virus and can contract the measles.

Measles is highly contagious making crowded places like schools a ripe environment for its transmission. A widespread measles outbreak in a highly vaccinated population (98 percent of the school had a history of full or partial vaccination) was documented in a Massachusetts high school.[632] Seventy percent of individuals who contracted measles at the school had a history of age-appropriate measles vaccination, suggesting a very high vaccine failure rate. Interestingly, the study noted that waning immunity was not a contributing factor among the vaccine failures. An Illinois high school with a documented vaccination level of 99.7 percent (according to school records) also experienced a measles outbreak in 1985.[633] Despite the high vaccination levels at the school, sixty-nine measles cases occurred. Evaluation of the data showed that students who were vaccinated before the age of 14 months were most likely to develop measles illness. Both outbreaks documented that children vaccinated before 12 months of age were far more likely to be infected. Based on this, it is possible that the measles vaccine provides inadequate long-term immunity to children who receive the vaccine at younger ages.

Military environments, such as barracks and ships, create an environment favorable for the rapid spread of certain infectious illnesses. For the sake of public health and the military operational consequences of infectious illnesses, members of the military must have evidence of immunity against multiple infections. From late December 2018 to early April 2019, a US Navy ship, the USS *Fort McHenry* was quarantined because of an outbreak of mumps (twenty-eight cases on the ship).[634] All service members aboard had been vaccinated with the MMR vaccine, which suggests that the vaccine failed to provide protection against the mumps and that the infection was transmitted from fully vaccinated individuals to fully vaccinated individuals.

The United States is not the only country that has experienced MMR vaccine failures. Despite only 3–5 percent of the population being unvaccinated, a large measles epidemic occurred in Quebec, Canada, during 2011.[635] The person who started the outbreak was reportedly vaccinated in childhood. In 2017, a measles outbreak occurred among a highly vaccinated population of Israeli soldiers.[636] The two soldiers that were the source of the outbreak self-reported a history of two doses of MMR vaccine. Nine additional cases of measles occurred among fully vaccinated soldiers. Despite a significant number of students who received age-appropriate measles vaccination, a measles outbreak occurred in a middle school in Beijing, China.[637] All eleven measles cases in students had received age-appropriate vaccinations according to Chinese domestic criteria, and eight were age-appropriately vaccinated according to US CDC/ACIP criteria. Elapsed time since the last vaccine played a significant role in measles risk. Children vaccinated five to nine and ten or more years previously had a 4.6 and 5.5 times greater risk of measles. More evidence that vaccinated individuals can infect vaccinated individuals. A more recent Japanese case at the end of 2018 also documented transmission of measles from a fully vaccinated individual to others.[638] The outbreak was traced to an individual who received two doses of measles vaccine who spread measles to three unvaccinated individuals and six fully vaccinated individuals. A report in China confirmed the spread of measles from a person with a documented record of vaccination to an unvaccinated individual, proving secondary vaccine failure.[639] A subsequent measles outbreak occurred because of the vaccine failure. It is possible that widespread vaccination reduced natural immunity (through infection by wild virus) sufficiently to contribute to reduced antibodies and decreased immunity in the overall population. It is very evident that fully vaccinated individuals pose a risk of spreading measles to vaccinated, unvaccinated, and undervaccinated individuals.

Loss of immunity to measles, mumps, and rubella over time can result in asymptomatic (subclinical) or a very mild case of measles. Asymptomatic people could unknowingly spread the infections to others. Subclinical infection is not uncommon for measles, mumps, and rubella infections.[640] The fact that individuals with subclinical infections can spread these infections caused the study authors to conclude "it is doubtful whether population immunity (herd immunity), which is necessary to eliminate the three diseases, can be attained in large populations." In addition, vaccinated individuals can shed the virus in respiratory secretions to infect others. A case of a child with fever eight days after MMR vaccination (the fever started four days after) found the vaccine-derived measles virus in the child's throat.[641] The study states "subcutaneous injection of an attenuated measles strain can result in respiratory excretion of this virus." The vaccine strain of the virus has also been identified in the urine of vaccinated individuals, suggesting it sheds this way also.[642,643] Vaccine virus in the urine is less of a risk than vaccine-derived virus in the throat as other people are more likely to come in contact with respiratory secretions than urine.

Mysteriously, observational studies connect receiving the MMR vaccine to increased emergency room visits. Analyzing the health records of nearly 414,000 children, scientists found that vaccinated children were significantly more likely to require an ER visit—including a sharp rise in febrile seizures—four to twelve days after receiving the MMR vaccine.[644] Evidence implies that girls may be more susceptible to adverse MMR reactions than boys.[645] Common reasons for an ER visit included ear infection, acute upper respiratory tract infection, viral infection, noninfectious gastroenteritis (inflammation of the gastrointestinal tract coupled with nausea, diarrhea, cramping, or vomiting that is not caused by a pathogen), and noninfectious colitis. Surprisingly, another study concluded that children from high-income families were less likely to require admission to a hospital following the MMR vaccine.[646] This contradicting study had a larger sample size (495,987 children), but both studies require replication in other populations to determine the actual risk of the MMR vaccine and ER visits or hospitalization.

Thrombocytopenia is a condition characterized by a low blood platelet count, which increases the risk of bruising and excess bleeding. Immune thrombocytopenia (IT), formerly called idiopathic thrombocytopenic purpura (ITP), occurs when the immune system produces antibodies against platelets. These platelets are marked for destruction and elimination by the spleen, which significantly reduces blood platelet count. Sometimes the immune system also interferes with the cells responsible for producing platelets, further diminishing platelet count. In children, IT usually develops after a viral infection.

Several independent studies confirm a relationship and possible causal association between IT development and the MMR vaccine.[647,648,649,650,651,652,653] IT typically develops within six weeks after vaccination and the increased risk of developing IT is up to six times greater, according to the studies. IT persists for more than one month in 26 percent of vaccine-related cases and 10 percent of children have IT for longer than six months.[654] The mechanism by which the MMR vaccine may trigger IT is through disruption of the immune system. Increased platelet-associated immunoglobulin (PAIg) and platelet autoantibodies have been observed in children with MMR vaccine-related IT.[655] Elevated PAIg and autoantibodies are signs of increased platelet destruction. Both the increased immunoglobulin and the autoantibodies play major roles in the development of IT.

Evaluation of the health records of 1.8 million children also found a strong correlation between the MMR vaccine and IT occurrence within forty-two days following vaccination. Indeed, the research reported a link between not only the MMR vaccine, but also hepatitis A, varicella, and Tdap vaccines as well.[656] On average, vaccine-related IT was five times more likely in children 12–19 months old. In children 11–17 years old, varicella increased the risk of IT twelve times, while Tdap increased IT risk by twenty times. The hepatitis A vaccine was the worst offender, increasing IT development in children 7–17 years old by twenty-three times. Other studies linked IT cases, some severe and causing internal hemorrhaging, to hepatitis A, hepatitis B, MMR, pertussis, varicella, and influenza vaccines.[657,658,659,660,661] The research also suggests that IT may be more severe in children with a recent history of vaccination.[662] Since IT is linked to viral and bacterial infections, it may be that vaccine antigens cause the immune system to mistakenly attack platelets.

It should be noted that some evidence demonstrates that the occurrence of vaccine-related IT is lower than the number of cases that occur as a consequence of measles, mumps, or rubella infections, meaning IT naturally occurs more than vaccine-related IT.[663] It is estimated that the MMR vaccine causes about one case of IT per 30,000 shots (not likely reflective of actual numbers because mild cases without bleeding are unlikely to be reported); whereas rubella is estimated to cause one case per 3,000 natural infections, higher incidence is reported after measles infection, and rubella 6 to 1,200 cases per 100,000 infections.[664,665] Based on this, a child is more likely to develop IT after an infection with measles, mumps, or rubella than after the MMR vaccine.

Observational studies also suggest a link between the MMR vaccine and autism. Many autistic children have elevated levels of antibodies to the measles virus, suggesting an overactive immune response.[666] Antibodies were identified in 83 percent of autistic children but none of their nonautistic siblings or the control group consisting of nonautistic children. The same authors also reported that an autoimmune reaction in the central nervous system to MMR antibodies, especially to myelin basic protein (MBP), might be associated with autism.[667] Again, unusual MMR antibodies positive for measles were found in 60 percent of

189

autistic children and none of the controls. Moreover, 90 percent of the autistic children who tested positive for MMR antibodies were also positive for MBP autoantibodies. In other words, the body was targeting healthy neurons for destruction after MMR vaccination. The study authors suggest that an unusual response to the MMR vaccine, which causes an abnormal measles virus infection, may trigger neurological symptoms that increase the risk of autism.

Researchers from the Sound Choice Pharmaceutical Institute postulate that DNA fragments from fetal cells used in the manufacture of some vaccines may trigger autoimmune reactions that provoke genetic mutations and increase the risk of autism.[668] Foreign DNA—like that which exists in some vaccines—can integrate into the cell nucleus and genome of vaccine recipients.[669] However, other researchers refute the connection between autism and the MMR vaccine and argue that not all autistic children have elevated measles antibodies.[670] Correlation and a plausible contribution of MMR vaccine ingredients to autism warrants further research.

See the *Reactions Observed and Documented in Published Research* section of chapter 4 for a discussion on vaccine-associated seizures and the MMR and MMRV vaccine.

See the *Reactions Observed and Documented in Published Research* section of chapter 5 for a discussion on MMR vaccine-associated type 1 diabetes risk.

INFECTION RISKS	VACCINE RISKS
Measles	Increased risk of chronic
Ear infection	conditions later in life:
Pneumonia (5%)	cardiovascular disease, cancer,
Secondary infections (<0.3%)	allergies, and eczema
Encephalitis (<0.1%)	Leukemia
Heart inflammation (very rare)	ER visits
Thrombocytopenia (very rare)	Febrile seizure
Sclerosing panencephalitis (very	Immune thrombocytopenia
rare)	Autism

Mumps
Testicular inflammation (≤10%)
Cerebrospinal fluid pleocytosis
Ovarian inflammation (≤1%)
Meningitis (<1%)
Encephalopathy (≤0.3%)

Rubella
Congenital rubella syndrome (first
16 weeks of pregnancy)
Joint pain
Thrombocytopenia (≤0.02%)
Encephalitis (≤0.02%)

Cancer
Type 1 diabetes

10

Varicella (Chickenpox)

What Is Varicella Infection?

More commonly known as chickenpox, varicella is a highly contagious illness caused by the varicella-zoster virus—a human herpesvirus. It causes a blister-like rash that normally begins around the hairline on the face and then appears on the trunk and extremities over the next five to seven days. Aside from the distinctive rash, chickenpox includes itching, fever, general malaise, and fatigue. Time from infection to symptom appearance varies between ten and twenty-one days (called the incubation period). The lesions usually crust over in about a week to ten days and then the child fully recovers. Children are contagious about two days prior to the appearance of the rash and until all lesions have crusted over. Chickenpox is self-limiting and rarely causes complications except in infants and individuals with a weakened immune system.

Like many other infectious illnesses, chickenpox is spread via respiratory droplets or direct contact with the skin lesions of an infected person. The virus easily spreads from one person to the next when in close proximity (within three to six feet). Chickenpox is widely recognizable by healthcare professionals because of the characteristic rash, but laboratory test by scraping a lesion may be requested if in doubt. Treatment typically involves oral acyclovir or valacyclovir—

antiviral drugs—for up to a week. Secondary bacterial infections are treated with antibiotics. However, most cases in otherwise healthy children can be managed at home with cool baths with added baking soda, uncooked oatmeal, or colloidal oatmeal and calamine lotion.

How Prevalent Is It?

Interestingly, chickenpox incidences differ between temperate and tropical climates. Peak incidence among children occurs in the winter and early spring in temperate climates, but in the dry, cool months in tropical climates. The reason for this is poorly understood, but it could be due to population density and climate. Annual incidence of chickenpox in industrialized nations is estimated at 300 to 1,291 cases per 100,000 population in Europe and 14.5 cases per 100,000 population in the United States[671] Chickenpox is a worldwide communicable illness, and few countries vaccinate for it today.

What Are the Health Risks of Varicella Infection?

The overwhelming majority of people completely recover from chickenpox without any complications, but rarely (less than 1 percent of cases) complications like secondary bacterial infections (cellulitis, pneumonia) and neurological conditions (encephalitis) occur, which may cause death. Severe complications most often affect people with a developing or weakened immune system. Chickenpox is more dangerous for adults over 45 than it is for children aged 5–14, resulting in a greater hospitalization rate and a 174-fold higher risk of dying.[672] Maybe the chickenpox parties thrown by moms of the prevaccine era were beneficial after all. Getting chickenpox between ages 5 and 14 provides a lifetime of immunity and is very low risk compared to being infected as an infant or middle-aged adult.

After infection, the virus lives permanently in a dormant state within nerve cells. Occasionally the virus is reactivated years after the chickenpox resolved and causes a secondary illness called shingles. Shingles is a painful rash that most often appears as a single stripe of blisters that wraps around either side of the torso. It most frequently occurs in adults over age 50 and causes a painful rash that can cause permanent nerve damage.

Varicella Vaccine

Description

Varicella virus was isolated from both chickenpox and zoster lesions in 1954. Further study led to the development of a live attenuated vaccine in Japan in the 1970s. The chickenpox vaccine became widely available in the United States in 1995. Children under 13 years of age are recommended to get two doses of varicella vaccine: one between 12 and 15 months and the second between 4 and 6 years of age. It is also recommended that those 13 and older who never had the chickenpox or never received the chickenpox vaccine get two doses, at least twenty-eight days apart. However, most children develop sufficient immunity—85 percent protection against any form of varicella and near 100 percent against severe cases—after only one dose of varicella vaccine.[673] Studies suggest that two doses of the vaccine provide 88–98 percent protection against any form of varicella, so on the low end, it is not a significant increase in protection to get a second shot. Despite being available for twenty-five years, only Japan, Canada, Australia, the United States, and a few European and Middle Eastern countries include it in their routine childhood vaccination programs as of this writing. This is likely because the vast majority of people, including healthcare professionals, consider it a mild, self-limiting illness with very little risk of complications.

Note: Because this is a live attenuated virus vaccine, people who have a weakened immune system, undergoing immunosuppressive treatment, or have conditions that affect cell-mediated immunity should not receive this vaccine.

Vaccine Manufacturing Process

Varivax is a preparation of the Oka/Merck strain of live, attenuated varicella virus, which was obtained from an infected child. The virus is introduced into human embryonic lung cell cultures, adapted to and propagated in embryonic guinea pig cell cultures and finally grown in lung cells from an aborted female of three months' gestation (WI-38 human diploid lung fibroblasts). Furthermore, the virus is passed through MRC-5 cells (diploid—containing two complete sets of chromosomes, one from each parent—human cells obtained from a 14-week-old aborted Caucasian male). The vaccine is freeze-dried with sucrose, phosphate, glutamate, gelatin, and urea as stabilizers.

Pregnant women should not receive the varicella vaccine because it contains live attenuated varicella virus, which may cause congenital varicella syndrome. People with a compromised immune system or with current illness with fever should not receive this vaccine either. In addition, the use of salicylates (aspirin) or salicylate-containing products should be avoided in children and adolescents aged 12 months to 17 years for six weeks following vaccination because of the association with Reye syndrome and aspirin therapy.

Ingredients[674]

- Varicella virus, live, attenuated (1350 plaque-forming units)
- Sucrose (18 mg)
- Hydrolyzed gelatin (8.9 mg)
- Sodium chloride (2.3 mg)
- Monosodium L-glutamate (0.36 mg)
- Sodium phosphate dibasic (0.33 mg)
- Potassium phosphate monobasic (57 mcg)
- Residual human cells (DNA and protein fragments)
- Bovine calf serum

Controversial Ingredients

- Aborted fetal cells
- Guinea pig cells
- Cow blood
- Monosodium glutamate (MSG)

Children aged 1–12 years: Injection-site reactions (19.3%), fever (14.7%), generalized varicella-like rash (3.8%), and injection-site varicella-like rash (3.4%). Adolescents and adults: Injection-site reactions (24.4%), fever (10.2%), generalized varicella-like rash (5.5%), and injection-site varicella-like rash (3.1%).

ProQuad and Priorix-Tetra include the varicella vaccine as part of the MMR combination shot. See chapter 9 for more information.

Parent or Healthcare Provider Adverse Events Reported through VAERS

Anaphylaxis, facial swelling, angioneurotic edema (swelling of the subcutaneous and submucosal tissue due to a deficiency in C1 inhibitor gene), peripheral swelling, necrotizing retinitis (immunocompromised individuals), aplastic anemia, thrombocytopenia, chickenpox (vaccine strain), encephalitis, cerebrovascular accident, transverse myelitis, Guillain-Barré syndrome, Bell's palsy, lack of voluntary coordination of muscle movements (ataxia), meningitis, aseptic meningitis, feelings of pins and needles, pharyngitis, pneumonia/pneumonitis, Stevens-Johnson syndrome, erythema multiforme, Henoch-Schönlein purpura, shingles, impetigo, cellulitis, and secondary bacterial infections of the skin and soft tissue.

Reactions Observed and Documented in Published Research

Evidence indicates that people who receive the varicella vaccine are substituting a mild childhood illness, chickenpox, for a more severe and costly teen/adult condition called shingles. Once a person has been infected by the varicella virus, it lives dormant in the nerves, especially the trigeminal ganglia, and can reemerge when the immune system is in a weakened state. Shingles is a very painful rash—usually on the torso—due to a reactivation of the dormant varicella-zoster virus. It is characterized by pain, burning, numbness, or tingling, a red rash that begins a few days after the pain, itching, sensitivity to touch, itching, and fluid-filled blisters that break open and crust over. Less commonly,

headache, fever, fatigue, and sensitivity to light accompany shingles. Exposure to wild varicella virus and a subsequent chickenpox illness can significantly reduce the incidence of shingles.[675] The rash typically resolves within one to two weeks, but the pain can persist for four to six weeks and possibly longer. Oral antiviral drugs may be used to shorten the duration of symptoms.

Routine vaccination against varicella has proven to be less effective than natural immunity gained from wild varicella virus infection and corresponded with an increase in shingles cases. Shingles cases have dramatically increased in direct relation to varicella vaccine rates and have negated the cost savings associated with a reduction in chickenpox illnesses.[676,677,678,679,680,681,682,683] Cases of shingles in all age groups increased by 90 percent as the varicella vaccination rate climbed to 89 percent.[684] More recent estimates report that shingles has almost doubled from 1998 to 2012.[685] The varicella vaccine was licensed for use in the United States in 1995. Estimates suggest that giving a 100 percent effective chickenpox vaccine to 1-year-olds could increase the incidence of shingles almost twofold thirty-one years after implementation.[686] When adults and teens are regularly exposed to children who are infected with chickenpox it provides a natural immunity boost against the varicella virus and therefore reduces the risk of shingles. Including the varicella vaccine in the routine vaccine schedule deprives teens and adults of this natural immunity boost and places future generations receiving the vaccine at the same risk of shingles as they age. Ironically, the vaccine industry's answer to an increase in shingles cases was to create a shingles vaccine that is recommended for all healthy adults fifty years and older.

Evidence indicates that the varicella vaccine is also becoming less effective as more people are vaccinated.[687] In fact, a Korean study showed that despite a 97 percent vaccine rate in 2011, the number of chickenpox cases reported to the Korean Centers for Disease Control and Prevention tripled.[688] A large portion of children who contracted chickenpox were vaccinated, indicating vaccine failure. During their

evaluation, Korean researchers also reported that 12 percent of vaccinated children experienced systemic adverse reactions to the vaccine. Outbreaks of chickenpox are reported among vaccinated children and vaccine effectiveness rates as low as 44 percent have been observed.[689] The poor efficacy of the varicella vaccine seems to be primarily due to primary vaccine failure.[690] Of 148 healthy children, the vaccine failed to generate sufficient antibodies to confer a protective effect in 24 percent of children.[691] Some evidence shows that age at vaccination can affect the protection that the vaccine provides. Receipt of the vaccine after 14 months of age reduces the immune response to the vaccine, increasing the risk of chickenpox in vaccinated children.[692] Other research found that vaccine efficacy was 64 percent for children vaccinated at 10–18 months, and 82 percent in those vaccinated at 10–24 months.[693] A second dose of varicella vaccine was recommended to increase protection because of waning immunity five years after the first dose of varicella vaccine. There is little doubt that the varicella vaccine has decreased chickenpox incidence and hospitalization due to varicella infection, but the increased risk of shingles and evidence of primary vaccine failure makes one question its value as a routine immunization.

Emerging evidence shows that the wild varicella strain may be in the process of genetically recombining with the vaccine strain and causing shingles in children vaccinated against chickenpox.[694,695,696] Incidences of shingles is significantly increasing in adolescents between 10 and 19 years old further validating this unfortunate trend.[697] Simply put, shingles may occur in children as a result of the vaccine strain of varicella.

Postherpetic neuralgia is a painful complication of shingles and chickenpox that affects the nerves and skin and causes a burning pain. It is logical that the increase in shingles cases in children will also result in an increased incidence of postherpetic neuralgia. Although very rare, children with postherpetic neuralgia are at risk of developing meningoencephalitis. Meningoencephalitis is inflammation of the brain and its surrounding protective membranes. Children with postherpetic neuralgia should be monitored for a few weeks for signs of the condition. Signs include flu-like symptoms, fever, disorientation, blurred vision, purple rashes, speech problems, or bulging forehead in infants initially; followed by seizure, vomiting, drowsiness, and unconsciousness in the later stages.

Very rarely, shingles can lead to serious problems like pneumonia, hearing problems, encephalitis, and death. Severe pain is long-lasting in about 20 percent of individuals after the rash clears up. One group of researchers projected that mass varicella vaccination could lead to a major shingles epidemic that lasts up to fifty years, affecting more than 50 percent of people aged 10–44 years and contributing to five thousand deaths.[698,699] Anyone who has had shingles and the chickenpox can tell you that chickenpox is easier and less painful to deal with. It makes no sense to continue to prevent chickenpox at the expense of an increase in shingles rates.

Transmission of the varicella virus vaccine strain is rare but does occur.[700] A varicella vaccine recipient with a rash can spread varicella vaccine virus to adults and children, which can cause chickenpox or shingles. This most commonly occurs among household members but only if the vaccine recipient exhibits a rash after vaccination. Anyone who gets a rash after the vaccine should stay away from people with a weakened immune system or young infants to avoid spreading the varicella vaccine virus to others.

Despite this increase in shingles cases because of varicella vaccination, some suggest that if we ride out the storm, shingles cases will decrease as the varicella-zoster virus is eradicated. Modeling shingles incidence, researchers suggest that the significant increase in shingles incidence will decline over decades of continued varicella vaccination.[701] The question is, will the public tolerate decades of increased shingles incidence to reduce a self-limiting and benign childhood illness?

Another type of shingles, ocular (eye) shingles, has also been on the rise. Ocular shingles, also called herpes zoster ophthalmicus, is also caused by the varicella-zoster virus and carries with it serious side effects that could permanently impair vision. Ocular shingles is characterized by a swollen upper eyelid (usually only one side), sensitivity to light, itchiness and irritation of the eye, blurred vision, burning pain, rash, and skin sensitivity. One study found that people are getting ocular shingles at younger ages—median age of onset declined from 61.2 to 55.8 years from 2007 to 2013.[702] While the researchers admitted that further study is necessary, they suggested "that varicella vaccination of children remains a possible explanation for the increased number of cases [of ocular shingles] and reduction in mean age." An increase in ocular shingles may not be associated with the vaccine though. Medical records show cases of ocular shingles increased before the varicella vaccine was introduced, beginning in 1993, with the greatest increase occurring from 1993 to 1996.[703]

Another eye condition associated with varicella vaccination is keratitis. Keratitis is inflammation of the cornea and causes eye redness and pain, excess tears, blurred or decreased vision, difficulty opening the eye because of irritation or pain, and sensitivity to light. Keratitis involving one eye has been observed within days of receiving a varicella vaccine.[704,705,706,707] It may happen if viral antigens remain in the cornea after vaccination. The occurrence of varicella vaccine-related keratitis is uncommon and usually self-limiting or resolves with treatment.

As with a childhood measles infection, experiencing the chickenpox during childhood may provide protection against heart disease and allergies. Adults who contracted chickenpox as children had significantly fewer coronary events—heart attack and angina pectoris (chest pain)—compared to controls.[708] Furthermore, each additional childhood infection, such as measles, mumps, and rubella, conferred an additional 14 percent protection against coronary events. Contracting shingles alone increases the risk of heart attack and stroke, so if varicella vaccination increases the risk of shingles it is highly likely to subsequently increase shingles-related heart disease.[709] Children who get the chickenpox by 8 years of age are far less likely than vaccinated children to develop asthma, allergic rhinitis, and eczema.[710] Childhood infections may suppress the production of antibodies (IgE) and alter white blood cell distribution to promote healthy development of the immune system and a reduced risk of allergies. The more we learn about vaccine-related alterations in immune function that contribute to increased chronic illness risk, the more we need to question the logic of a vaccine approach to preventing infectious illnesses.

See the *Reactions Observed and Documented in Published Research* section of chapter 9 for a discussion of immune thrombocytopenia associated with varicella vaccination.

See the *Reactions Observed and Documented in Published Research* section of chapter 9 for a discussion about how certain childhood infections may protect against cancer development later in life.

INFECTION RISKS	VACCINE RISKS
Secondary infections (≤1%)	Shingles
Encephalitis (≤1%)	Postherpetic neuralgia
Shingles	Ocular shingles
	Increased risk of allergies, asthma, and eczema later in life
	Meningoencephalitis (very rare)
	Pneumonia (very rare)
	Vision/hearing impairment (very rare)
	Death (very rare)

11

Hepatitis A (HepA)

What Is Hepatitis A Infection?

Like hepatitis B, hepatitis A is an infectious illness that causes inflammation of the liver. It is caused by the hepatitis A virus (HepA virus). Unlike the hepatitis B virus that is primarily spread by direct contact with body fluids (blood, semen, or other body fluids), the HepA virus can be spread by contact with infected feces, sexual contact, or consuming contaminated food or water. It is most commonly spread by the fecal-oral route—touching infected feces and then your mouth. A person is most contagious for about one week before symptoms begin, if symptoms appear. Infection with HepA confers lifelong immunity against the illness and it cannot re-infect a person.

HepA infection is a self-limiting illness that does not cause chronic infection, and is very rarely fatal. Symptoms include jaundice (or elevated bilirubin levels ≥ 3.0 mg/dL) or elevated liver enzymes (ALT >200 IU/L), with fever, headache, loss of appetite, general malaise, joint pain, nausea, vomiting, abdominal pain, diarrhea, clay-colored stool, and dark urine. The average incubation period for HepA is twenty-eight days. HepA infection is confirmed by positive immunoglobulin M HepA virus antibody or a positive nucleic acid amplification test for hepatitis A virus RNA.

About 70 percent of HepA infections in children under age 6 are not accompanied by symptoms.[711] If young children are symptomatic they usually don't exhibit jaundice. In contrast, most children 6 and over (about 70 percent) and adults who are infected do show symptoms, including jaundice.[712,713] Most symptoms resolve within two months, but a small percentage (10–15 percent) of people experience prolonged symptoms or recurring symptoms for up to six months.[714,715,716] The liver is fully healed within six months with no lasting damage in the overwhelming majority of cases. There are no specific medicines used in the treatment of HepA, and unless the illness becomes severe, the body clears the virus on its own. Instead, rest, proper hydration, and avoidance of alcohol and medications that damage the liver are all that is needed.

It is worth noting that preventive shots can be given to a person exposed to HepA during outbreaks. This is not a vaccine but a shot with actual antibodies, called immune globulin. The shot is made by filtering the antibodies out of donated blood units and chemically treating and filtering them to prevent HepA transmission. It can prevent HepA disease up to 85 percent of the time if it is given within two weeks of a person's exposure. This shot is recommended for infants and adults of any age who are suspected of being exposed to HepA.

How Prevalent Is It?

Worldwide, an estimated 1.4 million cases of HepA are reported each year, but this number is likely low because so many cases are asymptomatic and not reported.[717] Risk of infection is higher in areas with poor sewage treatment and that lack safe water. Countries in Africa and Southeast Asia have higher infection rates, while the Middle East, Central Asia, and South America experience moderate infection rates.[718] Ironically, the majority of children in developing countries get infected at an early age and acquire lifelong immunity, but children and adults in developed countries remain susceptible to infection because of low infection rates at a young age. Generally, developed countries have very low HepA infection rates, while developing countries have higher incidence. Sometimes beachgoers get it from sewage runoff that contaminates certain beaches. Past outbreaks have been caused by contaminated foods. HepA remains a global public health concern with the majority of those infected being unaware of their illness.

What Are the Health Risks of Hepatitis A Infection?

As suggested above, HepA infection rarely causes complications, and the overwhelming majority of people make a full recovery without complications. Seldom relapsing hepatitis, cholestatic hepatitis A (decreased bile flow), hepatitis A triggering autoimmune hepatitis (the body's immune system turns against liver cells), subfulminant hepatitis (liver disease for up to twenty-six weeks before the development of hepatic encephalopathy), and fulminant hepatitis (the development of encephalopathy within eight weeks of the onset of symptoms in a patient with a previously healthy liver) are reported. Fulminant hepatitis is the most severe complication, with a mortality rate of up to 80 percent.[719] Progression of HepA infection to severe complications may be due to preexisting liver damage, a clotting factor disorder, or age.

Less than 1 percent of cases result in acute liver failure,[720] and most HepA cases are not fatal. People with preexisting liver damage—nonalcoholic fatty liver disease or alcoholic steatohepatitis—are more susceptible to acute liver failure. If HepA does cause acute liver failure, the spontaneous survival rate is estimated at 69 percent—the rest of the cases require liver transplant or die.[721] HepA-related fatalities are estimated to be 0.1 percent in adolescents and young adults (15–39 years), 0.3 percent in children under 14, 0.4 percent in older adults (40–59 years), and highest in people over 60 (1.8%).[722] Overall, the mortality rate from hepatitis among all ages is 0.3 percent.

Hepatitis A Vaccine

Description

Two inactivated whole-virus monovalent vaccines are available: Havrix and Vaqta. Both monovalent vaccines are considered highly immunogenic (95 percent), meaning they effectively trigger the body to develop antibodies within four weeks of a single dose, and nearly 100 percent have antibodies after two doses. Havrix and Vaqta are available in both pediatric and adult formulas. The pediatric formulas are approved for persons 12 months to 18 years and the adult formula is used for adults 19 years and older. The first dose is typically administered around 12 months of age and the second dose six to thirteen months later, usually between 18 and 24 months of age. An additional vaccine, Twinrix, contains both HepA and HepB (bivalent) and is approved for adults 18 and over. This vaccine is given as a 3 or 4 dose series.

Note: live, attenuated HepA vaccines—manufactured in China—may be used in China and India. This is a single-dose vaccine.

Vaccine Manufacturing Process

The Havrix and Vaqta vaccines are produced by growing cell-culture-adapted HepA virus in MRC-5 cells (diploid—containing two complete sets of chromosomes, one from each parent—human cells obtained derived from a 14-week-old aborted Caucasian male), purified from cell lysates, inactivated with formalin, and adsorbed to an aluminum hydroxide adjuvant. The HepA portion of the Twinrix vaccine is manufactured the same way as the monovalent version. The hepatitis B surface antigen is obtained by culturing it in genetically engineered *Saccharomyces cerevisiae* yeast cells. HepA and HepB are individually adsorbed onto aluminum salts and pooled during formulation.

Ingredients

Havrix[723]

- HepA virus, inactivated and whole (Pediatric—720 EL.U.; Adult—1440 EL.U.)
- Amino acids (0.3% w/v)
- Phosphate-buffered solution
- Polysorbate 20 (0.05 mg/mL)

- Residual human cells, DNA and protein fragments ($\leq$0.05 mg/mL)
- Formalin ($\leq$0.1 mg/mL)
- Neomycin ($\leq$40 ng/mL)

Vaqta[724]

- HepA virus, inactivated and whole (Pediatric—25U of antigen; Adult—50U of antigen)
- Aluminum (Pediatric—0.225 mg; Adult—0.45 mg)
- Sodium borate (Pediatric—35 mcg; Adult—70 mcg)
- Residual human cells, DNA and protein fragments (<0.1 mcg)
- Bovine serum proteins (<0.1 mcg)
- Formaldehyde (<0.8 mcg)
- Neomycin (<10 PPB)

Twinrix[725]

- HepA virus, inactivated and whole (720 EL.U.)
- Hepatitis B surface antigen
- Aluminum (0.45 mg)
- Formaldehyde ($\leq$0.1 mg)
- Residual human cells, DNA and protein fragments (<2.5 mcg)
- Neomycin sulfate ($\leq$20 ng)
- Yeast protein ($\leq$5%)
- Amino acids
- Sodium chloride
- Phosphate buffer
- Polysorbate 20
- Water

EL.U.=Enzyme linked immunosorbent assay units.

Controversial Ingredients

- ➢ Residual human cells (DNA and protein fragments)
- ➢ Aluminum
- ➢ Formaldehyde
- ➢ Cow blood

Havrix: Irritability (33.3%), injection-site pain (23.8%), drowsiness (22.3%), injection-site redness (20.1%), loss of appetite (18.3%), injection-site swelling (8.7%), and fever (3.0%). Among four studies, 0.9 percent of subjects reported a serious adverse event, which included seizure, bronchial hyperreactivity, and respiratory distress. In addition, the following were observed between 1 and 9.9 percent of the time: nausea, fatigue, and general malaise.

Vaqta: Children 12–23 months of age—Injection-site pain (15.3%–27.4%), injection-site redness (11.7%–21.5%), injection-site swelling (7.0%–12.7%), fever (9.0%–12.4%), irritability (2.8%–8.8%), rhinorrhea (2.0%–6.2%), upper respiratory tract infection (2.3%–5.2%), diarrhea (3.8%–4.6%), and diaper rash (1.1%–2.4%). In addition, the following were observed between 1 and 9.9 percent of the time: conjunctivitis, constipation, vomiting, injection-site bruising, ear infection, cold involving swelling of the nasal passages and back of the throat, rhinitis, viral infection, croup, strep throat, nonspecific viral rash, viral gastroenteritis, roseola, loss of appetite, insomnia, excessive crying, cough, nasal congestion, respiratory congestion, measles-, rubella-, or varicella-like rash, vesicular rash, and morbilliform rash (rose-red flat or slightly elevated eruption). Across the five studies, 0.7 percent of subjects reported a serious adverse event—febrile seizure, dehydration, gastroenteritis, and cellulitis, of which 0.1 percent were judged to be vaccine related by the study investigator. Persons 2–18 years of age—Injection-site pain (3.4%–6.4%), injection-site tenderness (1.7%–4.9%), injection-site redness (0.8%–1.9%), injection-site swelling (1.5%–1.7%), injection-site warmth (0.6%–1.7%), abdominal pain (1.1%–1.2%), pharyngitis (0%–1.2%), and headache (0.4%–0.8%).

Twinrix: Injection-site pain (35%–41%), headache (13%–22%), fatigue (11%–14%), injection-site redness (8%–11%), diarrhea (4%–6%), injection-site swelling (4%–6%), nausea (2%–4%), fever (2%–4%), and vomiting (0%–1%). In addition, the following were observed between 1 and 9.9 percent of the time: upper respiratory tract infections and injection-site hardening.

Parent or Healthcare Provider Adverse Events Reported through VAERS

Havrix—Rhinitis, thrombocytopenia, anaphylaxis, serum sickness-like syndrome, seizure, dizziness, encephalopathy, multiple sclerosis, Guillain-Barré syndrome, reduce sense of touch or sensation, myelitis, neuropathy, pins-and-needles feeling, excessive tiredness or lack of energy, temporary loss of consciousness, vasculitis, hepatitis, jaundice, erythema multiforme, swelling beneath the skin (angioedema), excessive sweating, congenital anomaly, musculoskeletal stiffness, chills, flu-like symptoms, injection-site reaction, and local swelling.

Vaqta—Thrombocytopenia, Guillain-Barré syndrome, cerebellar ataxia (sudden, uncoordinated muscle movement due to disease or injury to the cerebellum), and encephalitis.

Twinrix—Shingles, meningitis, thrombocytopenia, allergic reaction (including anaphylaxis), serum sickness-like syndrome, Bell's palsy, seizure, encephalitis, encephalopathy, Guillain-Barré syndrome, myelitis, transverse myelitis, multiple sclerosis, neuritis, neuropathy, optic neuritis, paralysis, loss of sense of touch or sensation, muscle weakness caused by nerve damage or illness (paresis), conjunctivitis, visual disturbances, earache, tinnitus, heart palpitations, tachycardia, vasculitis, bronchospasm, asthma-like symptoms, difficulty breathing, stomach upset, hepatitis, jaundice, hair loss, angioedema, eczema, erythema multiforme, erythema nodosum, excessive sweating, lichen planus, arthritis, muscle weakness, chills, immediate injection-site pain, stinging and burning sensation, injection-site reaction, general malaise, and abnormal liver functions tests.

Reactions Observed and Documented in Published Research

Thrombocytopenia—low blood platelet count that may cause excessive bleeding—is frequently reported as an adverse reaction following the hepatitis A vaccine by parents and healthcare professionals. Research also documents an increased risk of thrombocytopenia after the HepA vaccine. Evaluation of the health records of 1.8 million children found that children aged 12–19 were twenty-three times more likely to develop immune thrombocytopenia (IT; formerly called immune thrombocytopenia purpura) after receiving the HepA vaccine.[726] IT occurs when your immune system mistakenly attacks or destroys platelets that help your blood clot. Having IT can lead to easy or excessive bruising and bleeding. However, some research suggests that the HepA vaccine itself doesn't cause IT and that it is only exacerbated in children who already have IT or are predisposed to it.[727] Strictly speaking, these researchers contend that the individual would have developed IT anyway but the vaccine somehow initiated a series of events that hastened its development. Some researchers also suggest that this risk is limited to the MMR vaccine. IT is typically successfully treated with platelet concentrates and intravenous immunoglobulin therapy.

See the *Reactions Observed and Documented in Published Research* section of chapter 9 for further discussion of immune thrombocytopenia associated with vaccinations.

INFECTION RISKS	VACCINE RISKS
Relapsing hepatitis	Immune thrombocytopenia
Autoimmune hepatitis	
Fulminant hepatitis	
Subfulminant hepatitis	
Acute liver failure (<1%)	
Death (0.3%)	

12

Human Papilloma Virus (HPV)

What Is Human Papilloma Virus Infection?

Human papillomavirus, or HPV, is a common virus and cause of sexually transmitted infections. Human papillomaviruses are a group of over a hundred related viruses, of which thirty to forty affect the genitals (genital herpes), and about ten (16, 18, 31, 33, 35, 39, 45, 51, 52, and 58) are considered high risk for causing cancer.[728] HPV 16 accounts for nearly half of all cervical cancers, and HPV 16 and 18 together account for approximately 70 percent of cervical cancers.[729] HPV 6 and 11 account for about 90 percent of HPV-caused genital warts. The virus causes epithelial cells to grow and accumulate more rapidly than normal in the skin and mucous membranes. HPV frequently lives silently in the cervix or on the penis without any symptoms to make the infected individual aware they are infected.

HPV is spread through intimate skin-to-skin contact during vaginal and anal sex with an infected person, and less commonly via oral sex. People who have sex with more than one person or have sex with a single person who has had sex with more than one person can get HPV. The risk of HPV directly correlates with the number of sexual partners a person has.[730,731] Correct usage of a condom during sexual intercourse significantly reduces the risk of HPV infection. Most cases (90 percent) of HPV resolve without any treatment and do not cause health problems.[732] The clearance of HPV is dependent on the strain a person is infected with. Some HPV types are cleared in approximately 70 percent of infected women within one year, with as many as 91 percent of women HPV negative after two years.[733] Men may clear HPV infection more rapidly than women, based on research that suggests 94 percent of men clear HPV within a one-year period.[734] The same research found that 72 percent of women infected with HPV 16 were negative for HPV after two years. If HPV does cause symptoms, it is often genital warts—a small bump or group of bumps in the genital area. Symptoms can develop years after being infected with the virus. Given that the majority of people infected with HPV don't have any noticeable symptoms, many individuals unknowingly spread the virus to others.

How Prevalent Is It?

Most sexually active women are carriers of the virus in their early twenties, and most sexually active men will also come in contact with it by their early twenties and perhaps carry it as well. About 291 million women worldwide are carriers of HPV, of which 32 percent are infected with HPV 16 or 18—the types responsible for most cervical cancers.[735] HPV is so common that a significant number of the population (about 40 percent) acquires the infection within two years of their first sexual experience.[736] It is estimated that around 80 percent of sexually active women will get infected with at least one HPV virus during their lifetime.[737] Approximately 20 percent of men are infected, but this is an average of estimates that range as high as 72.9 percent.[738] Research suggests that having five or more children, smoking, being infected with multiple types of HPV, a weakened immune system, and, to a lesser degree, oral contraceptive use increases the risk of HPV infection in women.[739] A higher burden of HPV is found in less developed countries than in developed countries. Higher rates of HPV infection are found in sub-Saharan Africa, Eastern Europe, and Latin America.

What Are the Health Risks of Human Papilloma Virus?

Long-lasting HPV infections—those that don't clear on their own—can cause certain types of cancer: cervical, vaginal, and vulvar cancer in women, penile cancer in men, and anal and throat cancer in both men and women. Globally, HPV accounts for about 570,000 cancer cases in women and sixty thousand cancer cases in men per year.[740] Men most commonly develop throat cancer after infection, while women are most likely to develop cervical cancer. More than 90 percent of cervical cancer cases are caused by HPV. These cancers may take years or decades after infection to develop. However, it should be noted that nearly 90 percent of cervical cancer deaths occur in countries where regular Papanicolaou test (also called a Pap test or Pap smear) tests are not routine, and that Pap testing has decreased cervical cancer mortality by 70 percent.[741,742] Regular Pap smear tests are intended to detect precancerous and cancerous processes in the cervix.

Human Papilloma Virus Vaccine

Description

The HPV vaccines, Gardasil, Gardasil 9, and Cervarix, protect against HPV infection by types that cause cancer and genital warts. All three protect against HPV 16 and 18. Gardasil also protects against HPV 6 and 11, which cause the majority of genital warts cases. Gardasil 9 protects against the same types of HPV as Gardasil, but includes additional protection against HPV 31, 33, 45, 52, and 58. The HPV vaccine is recommended for children and adults ages 9 to 26 years, and routinely administered at age 11 or 12 before a teen is likely to be sexually active. Women who are pregnant should not receive the vaccine. The vaccine is not routinely recommended for adults 27 through 45 years because most people have already been exposed to HPV by these ages. The vaccine is received as a series of shots depending on the age of the person. Children who receive their first dose before their 15th birthday get two doses and those who receive their first dose at 15 or older get a three-series dose.

Vaccine Manufacturing Process

Both Gardasil and Gardasil 9 HPV vaccines are prepared from virus-like particles (VLPs) produced by recombinant (produced by inserting the DNA encoding of an antigen to stimulate an immune response) technology. Protein (L1) that resides on the surface of the vaccine is grown in a lab in *Saccharomyces cerevisiae* yeast cells on a chemically defined fermentation media that includes vitamins, amino acids, mineral salts, and carbohydrates. The protein assembles itself to look like the HPV within the culture medium. It does not contain HPV genetic material, so the protein cannot reproduce itself. Depending on the vaccine, the vaccine will contain from two to nine different types of HPV proteins. The L1 proteins are released from the yeast cells by cell disruption and purified by chemical and physical methods. The purified VLPs are adsorbed on an aluminum-containing adjuvant (amorphous aluminum hydroxyphosphate sulfate). The resulting vaccine is a sterile liquid suspension that combines the adsorbed VLPs from each type of HPV with additional aluminum adjuvant and a buffer.

Cervarix is produced similarly but the VLPs are self-assembled in recombinant baculovirus in a serum-free culture medium composed of chemically defined lipids, vitamins, amino acids, and mineral salts. Following replication of L1 proteins in cabbage looper (*Trichoplusia ni*) insect cells, the L1 proteins are released from the cytoplasm of the cells by disruption and then purified and filtered. They are then adsorbed onto aluminum and combined with sodium chloride, sodium dihydrogen phosphate dihydrate, and water for injection.

Ingredients

Gardasil[743]

- HPV 6 VLPs (20 mcg)
- HPV 11 VLPs (40 mcg)
- HPV 16 VLPs (40 mcg)
- HPV 18 VLPs (20 mcg)
- Aluminum (225 mcg)
- Sodium chloride (9.56 mg)
- L-histidine (0.78 mg)
- Polysorbate 80 (50 mcg)

- Sodium borate (35 mcg)
- Yeast protein (<7 mcg)
- Water

Gardasil 9[744]

- HPV 6 VLPs (20 mcg)
- HPV 11 VLPs (40 mcg)
- HPV 16 VLPs (60 mcg)
- HPV 18 VLPs (40 mcg)
- HPV 31 VLPs (40 mcg)
- HPV 33 VLPs (20 mcg)
- HPV 45 VLPs (20 mcg)
- HPV 52 VLPs (20 mcg)
- HPV 58 VLPs (20 mcg)
- Aluminum (500 mcg)
- Sodium chloride (9.56 mg)
- L-histidine (0.78 mg)
- Polysorbate 80 (50 mcg)
- Sodium borate (35 mcg)
- Yeast protein (<7 mcg)
- Water

Cervarix[745]

- HPV 16 VLPs (20 mcg)
- HPV 18 VLPs (20 mcg)
- 3-O-desacyl-4'-monophosphoryl lipid A (50 mcg)
- Aluminum hydroxide (0.5 mg)
- Sodium chloride (4.4 mg)
- Sodium dihydrogen phosphate dehydrate (0.624 mg)
- Insect cell and baculovirus viral protein (<40 ng)
- Bacterial cell protein (<150 ng)

Controversial Ingredients

- ➤ Aluminum
- ➤ Monophosphoryl lipid A adjuvant

215

> - Polysorbate 80
> - Insect cell proteins
> - Baculovirus proteins

Package Insert Adverse Reactions

Gardasil: Injection-site pain (61.4%–83.9%), injection-site swelling (13.9%–25.4%), injection-site redness (16.7%–24.7%), fever (8.3%–13.0%), headache (12.3%), nausea (2.0%–6.7%), dizziness (1.2%–4.0%), diarrhea (2.7%–3.6%), injection-site itching (3.2%), sore throat (2.8%), injection-site bruising (2.8%), common cold (2.6%), vomiting (1.0%–2.4%), cough (2.0%), toothache (1.5%), upper respiratory tract infection (1.5%), abdominal pain (1.4%), general malaise (1.4%), muscle aches (1.3%), joint pain (1.2%), insomnia (1.2%), nasal congestion (1.1%), and injection-site hematoma (1.0%). Less than 1 percent reported serious adverse events in the clinical trials. Across the clinical trials, forty deaths occurred that were deemed "consistent with events expected in healthy adolescent and adult populations." In addition, 245 systemic autoimmune disorders (about 3.3 percent of total vaccine recipients) were reported in one clinical trial of girls and women aged 9 to 26 years, of which joint pain, arthritis, and joint diseases made up the majority of cases, followed by thyroid disorders. Another study found that boys were less likely to experience these systemic autoimmune conditions, but similarly joint-related disorders were the most common observed.

Gardasil 9: Injection-site pain (63.4%–89.9%), injection-site swelling (20.2%–47.8%), injection-site redness (20.7%–34.1%), headache (7.3%–14.6%), fever (4.4%–8.9%), injection-site itching (4.0%–5.5%), nausea (3.0%–4.4%), injection-site hematoma (0.9%–3.7%), nausea (0.7%–3.0%), sore throat (1.0%–2.7%), fatigue (0.0%–2.3%), and injection-site hardening (0.8%–2.0%). Serious adverse events were reported 2.3 percent of the time across several studies. Of ten deaths that occurred during the trials, none were deemed vaccine related. In all clinical trials, 2.2 percent of vaccine recipients reported new systemic autoimmune disorders following vaccination.

Cervarix: Injection-site pain (86.9%–91.8%), fatigue (55.0%), headache (53.4%), muscle aches (49.1%), injection-site redness (27.8%–48.0%), injection-site swelling (22.7%–44.1%), gastrointestinal symptoms (27.8%), joint pain (20.8%), fever (12.8%), rash (9.6%), hives (7.4%), common cold (3.6%), flu (3.2%), sore throat (2.9%), dizziness (2.2%), upper respiratory infection (2.0%), chlamydia infection (2.0%), and painful menstruation (2.0%). Unlike Gardasil, the most commonly reported autoimmune condition post-vaccination for Cervarix was hypothyroidism followed by hyperthyroidism. In pooled data (including controlled and uncontrolled studies), 5.3 percent of subjects aged 10–72 years reported at least one serious adverse event, while this number increased to 6.4 percent among females aged 10–25 years. Completed and ongoing studies reported twenty deaths among people who received Cervarix, but this includes motor vehicle accident, homicide, and other unrelated deaths in the total.

Parent or Healthcare Provider Adverse Events Reported through VAERS

Most concerning for all HPV vaccines is a greater incidence of mortality and neurocognitive syndromes among those receiving the vaccine compared to placebo—despite the placebo being aluminum.[746] From June 2006 to December 2007, 183 deaths were reported after people received Gardasil, the vast majority of which were written off by CDC researchers stating that "the evidence did not suggest a causal link between Gardasil and the reported deaths."[747] A notable number of seemingly healthy girls are injured following HPV vaccination and some of these die. Although researchers don't always attribute their deaths to vaccination, the number of parents claiming vaccine-related injury or mortality is striking for the HPV vaccine.

Gardasil—Death, autoimmune diseases, autoimmune hemolytic anemia, enlarged lymph nodes, idiopathic thrombocytopenic purpura, pulmonary embolism, nausea, pancreatitis, vomiting, joint pain, muscle aches, chills, hypersensitivity reactions, anaphylaxis, hives, bronchospasms, abnormal lack of energy or weakness, general fatigue or malaise, acute disseminated encephalomyelitis, dizziness, Guillain-Barré syndrome, headache, motor neuron disease, paralysis, seizure, temporary loss of consciousness (including with associated seizure), transverse myelitis, cellulitis, and deep vein thrombosis.

Gardasil 9—Death, autoimmune diseases, autoimmune hemolytic anemia, enlarged lymph nodes, idiopathic thrombocytopenic purpura, pulmonary embolism, nausea, vomiting, pancreatitis, chills, lack of energy or weakness, fatigue, general malaise, hypersensitivity reactions, anaphylaxis, bronchospasms, hives, joint pain, muscle aches, acute disseminated encephalomyelitis, dizziness, Guillain-Barré syndrome, headache, motor neuron disease, paralysis, seizures, temporary loss of consciousness (including with associated seizure), transverse myelitis, cellulitis, and deep vein thrombosis.

Cervarix—Swollen lymph nodes, allergic reactions (including anaphylaxis), erythema multiforme, angioedema (swelling beneath the skin similar to hives), and temporary loss of consciousness.

Reactions Observed and Documented in Published Research

As the VAERS reports suggests, the HPV vaccine has been linked to several serious adverse events, particularly in females under 30 years of age.[748] A preponderance of evidence indicates that manufacturers of the HPV vaccines unduly influenced vaccine policy and that their safety and efficacy studies were largely inadequate and foolishly misinterpreted or intentionally misrepresented. Researchers from Harvard and Columbia universities discovered that legislators heavily relied on Merck (the manufacturer of an HPV vaccine) to establish HPV vaccine recommendations, who acted "too aggressively and nontransparently" to promote their vaccine as a requirement for school entry.[749] Furthermore, the study authors found that Merck was financially entangled with legislators and special interest groups to push the HPV vaccine mandates, many of which were not disclosed publicly. Another study evaluating Merck's aggressive practices concluded that "the past two decades the pharmaceutical industry has gained unprecedented control over the evaluation of its own products."[750] The same study concluded that given the remarkable success of Pap screening programs, "it is unlikely that vaccination with Gardasil would have a notable impact in reducing further the global cervical cancer burden beyond that accomplished by Pap screening." It is readily apparent that some vaccine manufacturers engage in unethical and aggressive campaigns to influence public health policies despite obvious conflicts of interest, and legislators rely too heavily on these manufacturers or permit themselves to be unduly influenced by industry lobbyists to establish rational vaccination policies.

Published commentaries call into question the safety and efficacy of the HPV vaccine and contend that HPV vaccine safety data published by manufacturers is at odds with unbiased scientific evidence. A commentary from scientists who conducted histological analysis of brain samples from a Gardasil-suspected death case published in the *Journal of Internal Medicine* states "whilst 12-year-old preadolescents are at zero risk of dying from cervical cancer, they are faced with a risk of death and a permanently disabling lifelong autoimmune or neurodegenerative condition from a vaccine that thus far has not prevented a single case of cervical cancer, let alone cervical cancer death."[751] Another commentary mistrusts Merck's safety trials because "their design, as well as data reporting and interpretation, were largely inadequate."[752] These scientists are not alone in questioning the safety and efficacy data presented by Merck.[753,754] A later commentary determined careful examination of data from clinical trials prior to the approval of the HPV vaccine and reported adverse events since its approval reveal that HPV vaccine efficacy and safety claims "are at odds with factual evidence and are largely derived from significant misinterpretation of available data."[755] While another commentary concluded that "cervical cancer is a rare disease with mortality rates that are several times lower than the rate of reported serious adverse reactions (including deaths) from HPV vaccination" in developed countries.[756] On top of that, research strongly indicates that cervical screening is safer and likely more effective than HPV vaccination in preventing cervical cancer.[757] In the end, the preponderance of evidence suggests that there are greater risks of serious harm than protective benefits when it comes to the HPV vaccine.

But these seemingly unethical practices shouldn't be a surprise coming from a company with a recognized history of alleged unethical behavior. Merck paid $4.85 billion to settle lawsuits filed by people who suffered injury or death after taking the arthritis drug Vioxx because Merck allegedly hid evidence that Vioxx increases the risk of heart attack.[758] Stephen Krahling, a virologist and former Merck employee also accused the company of falsifying data—by adding animal antibodies to a blood sample to give a false impression of efficacy—related to its MMR vaccine.[759]

Even more recently, an analysis of twelve published Phase 2 and 3 randomized, controlled efficacy trials of the HPV vaccines Cervarix and Gardasil raised doubts about the vaccines' effectiveness.[760] The scientists concluded that vaccine efficacy may have "overestimated" cervical cancer reductions because cervical tests were performed earlier than established standards of care—at 6–12 months instead of 36 months. Vaccine manufacturer studies combined low-grade cervical cell changes that frequently self-resolve with high-grade cervical disease causing the researchers to conclude "we found insufficient data to clearly conclude that HPV vaccine prevents the higher-grade abnormal cell changes that can eventually develop into cervical cancer." Substantial flaws in safety and efficacy assessment trials combined with the significant number of reported injuries following HPV vaccine should cause both parents and healthcare professionals concern. Evidence-based healthcare practices of providing high-quality and safe care with transparency and accountability must be applied to vaccines.

A large amount of data connects the HPV vaccine to serious autoimmune disorders or exacerbation of existing autoimmune diseases.[761] This research indicates that some individuals sharing common features—personal or family history of autoimmune disorder (especially lupus) and genetic or epigenetic vulnerability—may be at a greater risk of HPV vaccine injury. A case-control study found that women diagnosed with systemic lupus erythematosus were five times more likely to have received the HPV vaccine.[762] The study also observed an increased risk of alopecia, gastroenteritis, vasculitis, arthritis, and central nervous system conditions in HPV vaccine recipients. On average, the start of adverse symptoms occurred six days after vaccination for vasculitis, nineteen days after vaccination for lupus, and fifty-five days after vaccination for arthritis. Vasculitis, gastroenteritis, and lupus were associated with the highest percentage of life-threatening adverse events. Central nervous system conditions, arthritis, and vasculitis were strongly associated with permanent disabilities. HPV vaccines may be disrupting inflammatory control and immune system guards against autoimmune conditions.

A significant number of deaths have also been reported after HPV vaccination.[763] Careful evaluation and autopsies reveal that autoimmune vasculitis potentially triggered by cross-reactivity of HPV-16L1 antibodies with the wall of blood vessels in the brain (cerebral vasculature) and the adherence of these HPV-16L1 particles to blood vessel walls contributed to the death.[764] HPV-16L1 antibodies are virus-like particles contained in HPV vaccines. Cross-reactivity describes when an infectious agent produces antigens so similar to antigens produced on normal cells (self-antigens) that the antibodies created to react against the foreign antigen also recognize self-antigens and disrupt normal cellular function and damage healthy tissues. This phenomenon can be explained by using the analogy of counterfeit consumer goods. Sellers of counterfeit products seek to pass off their goods as one made by the actual brand owner. In some cases, the counterfeit product can so closely resemble the original brand-name product that only a well-trained person can tell the difference. Similarly, pathogens can create counterfeit antigens that so closely resemble antigens normally produced by healthy cells that they body can't tell the difference. In the case of autoimmune vasculitis, the immune system perceives its own blood vessel cells that present HPV-16L1 antibodies as foreign and attacks and destroys them leading to blood vessel inflammation, narrowing, and weakening. This can cause small clots to form and damage tissues and organs supplied by those blood vessels, including the kidneys, lungs, nerves, skin, and brain. Another study reported that it is very rare to develop vasculitis after the HPV vaccine, but could not rule out the HPV vaccine as a triggering cause of vasculitis.[765] Nevertheless, parents and individuals should be informed by their health care professional of the potential risk and make informed decisions.

Serious adverse reactions to HPV vaccination appear to be more frequent than other vaccines. Various reports describe the development of complex regional pain syndrome (CRPS), postural orthostatic tachycardia syndrome (POTS), myalgic encephalomyelitis/chronic fatigue syndrome (ME/CFS), and fibromyalgia after HPV vaccination.[766,767,768,769,770] A Japanese report determined that of 120 adverse events—including CRPS and autonomic and cognitive dysfunctions—after HPV vaccine, 25 percent were definitely vaccine caused and another 35 percent were considered probably vaccine caused.[771] This means an astonishing 60 percent of all adverse reactions were caused or likely caused by HPV vaccines—far greater than manufacturer reports admit. The significant number of adverse events in Japan caused the Japanese Ministry of Public Health, Labour, and Welfare to withdraw its recommendation for the HPV vaccine in 2013. Evidence collected since its discontinuation in Japan shows that the episodes of nervous system disorders in adolescent and teem girls have declined since vaccine withdrawal.[772,773] It is hard to argue with the evidence on the timing of adverse events, both their beginning when the vaccine was introduced and their decline when it was withdrawn.

Many adverse events occur within days of the HPV vaccine, but some take months or even years to develop. Generally, onset of symptoms occurs about eleven days after HPV vaccination (but ranged from one to 1,532 days), and includes headache, fainting, fatigue, cognitive dysfunction, insomnia, sensitivity to light, abdominal pain, neuropathic pain, chest pain, tremors or twitching, muscle weakness, trouble walking, dry mouth, rapid breathing, and irregular periods.[774,775,776,777] These symptoms cause a significant disruption in quality of life. Approximately 98 percent of those harmed after receiving an HPV vaccine are unable to continue daily activities and two-thirds have to quit school or work for at least two months.

Dysfunction of the sympathetic nervous system—the division of the autonomic nervous system that controls rapid involuntary responses (the release of large quantities of epinephrine, increased heart rate and cardiac output, changes in blood vessel constriction, and increased respiratory capacity) to dangerous or stressful situations—appears to play a major role in the development of these disorders. In addition, small fiber neuropathy—severe stabbing or burning pain attacks that usually start in the feet or hands often due to decreased nerve fiber density—and nerve demyelination are contributing factors.[778,779] Mutations in the SCN9A or SCN10A gene can cause small fiber neuropathy. Although no studies to date have connected an increased incidence of neurological adverse events after HPV vaccine to mutations in these genes, it may be a contributing factor and warrant further study. Interestingly, examination of thirty-five females with symptoms of nervous system dysfunction following HPV vaccination, noted that the majority of the females had a high level of physical activity prior to vaccination. Furthermore, all thirty-five females reported irregular periods prior to vaccination.[780] Physical activity is known to cause changes in antibodies and white blood cells, resulting in a heightened state of immune surveillance and immune regulation.[781] In addition, sex hormones like estrogen and progesterone are involved in immune responses. Indeed, women have an enhanced capacity to produce antibodies, which provides them greater protection against viral infections but, at the same time, increases the likelihood of excessive immune responses and autoimmunity.[782] Preexisting reproductive abnormalities involving abnormal sex hormone levels may be a risk factor for HPV vaccine injury.

Other research implicates the adjuvants used in HPV vaccines with autoimmune and autoimmune syndromes. They theorize that the vaccine adjuvant triggers abnormal activation of the immune system, involving glia cells in the nervous system.[783] These conditions are difficult to diagnose making it important for clinicians to be aware of the possible association between HPV vaccination and CRPS, POTS, fibromyalgia, and other disorders.

Guillain-Barré syndrome (GBS) is a neurological disorder where the immune system mistakenly attacks the peripheral nervous system. Symptoms include prickling, pins-and-needles sensation in the extremities, weakness in the legs and upper body, unsteady walking, difficulty speaking, swallowing, chewing, or moving the face, severe pain, rapid heart rate, difficulty breathing, abnormal blood pressure, and loss of bladder or bowel control. An elevated risk of GBS has also been observed in HPV vaccine recipients.[784] The onset of symptoms usually occurred within six weeks of vaccination. Although significant association has been made with nervous system disorders and HPV vaccination, Australian researchers funded by the Australian government and involved in immunization policy in the country, published a review stating there was no consistent evidence of increased adverse events, including neurological symptoms, following HPV vaccination.[785] At the very least, the timing of symptoms in relation to vaccination and mounting evidence warrants "well-designed case-control studies to determine the prevalence and possible causation between these symptom clusters and HPV vaccines" as one study put it.[786]

Premature ovarian insufficiency (POI), or premature ovarian failure, is a condition where a women's ovaries stop working normally—don't produce typical amounts of estrogen or release eggs regularly—before age 40. POI can cause a lack of menstruation (amenorrhea) and lead to difficulty becoming or the inability to become pregnant. Women with POI may be at a greater risk of heart attack and stroke.[787] Several reports of POI emerged shortly after the HPV vaccine was introduced. Scientists attempted to identify a cause of this increased number of POI cases after HPV vaccination. The mechanism responsible for POI after HPV vaccination was not identified but theories included abnormal immune responses to the adjuvant or toxicity caused by polysorbate 80.[788,789] A study reports three cases of POI in girls aged 16, 16, and 18 after HPV vaccination.[790] Abnormal hormone levels were identified through lab testing in the three cases. Unfortunately, three additional cases of POI and amenorrhea following HPV vaccination did not resolve after treatment with hormone replacement therapy.[791] These authors concluded "the increasing number of similar reports of post HPV vaccine-linked autoimmunity and the uncertainty of long-term clinical benefits of HPV vaccination are a matter of public health that warrants further rigorous inquiry." Another case report in a 16-year-old girl with amenorrhea determined that the HPV vaccine was the plausible cause of her POI after the primary identifiable causes of the condition were all excluded.[792] Another observational study correlated the HPV vaccine to a lowered probability of becoming pregnant.[793] Although case reports can't sufficiently establish HPV vaccines as the cause of POI, some HPV vaccine ingredients are known to cause ovarian toxicity and possibly autoimmune ovarian damage. Further research that monitors hormone levels is needed to determine if HPV vaccines contribute to POI.

Despite these documented case reports and accounts in VAERS, a study evaluating POI and its association with vaccines, concluded that "we did not find a statistically significant elevated risk of POI after HPV."[794] Another study concluded physicians should acknowledge the case reports but emphasize the lack of causation found in an epidemiological study.[795] Others are quick to dismiss the association of HPV vaccines with POI as a belief rather than based on actual evidence.[796] Further monitoring and evaluation is necessary to confirm or exclude HPV vaccine as a cause of POI in females potentially predisposed to ovarian damage after vaccination.

INFECTION RISKS	VACCINE RISKS
Cancers: cervical, vaginal, vulvar, penile, anal, throat	Autoimmune disorders (multiple)
Genital warts	Neurological disorders (multiple)
	Death
	Alopecia
	Gastroenteritis
	Vasculitis
	Arthritis
	Postural orthostatic tachycardia syndrome
	Premature ovarian insufficiency
	Infertility

13

Meningococcal

What Is Meningococcal Infection?

Meningococcal illness, also known as meningococcus, is a group of illnesses caused by the *Neisseria meningitidis* bacteria. They include infections of the brain and spinal cord (meningitis) and bloodstream infections (septicemia), which account for more than 90 percent of meningococcal illnesses. Although the bacteria can travel through the bloodstream to various places in the body, infections of the heart, joints, and lungs are less common. There are six serotypes (strains) of *Neisseria meningitidis*: A, B, C, W, X, and Y that are responsible for meningococcal illness worldwide. Different areas of the world are burdened with different types of the bacteria.

The bacteria spreads through direct contact with respiratory and throat secretions (saliva or spit) of an infected individual. Fortunately, these bacteria are not as contagious as pathogens that cause other illness, like the common cold or flu. It usually requires close (e.g., kissing or coughing) or prolonged contact with an infected person to catch these bacteria. People do not get infected by breathing the air where an infected person has been like other infectious diseases we have previously discussed. However, once infected, symptoms caused by the bacteria can spread rapidly (often within twenty-four hours).

Meningococcal illness can be very serious, even deadly, and requires prompt medical attention.

Generally, signs of meningococcal illness begin with flu-like symptoms that rapidly get worse. A characteristic sign of meningococcal infection is a rash of red pinpoint dots that progressively turn larger and purple. A small percentage of the population, about 10 percent, are carriers of the bacteria—have the bacteria in their nose and throat—without showing any symptoms. If symptoms do occur, they are not mild. The symptoms vary based on what part of the body is infected. Meningococcal meningitis (infection of the brain and spinal cord) commonly causes a high fever, stiff neck, and headache. These characteristic symptoms of meningitis may be accompanied by eye sensitivity to light, confusion, nausea, and vomiting. Infants and babies may have atypical symptoms, such as inactivity, slow movement, excessive irritability, vomiting, loss of appetite, a weak cry, or a bulging area in the soft spot on the skull. Young children may exhibit poor reflexes. Unlike viral meningitis, which often clears up on its own, bacterial meningitis is life-threatening, and medical treatment is required immediately.

Meningococcal septicemia (meningococcemia; a bloodstream infection) occurs when the bacteria enters the bloodstream, multiplies, and damages the walls of blood vessels. It is characterized by fever, chills, cold hands and feet, vomiting, severe aches or pain in the muscles, chest, joints, or abdomen, rapid breathing, diarrhea, and in the later stages, a dark purple rash. Immediate medical attention should be sought if these symptoms are witnessed.

Similar symptoms to other illnesses can make meningococcal illness difficult to diagnose. Meningococcal illness is confirmed by laboratory analysis to check for the presence of *Neisseria meningitidis* in the blood or cerebrospinal fluid. Various intravenous antibiotics are the primary treatment if the bacteria is found in the body fluids, which may be adjusted based on the type of bacteria a person is infected with. Antibiotics are frequently started prior to laboratory confirmation of the illness because time is of the essence when it comes to the treatment of meningococcal illness. The body systems stabilize and gradually return to normal if the antibiotics can get ahead of the infection. Meningococcal illness is so dangerous that anyone exposed to the individual before they sought treatment—including hospital personnel that encountered the patient before meningococcus was suspected—should receive oral antibiotics as a precautionary measure. Additional treatment, such as breathing support, surgery to remove dead tissue, wound care, and medications to treat low blood pressure may also be necessary depending on the severity of the illness.

How Prevalent Is It?

The incidence of meningococcal illness varies significantly by region of the world. In temperate climates, most meningococcal infections occur in the spring and summer. Meningitis infections are prevalent in sub-Saharan Africa between Senegal and Ethiopia (an area known as "the meningitis belt"). In this region, outbreaks that can affect up to 1 percent of the population occur every five to twelve years. There are no reliable estimates of global meningococcal illness cases because of poor reporting and inadequate surveillance in several parts of the world, but cases are estimated to eclipse 1.2 million each year.[797] MenA is a common cause of meningococcal infection in Africa and parts of Asia, whereas MenB, MenC, and MenY are predominant in other areas of the world, including Europe and North America. A substantial percentage of meningococcal infections are caused by MenB, including prolonged epidemics.[798,799,800] Children aged 6 months to 3 years are at greatest risk of infection, but infections are also common among college students living in dorms, military personnel, people with a compromised immune system, people with a damaged or removed spleen, people taking immunosuppressive medications, and adolescents.

What Are the Health Risks of Meningococcal Infection?

Invasive meningococcal disease, involving septicemia or meningitis, is a severe complication of meningococcal infection. Death occurs in approximately 6–10 percent of meningococcal infections, and long-term complications happen in 4.3–11.2 percent of cases.[801] As mentioned earlier, two of the most severe and life-threatening complications of meningitis infection include meningitis and septicemia. Worldwide, meningococcal illness is estimated to cause around 135,000 deaths annually.[802] Meningococcal meningitis has a high fatality rate (up to 50 percent) when untreated and a high frequency of chronic complications (more than 10 percent).[803] Even with prompt antibiotic treatment, 10–15 percent of people with meningococcal illness die and up to 20 percent of survivors have long-term disabilities (loss of limbs, brain damage, deafness, visual impairment, seizures, and other nervous system disorders).[804] The risk of complications is quite high with meningococcal infections, particularly the longer a person waits to seek treatment.

Meningococcal Vaccine

Description

There are two primary meningococcal vaccines: MenACWY (protects against types A, C, W, and Y) and MenB (protects against type B). Bivalent (A and C) and trivalent vaccines (A, C, and W) may also be available internationally. MenACWY is routinely given to children aged 11–12, with a booster at age 16, but can be given as young as 2 months old. The CDC suggests that children at an increased risk of meningococcal infection (children with HIV or poor spleen function) not receive MenACWY before age 2 because of possible interference with the response to the pneumococcal vaccine.[805] MenB is approved for children 10 years of age and older and given to people who are at increased risk of meningococcal infection—exposed during an outbreak, work in laboratories that handle meningococcal bacteria, people with certain immune disorders, people taking immunosuppressants, and people without a spleen or a damaged spleen. Teens and adults may receive the MenACWY and MenB vaccines for increased protection.

Menveo (MenACWY) is given as a four-dose series administered at 2, 4, 6, and 12 months of age in children who begin the vaccine at 2 months. In children initiating vaccination at 7–23 months of age, Menveo is given as a two-dose series with the second dose given during the second year of life but at least three months after the first dose. Individuals 2–55 years of age receive a single dose with a single booster dose recommended between the ages of 15 and 55 in persons with an increased risk for meningococcal infection if at least four years have passed since the first dose.

Menactra (MenACWY) is given as two doses in children 9–23 months, three months apart. Individuals 2–55 years of age receive a single dose. A booster dose may be given to individuals aged 15–55 at continued risk of meningococcal infection as long as four years have elapsed since the prior dose.

Bexsero (MenB) is given as a two-dose series at least one month apart. It is approved for individuals aged 10–25 years.

Trumenba (MenB) is given as a two- or three-dose series. The three-dose series is administered at birth, 1–2 months, and 6 months of age, while the two-dose series is given at birth and 6 months unless the second dose is received earlier than 6 months of age. In this case, a third dose is given at least four months after the second dose.

Vaccine Manufacturing Process

Menveo conjugates *Neisseria meningitidis* sugars (oligosaccharides) individually with diphtheria (*Corynebacterium diphtheriae*) protein. Meningococcal sugars are produced by fermentation of *Neisseria meningitidis* types A, C, Y, and W-135, which are cultured in Franz Complete medium. Each type is treated with formaldehyde and then purified by several extraction and precipitation steps or by chromatography and precipitation. The diphtheria protein is produced by bacterial fermentation in a CY medium containing yeast extracts and amino acids then purified. After preparation for conjugation and

231

activation, each meningococcal sugar is covalently bonded to the diphtheria protein. The resulting glycoconjugates are purified and the vaccine is created without preservative or adjuvant.

Like Menveo, Menactra contains meningococcal sugars (polysaccharides) individually conjugated to diphtheria toxoid protein. *Neisseria meningitidis* types A, C, Y, and W-135 are cultured on Mueller Hinton agar and grown in Watson Scherp media containing casamino acid. The meningococcal sugars are extracted from the bacterial cells and purified by centrifugation, detergent precipitation, alcohol precipitation, solvent extraction, and diafiltration. The sugars are prepared for conjugation using a multistep process. Diphtheria toxoid is derived from *Corynebacterium diphtheriae* grown in a modified culture medium with hydrolyzed casein and detoxified using formaldehyde. Diphtheria toxoid is purified by ammonium sulfate and then the meningococcal sugars are covalently bonded to the diphtheria toxoid.

Bexsero is a recombinant vaccine that contains manufactured meningococcal proteins: Neisserial adhesin A (NadA), Neisserial heparin binding antigen (NHBA), and factor H binding protein (fHbp). NadA is a fragment of the full-length protein derived from *Neisseria meningitidis* B (strain 2996). NHBA is a recombinant fusion protein comprised of NHBA and accessory protein 953 derived from *Neisseria meningitidis* B (strains NZ98/254 and 2996). fHbp is a recombinant fusion protein comprised of fHbp and the accessory protein 936 derived from *Neisseria meningitidis* B (strains MC58 and 2996). These three recombinant proteins are produced in the bacteria *Escherichia coli* and purified. The outer membrane vesicles (OMV)—small fluid-filled sacs released from the outer membrane of the meningococcal bacteria— portion is produced by fermentation of *Neisseria meningitidis* and inactivated with deoxycholate. The antigens are adsorbed onto an aluminum hydroxide adjuvant.

Trumenba is composed of two recombinant lipidated fHbp variants from *Neisseria meningitidis* serogroup B—one from fHbp subfamily A

(A05), and one from fHbp subfamily B (B01). The proteins are individually produced in *E. coli* and grown in defined fermentation growth media. The proteins are extracted and purified then combined together. Polysorbate 80 is added as a preservative.

Ingredients

Menveo (MenACWY)[806]

- MenA sugars (10 mcg)
- MenC sugars (5 mcg)
- MenY sugars (5 mcg)
- MenW-135 sugars (5 mcg)
- Diphtheria toxoid protein (32.7–64.1 mcg)
- Formaldehyde (< 0.3 mcg)

Menactra (MenACWY)[807]

- MenA sugars (4 mcg)
- MenC sugars (4 mcg)
- MenY sugars (4 mcg)
- MenW-135 sugars (4 mcg)
- Diphtheria toxoid protein (48 mcg)
- Formaldehyde (< 2.66 mcg)

Bexsero (MenB)[808]

- NadA recombinant protein (50 mcg)
- NHBA recombinant protein (50 mcg)
- fHbp recombinant protein (50 mcg)
- Outer membrane vesicles (25 mcg)
- Aluminum (0.519 mg)
- Sodium chloride (3.125 mg)
- Histidine (0.776 mg)
- Sucrose (10 mg)
- Kanamycin (0.01 mcg)

Trumenba (MenB)[809]

- fHbp recombinant protein, A05 (60 mcg)
- fHbp recombinant protein, B01 (60 mcg)
- Polysorbate 80 (18 mcg)
- Aluminum (0.25 mg)
- Histidine
- Sodium chloride

Controversial Ingredients

➢ Formaldehyde
➢ Aluminum
➢ Polysorbate 80

Package Insert Adverse Reactions

Menveo: Infants—Irritability (42%–57%), sleepiness (29%–50%), injection-site tenderness (24%–41%), persistent crying (21%–41%), change in eating habits (17%–23%), diarrhea (8%–16%), injecting site redness (11%–15%), vomiting (5%–11%), injection-site hardening (8%–9%), fever (3%–9%), and rash (3%–4%). Serious adverse events occurred between 0.3–3.8 percent of the time depending on the dose received and age at vaccination. Children 2–10 years—Injection-site pain (31%), injection-site redness (23%), irritability (18%), injection-site hardening (16%), sleepiness (14%), general malaise (12%), and headache (11%). Other adverse reactions noted included diarrhea, rash, joint pain, muscle aches, vomiting, chills, and fever. Children and adults 11–55 years—Injection-site pain (41%), headache (30%), muscle aches (30%), general malaise (16%), and nausea (10%). Other adverse reactions noted included chills, joint pain, rash, and fever.

Menactra: Infants—Irritability (56.8%), injection-site tenderness (37.4%), abnormal crying (33.3%), injection-site redness (30.2%), drowsiness (30.2%), appetite loss (30.2%), injection-site swelling (16.2%), vomiting (14.1%), and fever (12.2%). These reactions tended to increase in occurrence when given at the same time as other vaccines

(PCV7, MMRV, and HepA). Serious adverse events were reported up to 2.5 percent of the time, which increased to up to 3.6 percent when given with other vaccines. Children 2–10 years—Injection-site pain (45.0%), injection-site redness (21.8%), injection-site hardness (18.9%), injection-site swelling (17.4%), irritability (12.4%), diarrhea (11.1%), drowsiness (10.8%), appetite loss (8.2%), joint pain (6.8%), fever (5.2%), rash (3.1%), and vomiting (3.0%). Serious adverse events occurred at a rate of 0.6 percent. Aged 11–18 years—Injection-site pain (59.2%), headache (35.6%), fatigue (30.0%), general malaise (21.9%), joint pain (17.4%), injection-site hardness (15.7%), diarrhea (12.0%), injection-site redness (10.9%), injection-site swelling (10.8%), appetite loss (10.7%), chills (7.0%), fever (5.1%), vomiting (1.9%), and rash (1.6%). Serious adverse events occurred at a rate of 1.0 percent. Adults aged 18 to 55 years—Injection-site pain (53.9%), headache (41.4%), fatigue (34.7%), general malaise (23.6%), joint pain (19.8%), injection-site hardness (17.1%), injection-site swelling (12.6%), diarrhea (11.8%), chills (9.7%), vomiting (2.3%), fever (1.5%), and rash (1.5%). Serious adverse events occurred at a rate of 1.3 percent.

Bexsero: Injection-site pain (83%–90%), injection-site redness (45%–50%), muscle aches (48%–49%), fatigue (35%–37%), headache (33%–34%), injection-site hardening (28%–32%), nausea (18%–19%), joint pain (13%–16%), and fever (1%–5%). Adverse reactions tended to occur more frequently for most reported reactions after the first dose when compared to the booster dose. Serious adverse reactions occurred 0.8–2.1 percent of the time.

Trumenba: Children 10–18 years—Injection-site pain (76.0%–86.7%), fatigue (35.9%–54.0%), headache (35.4%–51.8%), chills (13.1%–25.3%), muscle aches (17.6%–24.4%), joint pain (16.0%–21.9%), injection-site swelling (13.9%–18.0%), injection-site redness (12.5%–16.2%), diarrhea (7.6%–10.6%), fever (2.0%–6.4%), and vomiting (1.7%–3.7%). Adults 19–25 years—Injection-site pain (79.3%–84.2%), fatigue (39.2%–50.9%), headache (32.5%–43.9%), muscle aches (15.6%–25.9%), joint pain (12.6%–19.6%), chills (12.4%–18.1%), injection-site redness (11.8%–17.1%), injection-site swelling (14.0%–16.6%), diarrhea (7.5%–12.7%), vomiting (2.0%–2.6%), and fever (1.2%–2.4%). Serious adverse events occurred in 1.8 percent of subjects in both age groups.

Parent or Healthcare Provider Adverse Events Reported through VAERS

Menveo—Hearing impairment, vertigo, vestibular disorder, eyelid drooping, injection-site reactions (including extensive swelling), fatigue, general malaise, fever, hypersensitivity reactions, anaphylaxis, injection-site cellulitis, fall (including with head injury), elevated alanine aminotransferase (a sign of liver injury), joint or bone pain, dizziness, temporary loss of consciousness, tonic convulsion, headache, facial paralysis, balance disorder, sore throat, skin exfoliation, and Bell's palsy (2.9% risk, which appears to be higher if other vaccines—Tdap, HPV, and influenza—are received at the same time).

Menactra—Enlarged lymph nodes, hypersensitivity reactions, anaphylaxis, wheezing, difficulty breathing, upper airway swelling, hives, erythema, itching, low blood pressure, Guillain-Barré syndrome, feelings of pins and needles, temporary loss of consciousness, dizziness, seizure, facial palsy, acute disseminated encephalomyelitis, transverse myelitis, muscle aches, large injection-site reactions, and extensive swelling of the injected limb.

Bexsero—Injection-site reactions (including extensive swelling of the vaccinated limb), allergic reactions, anaphylaxis, rash, eye swelling, temporary loss of consciousness, and vasovagal responses to injection.

Trumenba—Hypersensitivity reactions, anaphylaxis, and fainting.

Reactions Observed and Documented in Published Research

Reports suggest that adolescents and teens (aged 11–18) are most likely to suffer from adverse events after the meningococcal vaccine, which makes sense since this is the recommended age range to receive the vaccine.[810] Anaphylaxis, temporary loss of consciousness, seizure, cellulitis, and Guillain-Barré syndrome (GBS) were the most commonly reported serious adverse events. GBS seems to be a very rare occurrence with 5.4 cases reported per one million persons during the time evaluated.[811] The actual risk attributed to the vaccine is 1.5 cases per one million doses. A CDC report concluded that the data "suggest a small increased risk for GBS after MCV4 [Menactra] vaccination."[812] Another group of researchers looked at the risks versus benefits of the meningococcal vaccine as they relate to quality-adjusted life years, which is a measurement of disease burden, including both quality and length of life lived. They found that the vaccination could save 2,397 quality-adjusted life years (QALYs) while vaccine-attributable GBS could result in 5 QALYs lost.[813] In other words, the benefits of the vaccine far outweigh the risks of GBS.

Bell's palsy is temporary paralysis of the facial muscles that makes half of your face appear to droop. The exact cause of Bell's palsy is unknown, but it is believed to be due to swelling and inflammation of the nerve that controls the muscles of the face (cranial nerve VII) following a viral infection. Viruses linked to Bell's palsy include varicella-zoster, herpes simplex, adenovirus, Epstein-Barr, rubella, mumps virus, influenza, coxsackievirus, and cytomegalovirus. For most people, it is temporary—lasting a few weeks—with complete recovery by six months. Reports show that Bell's palsy occurs more frequently within close proximity to vaccination that it could be associated with the vaccine.[814] However, since the meningococcal vaccine is frequently given at the same time as other vaccines—one study found 63 percent of the time— and a serious adverse event was documented, it is difficult to tell if these were solely related to the meningococcal vaccine. Additionally, epidemiological evidence suggests "there is no association between immunization and [Bell's palsy] in children."[815] A possible explanation of Bell's palsy after viral vaccines could be that vaccine viruses or virus-like particles infect the cranial nerve VII. Infection leads to swelling, compression, and irritation of the nerve and a loss of facial control.

INFECTION RISKS	VACCINE RISKS
Septicemia	Anaphylaxis
Meningitis	Temporary loss of consciousness
Long-term complications (4.3%–11.2%)	Seizure
	Cellulitis
Death (6%–10%)	Guillain-Barré syndrome
	Bell's palsy

14

People with a Greater Risk
of Vaccine Injury

Before we discuss individuals who may be at an increased risk of vaccine injury or serious adverse events, it is interesting to make a comparison of the health of vaccinated versus unvaccinated individuals. A US study that compared a broad range of health outcomes reported that vaccinated children were less likely to have been diagnosed with childhood infectious illnesses like pertussis or chickenpox, those illnesses for which a vaccine exists.[816] Conversely, vaccinated children were considerably more likely to be diagnosed with pneumonia, middle ear infection, allergies, eczema, neurodevelopmental disorders—a learning disability, attention deficit hyperactivity disorder (ADHD), and autism spectrum disorder (ASD)—and any chronic condition when compared to unvaccinated or partially vaccinated children. Neurodevelopmental disorders continued to be associated with vaccination even after adjustment for other measured factors. In a nutshell, the evidence suggests that vaccines are reducing childhood infectious illnesses but may be trading these illnesses for chronic conditions primarily involving the immune and nervous systems. Children born prematurely who were vaccinated fared much worse with an even higher risk of neurodevelopmental disorders. Although the data did not expressly blame vaccines as a cause of chronic childhood conditions, the statistics are hard to argue with as far as the overall health of fully vaccinated children in comparison with their partially vaccinated and unvaccinated peers. It is also possible vaccines are just one contributing factor in the heavy toxic burden children face today via chemicals in personal care products, household cleaners, food, water, air, medicines, and others.

Biological diversity, immunocompetence (the ability of the body to respond normally after exposure to an antigen), genetics and epigenetics, nutrition, lifestyle, environmental factors, and vaccine timing (both number and age) all need to be considered when it comes to risk of vaccine injury. It is well known that immune responses to vaccination vary substantially among individuals, so it is common sense that some will be more susceptible to vaccine harm.[817] Without a doubt, some people are predisposed or more prone to vaccine injury because of these differences.

Premature and Low-birth Weight Babies

Approximately 11 percent of births globally are premature—babies born before the end of the full term of gestation, especially three or more weeks before. One of the consequences of premature birth is an immature immune system. Reduced innate (nonspecific physical, chemical, and cellular defenses that are activated immediately or within hours of a pathogen's presence in the body) and adaptive (immune responses that are activated in response to specific pathogens that also leave a "memory" that makes future responses against the same pathogen more efficient) immunity limits the immune system's ability to fight bacteria and viruses.[818] In addition, data and experience indicate that premature infants may be hampered by poor development of the brain, lungs, eyes, liver, and cardiovascular system.[819,820,821,822,823,824] Underdeveloped kidneys and liver are of particular concern since these organs play crucial roles in the metabolism, detoxification, and excretion of substances that enter the body. Poor immune function, combined with other organs that aren't working efficiently yet, makes premature infants more susceptible to toxicity and harm caused by the same amounts of substances that would not normally hurt their fully developed peers.

In reality, premature and low-birth-weight infants may be at a greater risk of vaccine injury because vaccines are given during vulnerable times when the infant is developmentally delayed and they have an immature immune system.[825] In the majority of cases, premature infants are vaccinated according to the same schedule as full-term infants, regardless of birth weight or how prematurely they were born. With the exception of hepatitis B vaccination, birth weight and size are not used as determining factors for immunization schedule or dosage. This is contrary to established practices in pediatric medicine where most drugs are dosed according to body weight or body surface area, which makes the dose more precise and safe. Instead, immunization practices ignore this tenet of medicine because, unlike medicines that require a specific level of the active ingredient be achieved for efficacy, vaccines typically require low doses of active ingredients to provoke an immune response that affords protection against the infectious agent. However, this ignores the fact that the smaller the child the greater the risk of toxicity from controversial vaccine ingredients like mercury, aluminum, polysorbate 80, and others. Put differently, the viral or bacterial antigens in vaccines aren't the concern; it's the potential toxicity caused by known toxic ingredients in such small and undeveloped children. Besides, preemies' immune systems could be so immature that vaccination may not always stimulate immune responses sufficient to protect them against the infections that vaccines prevent.[826] This documented phenomenon may depend on the type of vaccine that a preemie receives.[827,828] Both the increased toxicity risk and the possibility of an inadequate immune response in preemies suggest that preemies may need to follow an alternate vaccine schedule.

Cardiovascular and respiratory complications, some serious, have been observed in premature infants who receive vaccines according to the prescribed schedule.[829] A prospective study of 239 preterm infants who received a single or multiple vaccines simultaneously noted significantly elevated CRP levels—a marker of elevated inflammation—in 85 percent of preemies receiving multiple vaccines and 70 percent of those given a single vaccine.[830] In addition, cardiorespiratory events (temporary cessation of breathing, low heart rate, bluish discoloration of the skin from poor circulation, and oxygen desaturation) were observed in 16 percent of preemies who received only one vaccine, with that number doubling in those who received multiple vaccines. A significant increase in gastroesophageal reflux also occurred in preemies receiving multiple injections. The conclusion by the study authors was that "some vaccines, including DTaP, even if administered alone were associated with cardiorespiratory adverse events and abnormal CRP values in premature infants in the NICU" and "the incidence of these events was higher following simultaneous administration of multiple vaccines." While CRP levels are expected to be elevated for up to 48 hours following vaccination as the immune system responds to vaccine antigens, for comparison purposes only 31.4% of healthy full-term infants experienced elevated CRP levels after the HepB vaccine.[831] Again, more evidence that preemies may require adjustment in the recommended vaccination schedule.

Other researchers examined the relationship between following the normal vaccination schedule in preemies and the incidence of adverse cardiorespiratory events. Major cardiorespiratory events, such as temporary cessation of breathing, low heart rate, and oxygen desaturation, occurred in 35 percent of preemies.[832] In total, 44 percent of preemies experienced an adverse reaction, with more major events occurring than minor events—minor events like body temperature fluctuations and injection-site reactions. They also identified risk factors for complications that included low gestational age, a chronic lung disease (bronchopulmonary dysplasia), and the need for respiratory support prior to vaccination, including methylxanthine treatment. Another study concluded that an imbalance in the regulation of heart rate by the nervous system (sympathetic predominance in heart rate control), abnormal heart rate variability, and long-lasting immaturity of respiratory rate control in preemies contributes to the increased incidence of adverse cardiorespiratory events in response to vaccines.[833] Both the sympathetic and parasympathetic nervous systems regulate heart rate, but the sympathetic nervous system releases hormones to accelerate heart rate, and the parasympathetic nervous system releases hormones to slow heart rate. Age of 70 days or less, smaller size, lower current weight or illness at time of vaccination, and more severe illness at birth are also important risk factors for major vaccine-related adverse cardiorespiratory events.[834,835,836,837,838] Preemies of the mean gestational age of 30.8 weeks also experienced mild decreases in oxygen saturation, low heart rate, and moderate cardiorespiratory reactions after vaccination.[839] Adverse events occurred in almost one-third of the infants in one study, which caused the study authors to recommend hospitalized preemies receive their first vaccinations "under cardiorespiratory monitoring" to observe for adverse events that frequently occurred within twenty-four hours of vaccination. Other research recommends monitoring for forty-eight to seventy-two hours after vaccination of a preemie.[840,841] Adverse cardiorespiratory events have also been documented in preemies with stable respiratory function prior to immunization.[842] One of the worst adverse reaction rates was documented in a study that included sixty-four very low-birth-weight preemies. Of the sixty-four preemies, 51.6 percent experienced a cardiorespiratory event after the first vaccination, and 18 percent had a recurrence of an adverse cardiorespiratory event after the second vaccination.[843] Two additional studies reported that 12–18 percent of preemies experienced recurrent respiratory problems (apnea) after their second immunizations.[844,845] Nearly one-third of preemies may require respiratory support after immunization, some of which is so severe they require resuscitation.[846,847,848] It is clear that vaccines may be exacerbating or triggering cardiorespiratory dysfunction in preemies.

Even full-gestational children with a reduced birth weight are at a greater risk of adverse reactions. Full-term children who were in the lowest tenth percentile of weight for their gestational age experienced higher incidence of immediate adverse reactions because of the comparatively increased dose of the vaccine per pound of body weight.[849] This is suggestive of a toxic effect in children of small size regardless of gestational age at birth.

In contrast, a German study concluded that preemies should be vaccinated according to the same schedule as full-term infants regardless of gestational age or weight. They concluded this because preemies only have a "few adverse events after timely immunization," despite their own data demonstrating a 10.8 percent risk of cardiorespiratory events "related to earlier gestational age."[850] Another group of researchers concluded that "vaccines are immunogenic [trigger antibodies production], safe, and well tolerated in preterm infants" and "preterm infants should be vaccinated using the same schedules as those usually recommended for full-term infants."[851] One exception mentioned by these authors was "the hepatitis B vaccine…because of a documented reduced immune response." This caution is followed not for safety, but to ensure that a preemies' immature immune system responds adequately to the HepB antigen. When considering immunizations for preemies, the benefits of protection against infection and potential complications from those infections must be weighed against the higher risk of serious adverse reactions.

In addition to cardiorespiratory events, preemies are at an increased risk of admittance to an emergency room and sepsis following vaccination. A multicenter study evaluated the incidence of sepsis in 13,926 extremely low-birth-weight infants born at twenty-eight weeks' gestation or less (twelve weeks premature). Over 90 percent of the infants received three or more vaccinations between 53 and 110 days old. After vaccination, the incidence of sepsis evaluations—laboratory or imaging tests to determine if sepsis is present—nearly quadrupled, the need for respiratory support more than doubled, and intubation almost doubled.[852] Preemies born at twenty-three to twenty-four weeks, or with a prior history of sepsis, had the highest risk of sepsis evaluation after vaccination. Conflicting research confirmed an increase in cardiorespiratory events in preemies following vaccination but found no increased number of sepsis evaluations.[853] Sepsis occurs when the body releases too many chemicals into the bloodstream to fight an infection. Basically, the immune system freaks out and triggers an inflammatory response throughout the body that impairs blood flow, causes tissue damage, and shuts down multiple organs—called systemic inflammatory response syndrome (SIRS). It is plausible that vaccines trigger a similar systemic inflammatory and hyperactive immune response that causes sepsis in a very small group of susceptible individuals. Documented cases of sepsis in healthy individuals, both infants and adults, have been reported following vaccination.[854,855,856] Unfortunately, sepsis is so devastating it can cause loss of limb or death.

People with Genetic Predispositions

As has been noted in a few of the preceding chapters, genetics may predispose a person to vaccine injury. Some of the genes associated with an increased risk of vaccine injury or adverse effects have been previously discussed in the individual vaccine sections. A significant amount of research regarding genetic risk factors for autoimmune disorders has focused on human leukocyte antigen (HLA) genes. Various subtypes of HLA genes have been strongly linked to autoimmune disorders for decades.[857,858,859] The HLA region is the densest region of the human genome and includes several key genes related to innate and adaptive immune responses. Some of these genes create antigens that flag peptides from viruses—such as influenza and Epstein-Barr—for destruction by killer T cells. Disruption in this normal process may cause killer T cells to destroy healthy cells or trigger an inflammatory response that is at the root of autoimmune disorders. Systemic adverse reactions have been documented in people with HLA gene mutations after receiving various vaccines.

Human endogenous retroviruses (HERVs) are remnants of ancient retroviruses found in human DNA and passed down through generations. About 8 percent of the human genome contains sequences of viral origin, namely HERVs, and they are found in most healthy tissues.[860] Interestingly, they are involved in immune responses and the regulation of immune balance. HERVs have been implicated in certain cancers, autoimmune disorders, diabetes, schizophrenia, and preeclampsia.[861] They may even trigger adverse vaccine reactions, especially HERVs that are introduced into the human body as vaccine contaminants. Many live attenuated vaccines are manufactured in animal cells, which are known to produce infectious retroviruses.[862] These HERVs don't infect cells like normal viruses, but they can generate proteins that allow their genes to be expressed in certain tissues under specific circumstances, such as immune deficiency.[863,864] HERVs indirectly contribute to chronic diseases when a perfect storm exists wherein human DNA is disturbed by retroviruses during an infection, trauma, a hormones imbalance, or exposure to chemicals. In this state, the immune system may be weakened sufficiently for chronic disease to occur. It has also been proposed that HERVs can mimic brain proteins or antigens from viruses to induce autoimmunity.[865,866,867] Given their role in immune balance, and the possibility for vaccines to contribute to the perfect storm, HERVs may play a role in adverse responses to vaccines, particularly neurological and autoimmune conditions.

A 2008 study identified several genetic factors associated with the development of vaccine-related adverse events following smallpox vaccination. The study detailed the findings of two independent clinical trials where volunteers underwent genotyping for 1,442 single nucleotide polymorphisms (SNPs) and then evaluated for occurrence of both local and systemic adverse reactions. SNPs are variations in the DNA sequence at particular locations and the most common type of genetic variation among people. Nucleotides adenine (A), thymine (T), cytosine (C), or guanine (G) are the basic building blocks of DNA. Each SNP represents a difference in a single nucleotide. For example, a SNP may replace the nucleotide cytosine (C) with thymine (T) in a specific strand of DNA (see image below). SNPs that occur in the protein coding region of DNA can be synonymous or nonsynonymous. Synonymous SNPs do not alter the amino acid sequence, while nonsynonymous SNPs change the amino acid sequence of the protein. Nonsynonymous mutations have a much greater effect on an individual because they throw off the entire amino sequence. Nonsynonymous SNPs that happen at the beginning of the amino acid sequence can be lethal because they change the entire protein.

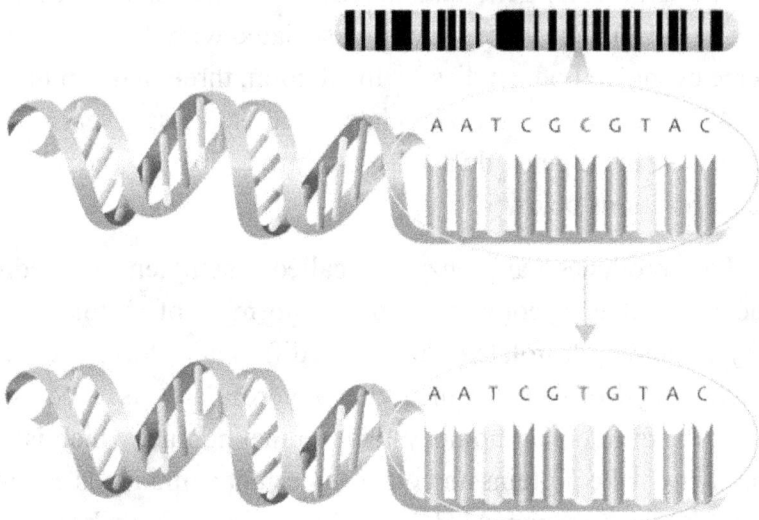

A A T C G C G T A C

A A T C G T G T A C

When an existing cell divides to make new cells, it first copies its DNA so that the new cells contain a complete set of genetic instructions (DNA). Cells sometimes make errors during this process that create variations in the DNA sequence, called SNPs (pronounced "snips"). A simple way to think about this is typos. You could intend to type "fantastic" and mistakenly type "fancastic." Like typos, SNPs represent mistakes where one nucleotide is inserted in the place of another.

SNPs are inherited from your parents. The more closely you are related to a person, the more your SNP versions will match. They can create biological variations among people because they influence the instructions for making proteins that are written into our genes. Sometimes these differences affect traits like appearance, disease susceptibility, and responses to drugs, supplements, and vaccines. However, most SNPs have no observable effect at all.

In the first study, thirty-six SNPs in twenty-six genes were associated with systemic adverse events after immunization. The second study tested these twenty-six genes, which resulted in three SNPs that were consistently associated with adverse events in both studies. The presence of a nonsynonymous SNP in the methylenetetrahydrofolate reductase (MTHFR) gene and two SNPs in the interferon regulatory factor-1 (IRF1) gene were strongly associated with the risk of systemic adverse events in both studies.[868] In addition, three SNPs in interleukin 4 (IL4) were moderately associated with adverse events. We will discuss what these genes do and how they may be involved with adverse vaccine reactions below.

MTHFR produces an enzyme called methylenetetrahydrofolate reductase that converts one form of folate, 5,10-methylenetetrahydrofolate, to a different form called 5-methyltetrahydrofolate. 5-methyltetrahydrofolate is necessary to convert the amino acid homocysteine to methionine, which is used by the body to make proteins and other important compounds essential for proper cellular function. MTHFR polymorphisms have been shown to influence responses to various pharmacologic agents and linked to adverse responses to drug therapies.[869,870,871] MTHFR (rs1801131, which causes a glutamic acid to alanine substitution at amino acid 429) also increases sensitivity to mercury possibly by impairing normal detoxification processes.[872] Just having an MTHFR mutation (SNP) may reduce your ability to create glutathione—a critical cellular antioxidant enzyme—and S-Adenosyl methionine (SAM), which means your body will experience more stress when exposed to heavy metals.[873,874,875] Conceivably, poor detoxification and increased oxidative stress may contribute to adverse vaccine reactions in individuals with this SNP. However, given how common MTHFR polymorphisms are, other factors may be contributing to adverse reactions to vaccination in combination with this SNP. If it were strictly the MTHFR mutation, we would likely see significantly more reactions to vaccines than we currently do.

IRF1 is important for the regulation of inflammatory and innate and adaptive immune responses. Essentially it makes a protein that activates genes involved in the body's response to viruses and bacteria. Many viruses attempt to disrupt IRFs to evade detection by the immune system.[876] SNPs at IRF1 can have profound effects on immune responses and the clearance of viruses.[877] IRF1 also suppresses the growth of tumors and stimulates immune responses against tumor cells. Given its important role in the immune system, it is no wonder that IRF1 gene mutations could affect responses—both positive and negative—to vaccines intended to induce an immune response.

IL4 is crucial to both innate and adaptive immune responses, including stimulation of activated B-cell and T-cell proliferation, and B-cell differentiation into antibody-secreting plasma cells. IL4 is also involved in regulation of allergic responses. SNPs in IL4 can increase the risk of allergies and even infections.[878,879] As with most biological processes, multiple factors can contribute to a positive or negative outcome after use of a pharmacologic substance. It is also possible that individuals with these genetic markers would have ultimately developed the adverse condition, but vaccination accelerated the timeline for development. Still, these identified genetic markers that may increase susceptibility to vaccine adverse events should not be ignored.

Environmental agents (foods, chemicals, drugs, foreign cells, pathogens, etc.) are frequently involved in the triggering of genes related to autoimmune disorders or the cause of the autoimmune disorder alone.[880,881,882,883] Vaccine ingredients may be acting as an environmental trigger and contributing to autoimmune disorders. Environmental triggers may alter or increase expression of autoantibodies (antibodies that target healthy cells for destruction), disrupt immune function, or use other mechanisms to initiate autoimmune reactions. Our current knowledge doesn't permit identifying every possible gene mutation or genetic factor that makes one person more susceptible to vaccine injury than others, but the evidence is slowly trickling in and there may come a day when people will need to undergo genetic testing before vaccination to prevent vaccine-related harm.

A strong correlation is emerging between vaccine adverse events and genetics that warrants further study. As the cost of genetic testing continues to decline, identifying genetic variants predictive for vaccine injury will become more feasible. Genetic testing for cancer risk is becoming more common, so why not perform genetic testing for potential vaccine injury? Including the above, published research has identified the following potential genetic susceptibilities to vaccine injury or an insufficient immune response to protect against infections after immunization.[884,885,886,887,888,889,890,891,892,893,894,895,896,897,898,899,900]

Vaccine	Gene (Variant)	Adverse Event
Rubella, live attenuated	HLA-DR1-10 (DR2, DR5)	Joint pain
MMR	SCN1a (rs6432860) SCN2a (rs3769955) IFI44L (rs273259) TMEM16 (rs114444506) Intergenic—between genes (rs11105468)	Febrile seizure
DTaP/DTP MMR Hib Polio, inactivated	SCN1A (not reported)	Seizures
Smallpox	IL1A (Haplotype 1, Haplotype 3) IL1B (Haplotype 7, Haplotype 8)	Fever

	IL1R1 (Haplotype 10) IL18 (Haplotype 1, Haplotype 9, Haplotype 10)	
Smallpox	MTHFR (1801133) IRF1 (9282736, 839) IL4 (Haplotype TCA)	Systemic adverse events
Aluminum adjuvant Hepatitis B HPV	HLA (DRB1, DRB2, DR4, DRQ8)	Autoimmune disorders
Measles	HLA (DRB1) HLA (DRB1*03, DPA*0701)	Reduced response to antigens
Hepatitis B	HLA (DRB1*0701, DQB1*0202)	Poor immune response
Mumps	HLA (DQB1*0303)	Inadequate antibody response
Mumps	HLA (DRB*0101, DRB*0301, DRB*0801, DRB*1001, DRB*1201, DRB*1302; DQA1*0101, DQA1*0105, DQA1*0401, and DQA1*0501; DQB1*0201, DQB1*0402, DQB1*0501)	Strong T-cell responses

Individuals with Mitochondrial Disorders

Related to genetics, mitochondrial disorders are a group of conditions that affect the energy-producing organelles found within almost every cell in the body called mitochondria. Since the primary function of mitochondria is to produce energy, substantial numbers of mitochondria are present in organs that demand considerable energy, such as the brain, heart, and muscles. Less energy is produced and organ dysfunction occurs if insufficient mitochondria are present or if they aren't functioning efficiently in cells. People who live in areas with high levels of environmental toxins are at an increased risk of mitochondrial disease. Moreover, physiological stress from external factors (e.g., fever, heat cold, sleep deprivation, and starvation) and inflammatory responses caused by infections may exacerbate mitochondrial disorder and subsequent organ damage.

Mitochondria are unique because they have their own DNA called mitochondrial DNA (mtDNA). Mutations in mtDNA or DNA inside the nucleus of a cell (nuclear DNA) can cause a mitochondrial disorder. Mitochondrial disease can be very difficult to diagnose because it affects each person differently and can produce a vast array of symptoms. Mitochondrial disease is estimated to affect one out of every 8,000 people, but one in 4,300 carry mtDNA or nuclear DNA mutations and have or are at an increased risk of mitochondrial disease.[901] In essence, people who carry these mutations have a ticking time bomb inside them just waiting for an opportunity to wreak havoc. Opportunities could present themselves because of poor nutrition, lack of exercise, age, heavy metal exposure, or another chemical stressor.[902] People with mitochondrial disease can have issues with the production of white blood cells and antibodies to fight infection.

Symptoms of mitochondrial disorders vary depending on the organ that is affected. If the heart is affected, cardiomyopathy, stroke, and arrhythmias may develop. Fatigue, growth impairment, loss of muscle coordination, and weakness may result if the muscles are affected, while cognitive disabilities, hearing impairment, autism, seizures, and vision impairment are symptoms of brain mitochondrial disease. Metabolic problems, diabetes, liver, gastrointestinal, thyroid, adrenal, and kidney problems are also possible.

Mitochondrial disorders change the way people respond to immunizations. Mitochondria play diverse and important roles in immune responses, including regulating the activation, differentiation, survival, and signaling of immune cells. The mitochondria produce energy—more energy is needed when these cells are activated—for immune cells to sustain an efficient immune response.

Because mitochondria are vital to appropriate immune responses, people with mitochondrial disorder are more likely to experience adverse events after vaccination. A vaccine could trigger systemic damage due to an impaired response to the immune challenge. It should also be noted that aluminum—used as an adjuvant in many vaccines—is known to cause mitochondrial disorder according to animal and laboratory studies.[903,904] Experts hypothesize that aluminum adjuvants act as reactive oxygen species (ROS) generators inside of cells. Derived from oxygen, which has two unpaired electrons in separate orbitals in its outer shell, ROS are highly reactive free radicals. ROS are produced by phagocytic immune cells in order to kill invading pathogens. They are also produced as a byproduct of mitochondrial metabolism. Despite their beneficial activities, ROS can cause significant damage to cells if not kept in check by antioxidant enzymes naturally produced by the body, such as glutathione peroxidase (GSH-Px), superoxide dismutase (SOD), and catalase. Each of these antioxidant enzymes acts as a protective mechanism against ROS damage. In addition, ethylmercury from thimerosal is a mitochondrial toxin capable of damaging mtDNA and proteins.[905,906] Mitochondrial dysfunction has even been linked to autism.[907,908] Theoretically, vaccine ingredients, or vaccine-caused fever and inflammation, could exacerbate mitochondrial disorders and cause a diversity of adverse events to occur. Presently, there are no definitive studies that say vaccines cause mitochondrial disorder, even those that contain aluminum adjuvants and thimerosal. The theory is plausible, but requires validation in scientific research.

The World Health Organization states, "While vaccines may cause fever, clinicians caring for children with mitochondrial disease recommend vaccinating their patients since the risk of developing an even more devastating clinical deterioration would be associated with natural infection."[909] The WHO has determined that the risk of childhood infection outweighs the risk of triggering or intensifying existing mitochondrial disease.

It may be a good idea to test children who have experienced adverse reactions to vaccines previously for mitochondrial disorder before receiving additional vaccinations. This is done through genetic testing, which starts with testing mtDNA. If the results are negative for mtDNA mutations, nuclear DNA may be tested for genes associated with mitochondrial disorder. If no mitochondrial disorder is found after these first two tests, whole exome sequencing—similar to whole genome sequencing but only the genes that code for proteins are analyzed—may be used to analyze your child's nuclear DNA. Unfortunately, most insurance companies don't cover this type of testing so it may cost between $400 and $1,500, as of this writing, to have the necessary testing down.

Immunocompromised Individuals

People with a weakened immune system caused by certain conditions (AIDS, cancer, diabetes, genetic disorders, and malnutrition) or medications (anticancer drugs, radiation therapy, DMARDs, high-dose corticosteroids, or drugs taken after stem cell or organ transplant) are considered immunocompromised. They have a reduced ability to fight infections. The degree and type of immune dysfunction can range from mild and limited to severe and widespread.

Generally speaking, severely immunocompromised individuals should not receive live viral vaccines (polio, measles, mumps rubella, varicella) due to an elevated risk of disease caused by the vaccine virus.[910,911] Vaccine strains may cause severe systemic reactions in these individuals. It should also be noted that individuals with immune deficiencies will not produce protective antibody levels achieved in healthy individuals after vaccination. Individuals who have a weak immune system should talk to their health professional about the risks versus benefits of receiving specific vaccines.

Overall, a small percentage of people may be predisposed to adverse effects following vaccination. Individuals should be aware of their susceptibility and discuss this with their healthcare provider to determine if an alternative vaccination schedule should be followed or certain vaccines declined.

15

Conflicts of Interest in Vaccinations

There are reasons to question the current vaccine recommendations and the standard for determining their safety. Like most things today, financial gain is at the root of vaccine policy. There is increasing concern that policy makers and advisers are not acting in the public interest, but instead emphasizing personal commercial interests. A growing erosion of public trust in vaccination policy and "independent" experts associated with vaccines is creating a general lack of confidence and undermining vaccination campaigns.

There has been an exponential increase in the number of vaccines children routinely receive since the 1940s and 1950s when vaccines became widely recommended. Smallpox and DTP were the only recommended vaccines during this era. Today, dozens of shots—some of which contain multiple vaccines with several antigens—are administered routinely throughout a child's life. The toll this takes on a child's health has not been fully investigated and this unknown risk is alarming to some parents.

There is also strong evidence that biomedical research has been compromised by industry manipulation and funding, conflicts of interest, and preconceived bias. An anonymous survey of 528 medical school faculty members at thirty-three top research institutions in the United States reported that industry sponsorship significantly influences scientific research.[912] Two-thirds of those surveyed received industry support and almost one-third acknowledged that part of their salary was paid for by industry. A significant number of scientists (61 percent) allowed their industry sponsor to review their scientific manuscript before publication and many agreed to present the data in a favorable way for their sponsor. The excessive influence of industry on scientists is steering findings and evidence in a direction that can only be favorable to industry, rather than evaluating the industry critically.

A more current survey analyzed the most recent 200 phase III and IV trials of vaccines, drugs, and devices fully funded by industry and at least one academic (nonindustry affiliated) author published in the top seven high impact general medical journals—*New England Journal of Medicine, Lancet, JAMA, BMJ, Annals of Internal Medicine, JAMA Internal Medicine*, and *PLoS Medicine*. Nearly all of the trials (92 percent) reported involvement of industry funders in the study's design, while 73 percent allowed the funder to be involved in data analysis, and 5 percent admitted to an unnamed funder or contract research organization employee being involved in data interpretation and reporting.[913] The study authors concluded that "the funders of industry-funded trials were usually involved in every step of the trial" and "few industry-funded trials were completely independently conducted by academics, and sometimes industry involvement was downplayed or omitted in trial publications." Simply put, industry funding of studies compromises research integrity and is not always reported.

Pharmaceutical companies don't just influence vaccine policy and government laws; they also unduly influence—some would say control—scientific journals. Doing so means that they can control the narrative that is being presented in published journals about their products and the industry as a whole. Because of growing concerns about the independence of academic medicine, a researcher evaluated the depth of control the pharmaceutical industry has over scientific societies and journals. The data demonstrated that the pharmaceutical industry has special interest groups acting as editors, reviewers, and consultants to medical journals, which allows them to block negative information from becoming public.[914] Another subtle form of censorship was identified. The industry uses the public relations industry to filter information, alter perception, engineer opinions, and marginalize dissenting individuals or organizations. Obvious financial incentives exist for the pharmaceutical industry to engage in these practices. "For a pharmaceutical company delaying or minimizing knowledge of a side effect of a medication has cash value," the paper stated. Similarly, not publishing negative studies can shift the findings of future meta-analyses. Meta-analyses are studies designed to assess the results of previous research to determine a reliable and valid conclusion about the existing research. Primary care physicians need good evidence for clinical practice and public health decisions, and many rely on meta-analyses to get this evidence. Shifting the narrative of a meta-analysis in favor of pharmaceuticals could lead to poor clinical outcomes and reduced safety. For example, out of seventy-four FDA-registered studies on antidepressants, thirty-seven studies that reported a positive effect of antidepressants were published and only one was not.[915] Of the remaining thirty-six studies that found antidepressants were not helpful, only three were published. If all seventy-four studies were published, a meta-analysis would conclude that nearly half of studies suggest antidepressants are not effective. Instead, the current published evidence suggests that 92.5 percent of published antidepressant studies suggest a positive outcome. This is a significant manipulation of the scientific narrative in favor of pharmaceuticals. If all of the studies were included, physicians who rely on these meta-analyses would choose other solutions for their depressed patients.

The top-five companies sponsoring studies in the *New England Journal of Medicine* and the *Journal of the American Medical Association (JAMA)* are all large vaccine/drug manufacturers. Data analysis uncovered the fact that authors with conflicts of interest (financial ties to industry) were far more likely to report favorable outcomes at the end of a trial and twenty times less likely to publish studies with negative findings.[916] The result is that pharmaceutical companies "heavily invest in 'independent' researchers" so that those researchers with conflicts of interest "are more likely to present positive findings." For all intents and purposes, researchers are being bribed to produce a specific outcome.

This unbridled control of medical journals by the pharmaceutical industry caused the editor of the *Lancet* to state "Journals have devolved into information laundering operations for the pharmaceutical industry" in 2004.[917] Later, that same year, a former editor of the *New England Journal of Medicine* criticized pharmaceutical companies for becoming "primarily a marketing machine" that co-opts institutions that stand in its way.[918] A study noted that medical journals are largely dependent on advertising dollars from the pharmaceutical industry but this was the least corrupting form of dependence between medical journals and the pharmaceutical industry.[919] Instead, the paper proposes that the bigger corruption in this incestuous relationship lies in the fact that about 70 percent of clinical trials published in major journals are drug industry–funded and these studies are four times more likely to have findings favorable to industry when compared to studies funded by other sources. Major journals appear to favor the publication of studies that sympathize with pharmaceutical companies.

Questionable and unethical practices, such as falsification or modification of data, is rampant in biomedical research. Analyzing data from twenty-one surveys asking scientists about research misconduct, a study showed how frequently unethical practices are engaged in during biomedical research. On average, 2 percent of scientists admitted to falsifying, fabricating, or modifying data to improve results.[920] This may not seem like much, but when asked if they had personal knowledge of colleagues who falsified data, an average of 14 percent responded that they did. People are inherently less likely to rat themselves out, so the 14 percent is likely a more reliable number. On top of that, up to 34 percent admitted they engaged in other questionable practices—altering design or methodology or eliminating data because of pressure from a funding source—and up to 72 percent knew about other questionable practices committed by their colleagues.

If you think that scientists at the US National Institutes of Health (NIH) are immune to this misconduct, you'd be wrong. Findings of another study determined that 33 percent of NIH scientists admitted to engaging in questionable scientific behavior and 16 percent admitted to changing study design, methodology, or results because of pressure from a funding source.[921] Fifteen percent excluded data points and 14 percent used inadequate or inappropriate research designs. In the end, the entire integrity of science is being damaged because of these unethical practices and behaviors.

Even worse, a meta-analysis of twenty-nine independent meta-analyses found that only two of 509 randomized controlled trials (RCTs) reported funding sources and zero disclosed the contributing authors' pharmaceutical industry ties or employment.[922] Remarkably, but not surprisingly, 100 percent of the included RCTs in seven of the twenty-nine meta-analyses had at least one conflict of interest in the form of financial ties to the pharmaceutical industry, but only one meta-analysis reported a monetary link between authors of the study and the pharmaceutical industry.

The Cochrane Collaboration is an organization that gathers and summarizes evidence from research to help healthcare professionals make informed choices about medical interventions. Systematic reviews and meta-analyses produced by them are widely recognized as a standard for the evaluation of healthcare interventions. However, a 2012 report found that most Cochrane reviews of drug trials did not report funding sources or author ties to the industry.[923] This suggests that study funding and author conflicts of interest that could influence the study outcome are rarely reported.

Conflicts of interest have the potential to decrease the validity of vaccine safety research. A researcher or adviser may receive financial gain for producing a favorable result versus a negative one. A controversy ensued when it was discovered that Juhani Eskola, a Finnish vaccine adviser on the World Health Organization board, had received $9 million for his research center, the Finnish National Institute for Health and Welfare, to research vaccines from vaccine manufacturer GlaxoSmithKline.[924] Similarly, Dr. Paul Offit, co-inventor of the rotavirus vaccine and former member of the CDC Advisory Committee on Immunization Practices, has been accused of receiving at least $29 million from royalties in Merck's Rotateq vaccine to leverage his position with the CDC to ensure the vaccine became part of the routine schedule.[925] While a member of CDC and FDA advisory committees, Dr. John Modlin also owned stock in Merck and served on Merck's immunization advisory board. Not surprisingly, he voted numerous times on matters relating to the rotavirus, including recommending it as a routine vaccine during childhood.[926] Dr. Patricia Ferrieri was granted a full conflict of interest waiver while serving as the chair of the FDA's advisory committee despite owning shares of Merck.[927] Other financial ties to the vaccine industry among advisers have been exposed, and these are just the ones that have been revealed. A 2009 report from the Office of the Inspector General of the Department of Health and Human Services found that vaccine advisers frequently have conflicts of interest and that the CDC has done a poor job screening medical experts for financial conflicts before hiring them to advise the agency.[928] Experts advising on vaccine safety and policy should be scrutinized better for financial ties to vaccines and vaccine manufacturers and those with conflicts should be excluded from advising agencies.

A paper published in 2012 summarizes noted conflicts of interest that are common in the vaccine industry.[929] One of the most glaring conflicts of interest is the number of vaccine industry lobbyists, particularly those who are former members of Congress. The paper shows that there are three vaccine industry lobbyists for every member of Congress—a significant number to potentially influence regulations indeed! According to Kaiser Health News, a nonpartisan congressional research company, almost 340 former congressional staffers now work for pharmaceutical companies or their lobbying firms.[930] Many of these former congressional staffers could wield undue influence as they return to Capitol Hill to lobby former colleagues to support legislation or government policy that is favorable to pharmaceutical companies. So rampant is the incestuous relationship between government and the drug industry that it is called a "'revolving door' that connects the drug industry to Capitol Hill and the Department of Health and Human Services."[931]

Vaccine manufacturers are also criticized for the fact that they have very little incentive to continue to research vaccine safety once they have met the expensive regulatory hurdles for vaccine approval because they are immune to injury lawsuits under current laws. The National Childhood Vaccine Injury Act of 1986 prevents injured parties from suing vaccine companies in the United States, which was largely implemented to reduce vaccine costs and prevent vaccine shortages because of increased litigation against vaccine manufacturers. Instead, alleged injuries are settled in a no-fault judicial system that provides compensation to people found to be injured by certain vaccines. The vaccine manufactures therefore have no financial risk.

Three major conflicts of interest are identified with the FDA. One is that their mission is to protect the public health by assuring the safety, efficacy, and security of drugs but they are also obliged to ensure the public gets accurate, science-based information necessary to use foods and medicines safely and effectively. Since the FDA approves vaccines for safety and efficacy, an alleged link between vaccines and a serious adverse outcome could greatly damage the FDA's reputation. Second, the FDA's budget largely relies on fees pharmaceutical companies pay to have their drugs evaluated for approval. While the law that allows this (the Prescription Drug User Fee Act of 1992) refers to drugs and not vaccines, many vaccine manufacturers also produce prescription drugs, incentivizing the FDA to be friendlier to companies it relies upon for funding. Lastly, The National Vaccine Injury Compensation Program (NVICP) and the FDA are both divisions of the US Department of Health and Human Services (DHHS). Therefore, if the FDA is mandated to provide information regarding vaccine injuries it would essentially be providing evidence for claims being filed against itself. In some ways the FDA would be forced to violate the Fifth Amendment that all citizens are granted by incriminating themselves in alleged vaccine injury cases.

The CDC also has conflicts of interest. Since the CDC is responsible for promoting vaccination programs for illness prevention as well as assessing vaccine risks, it could be reluctant to sponsor research that reports risks it may have created by recommending a particular vaccine. This is effectively what it did when investigating a link between vaccines and autism. Dr. Marie McCormick, the Chair of the Immunization Safety Review Committee of the Institute of Medicine, declared, "[We] are not ever going to come down that [autism] is a true side effect [of vaccines]" before the safety evaluation to determine whether a causal link existed even started. Similar to the FDA, the CDC falls under the DHHS and could potentially be forced to provide evidence for claims being filed against its own agency. Lastly, it is very common for CDC employees to use the government as a means to gain employment at a vaccine manufacturer. In 2009, Dr. Julie Gerberding, former director of the CDC, was named president of Merck's vaccine division. Conceivably, individuals could use their former authority in government positions to benefit their current employers.

Ironically, the CDC has a disclaimer on its website that states "CDC, our planners, content experts, and their spouses/partners wish to disclose they have no financial interests or other relationships with the manufacturers of commercial products" and furthermore that the CDC does not accept commercial support for educational content. However, this is contradicted by investigators that claim "the CDC does receive millions of dollars in industry gifts and funding, both directly and indirectly, and several recent CDC actions and recommendations have raised questions about the science it cites, the clinical guidelines it promotes, and the money it is taking."[932] Frankly, agencies that oversee vaccine safety should not be promoting vaccines.

Financial interests have led to the production and publication of biased and misleading research findings. A study seeking to identify bias in biomedical research called the extraordinary influence the pharmaceutical industry has on major medical journals "a culture of corruption."[933] Publication of skewed and biased research by researchers and their sponsors was commonly identified. Even data audits by the FDA show that up to 20 percent of research and development dollars are spent on questionable studies that contain biased, fabricated, and misrepresented data.[934] A culture of lying and cheating leads to greater motivation to lie and cheat because of a sense that everyone is doing it.

Bias that results in false findings can occur from any combination of a number of factors: study design, manipulation or intentional misinterpretation of data, or the selective reporting of data and findings. Findings can also be suppressed because of bias. For example, the peer-review process may be exploited to suppress the publication of studies that refute a reviewers' own findings or current beliefs, or represent a threat to his financial or other interests. Bias is so extensive in scientific research that one paper declared that "most current published research findings are false."[935]

Scientific consensus is a dangerous and false term that miscreants throw around to avoid debate by claiming the matter is already settled. It implies substantial, if not unanimous, agreement among scientists on a particular issue. Consensus is inconsequential in science, and truly, there is no such thing as consensus science. Science requires that only one researcher be right through verifiable results. The greatest scientists in history dissented from consensus, broke through paradigms, and discovered new demonstrable findings. The path to true knowledge is through challenging paradigms and open debate. Those scientists that invoke consensus science on vaccines know that their science is not solid enough to withstand full scrutiny and these individuals will go to great lengths to maintain their beliefs as the official narrative of society.

With all of the conflicts of interests involved in the vaccine industry—in vaccine manufacturers, medical journals, medical schools, and government agencies—one has to wonder if these organizations are working for the public or private interest. The pharmaceutical industry wields a great deal of power with the implicit help of government agencies at the expense of the public's health and wellness. Vaccine policy needs to get back to a disease prevention focus rather than a profit focus. This is a significant uphill battle—a modern-day David versus Goliath. But nothing will change for the better unless the worldwide public demands transparency, accountability, and justice be restored to the vaccine industry and the agencies charged to monitor it.

16

Concluding Thoughts

This is likely where you anticipated a list of vaccines you should have your children get and those you shouldn't. But informed medical care means that you need to learn the risks and benefits of whatever medical intervention is recommended by your healthcare professional and make a decision based on all available information. Providing a list of vaccines to get and not get takes decision-making authority away from where it belongs, with the parents and individuals. It also circumvents individualized approaches that consider your child's exact situation and what is best for him or her. Speaking about an inflammatory book, Thomas Jefferson was quoted as saying if "[it is] false in its facts, disprove them; if false in its reasoning, refute it. But...let us freely hear both sides, if we choose." That is what all parents deserve—the right to hear both sides and make an informed choice about vaccination. No government or organization—public or private—should force a human being to receive vaccinations without a choice and against their consent. Now that you better understand the risks of your child receiving or forgoing vaccinations, you are equipped to intelligently discuss your concerns and decision with your primary healthcare provider.

Vaccination is not an all-or-nothing decision. Some parents may choose to get a select group of vaccinations. Others will choose no vaccinations and still others will elect to have their child receive all applicable vaccinations. Furthermore, some parents may adjust the timing of when their child receives vaccines. You as the parent have the right to decide what is best for your child given her individuality, current state of health, and what is best for her.

We live during a time of marvelous scientific progress and genetic advancements. Our improved understanding of genetics permits detection of factors that influence our susceptibility for disease. There is a great urgency and necessity to practice individualized medicine that caters each preventive or treatment approach to the individual's unique situation, including genetic factors. Doing so will ultimately reduce health care costs and treatment-caused adverse reactions and illness.

As said in the very beginning, the idea of vaccines is a noble one. On the whole, physicians, nurses, and other healthcare professionals that administer them have the child's well-being in mind and at heart. They believe doing so protects them against devastating, and sometimes deadly, illnesses. However, most of them are unaware of the risks of vaccination and how frequently they happen. Actually, for most doctors, very little vaccine training is received during medical school or during postgraduate training programs.[936,937] Most physicians are taught about the vaccine schedule that should be followed but nothing about the contents of the vaccines and possible risks. Vaccines simply aren't featured prominently in medical school curriculums. This is an unacceptable practice since vaccines are routinely administered as part of a comprehensive standard of child health care. All pharmacologic agents have risks and benefits which should be weighed when making decisions about health care.

There is little doubt that vaccines save lives. The unresolved science and question is, what are the costs of vaccines on long-term health? While vaccinations appear safe in the short-term for most children, if and how much vaccines are contributing to long-term health conditions is undetermined. The preponderance of evidence also suggests that certain individuals are susceptible to adverse events, both acute (short-term) and chronic (long-term) after vaccination.

Vaccines are not a one-size-fits-all matter. An individualized approach to medicine is essential for the health and safety of our children. Parents are encouraged to have crucial conversations with their chosen healthcare professional after learning about the risks and benefits of vaccines and then, armed with evidence and information, to make an informed medical choice about what is best for their children. Avoid a debate with your healthcare professional. Each person is entitled to take a position on vaccines and you are not likely to change your doctor's chosen stance and perspective on vaccines. The worst thing you can do is go in unprepared. You need to be comfortable discussing the illnesses vaccines prevent and the risks of certain vaccines. Showing your doctor that you have carefully considered your options will help him or her be more willing to accept your choice. Some doctors refuse to keep patients who decline vaccines, so you should be prepared to find another doctor if this happens. Whatever you choose, hopefully, you now feel equipped to make a fully educated decision for your children.

Regardless of your opinion on vaccines, you should be an advocate for choice. For each individual to make an informed decision based on individual circumstances. It is not mine nor your place to tell anyone whether to vaccinate or not. You never know when you may be faced with a compulsory mandate that you disagree with and wish you had been more supportive of the choices of others. There are risks associated with all medical practices, including vaccines, making it extremely important that parents and health professionals have the full information to make an informed choice. This book is intended to raise awareness of the potential risks, small or great, as these risks are largely disregarded by public health officials. In the end, the information in this book is what parents deserve, health professionals should know, and may be critical to avoiding an undesirable outcome in our precious children.

SARS-CoV-2 (COVID-19)

What Is SARS-CoV-2 Infection?

Coronaviruses are a large family of common viruses that infect both animals and humans. They are zoonotic, meaning they circulate among animals but sometimes mutate to infect humans. These viruses typically cause mild to moderate upper-respiratory tract illnesses, like the common cold. They are divided into four major subgroups: alpha, beta, gamma, and delta. The viruses were originally sorted into these subgroups based on serology but more recently are subgrouped by phylogenic clustering—groups of genetically related viruses. People around the world are regularly infected with 229E (alpha coronavirus), NL63 (alpha coronavirus), OC43 (beta coronavirus), and HKU1 (beta coronavirus). Coronaviruses get their name "corona," meaning "crown" in Latin, from the characteristic spikes that project from the center of the virus. These spike proteins are critical for the virus to gain entry into cells and make copies of itself.

Coronaviruses are medium-sized enveloped positive-stranded viruses. They have the largest known viral genomes—genetic material to replicate the virus. Replication of the viruses' RNA (ribonucleic acid) occurs in the cytoplasm of the host cell. At the core of the SARS-CoV-2 virus is a single strip of ribonucleic acid (RNA) surrounded by a protein shell. Coronaviruses create structural proteins—spike (S), membrane (M), nucleocapsid (N), hemagglutinin-esterase (HE), and envelope (E)—based on their genome. The S protein binds to angiotensin-converting enzyme 2 (ACE2) receptors on the host cell and allows the virus to enter the cell and then replicate (spread).[938] ACE2 receptors are abundantly present in many cells and tissues throughout the body, including the heart, blood vessels, lungs, kidneys, liver, gallbladder, gastrointestinal tract, and bone marrow. Its wide expression in the body partly explains why the symptoms of COVID-19 are so diverse—a variety of organs and tissues can be infected.

Occasionally, new coronaviruses emerge from animals that jump to humans and cause serious and widespread illness. This is the case with SARS-CoV-1, MERS-CoV, and most recently, SARS-CoV-2. SARS-CoV-1 emerged from an as-yet-uncertain animal—possibly bats—and jumped to humans in the Guangdong province of southern China during November 2002 and disappeared by early 2004. It infected about eight thousand people, killing an estimated 10 percent of those infected. MERS-CoV emerged from camels and jumped to humans in Jordan in April of 2012, becoming more widespread in Saudi Arabia in September 2012. Another large MERS-CoV outbreak occurred in South Korea in 2015, but it now only causes sporadic and localized outbreaks. Estimates suggest that 35 percent of infections result in death, but this may be overestimated because mild cases of the illness are missed or not reported. Originating in Wuhan, China, beginning in late 2019, and allegedly originating from bats, SARS-CoV-2 spread across the globe in 2020. Of the three coronaviruses responsible for pervasive illness, it has been the most prolific. Governmental and organizational reactions to SARS-CoV-2 singlehandedly disrupted global economies and the lives of billions of people. Unprecedented restrictions were instituted in multiple countries in efforts to stop the spread.

The infection that SARS-CoV-2 causes is called coronavirus disease 2019 (COVID-19). COVID-19 is primarily spread from person to person through respiratory droplets released after a sneeze or cough. To a lesser degree, droplets can be spread by singing, talking, and breathing. Part of the reason scientists believe it has spread so quickly is its so-called silent transmission. Reports suggest that people who are presymptomatic (not displaying symptoms yet but eventually having symptoms) account for 47–48 percent of COVID-19 transmission, whereas asymptomatic (no symptoms) individuals account for 3.4–6.6 percent of COVID-19 transmission.[939] This means that people who don't currently have symptoms could be unknowingly infecting others who are around them. However, most experts believe it requires close contact with an infected individual for ten or more minutes to become infected.

Interestingly, data tracking the spread of SARS-CoV-2 in Utah found that the virus was only spread to another family member 12.4 percent of the time when one family member was infected.[940] This means the virus failed to transmit nearly 88 percent of the time despite close proximity and living in the same household. Experts attribute this fact to a phenomenon known as "superspreaders," which means that only a small percentage of the population is responsible for a large proportion of spread. It is possible that biological uniqueness makes some people more infectious for longer periods and, therefore, greater spreaders of the virus.

Based on this possibility, "social distancing" (better termed physical distancing) of six feet (two meters) was recommended by health organizations worldwide. The six-foot rule is based on outdated information that assumes viral transmission occurs through large droplets or small airborne particles. In reality, viral transmission is far more complex and depends on the type and size of droplets exhaled, the range they can travel, how long they stay in the air, the number of viral particles (viral load) in the air, air ventilation, and more. More recent evidence suggests that while droplets visible to the naked eye only travel up to six feet, other droplets can travel over twenty-six feet (eight meters).[941,942,943] Universal masking was also implemented despite conflicting evidence of its benefits and a poor understanding of the risks.[944,945] The collection of actions—some nonsensical such as wearing gloves while grocery shopping, covering credit card pads with plastic, and one-way shopping isles—taken to slow the spread of

COVID-19 were truly a grand research experiment that few knew they were participating in.

Although COVID-19 has a very wide range of symptoms associated with it, the primary symptoms are fever or chills, cough, shortness of breath, difficulty breathing, loss of sense of smell or taste, fatigue, headache, sore throat, body aches, and occasionally vomiting and diarrhea. Symptoms usually develop 2 to 14 days (average of 4 to 5 days) after infection with the virus. The overwhelming majority of COVID-19 cases are mild, many asymptomatic (between 5 and 80 percent depending on the research),[946] and most people recover spontaneously with self-care. Indeed, most cases are so mild that many don't even know they ever were infected. One challenge with knowing whether you have COVID-19 or another illness like the flu is that these illnesses share several common symptoms. A major difference is that COVID-19 has a more rapid onset of symptoms than the flu. Additionally, loss of taste or smell is a major differentiating characteristic of COVID-19. In the end, a nasal swab test remains the best way to distinguish the two illnesses.

How Prevalent Is It?

By the end of August 2020, more than twenty-five million people worldwide had been infected by SARS-CoV-2.[947] This number potentially grossly underestimates total actual cases because some studies have estimated that up to 45 percent of infected individuals experience no symptoms and therefore likely were never diagnosed with the illness and counted in official totals.[948,949] According to the data available, the hardest-hit countries were the United States, Brazil, India, and Russia. If you do experience symptoms, they will usually begin about two to fourteen days after infection. Infected individuals are encouraged to self-isolate for at least ten days after symptoms first appear and then at least three days after symptoms resolve.

What Are the Health Risks of SARS-CoV-2?

As previously stated, COVID-19 is a minor illness in the overwhelming majority of people. Pooled data from several countries suggests that 14 to 19 percent of people infected with SARS-CoV-2 are hospitalized, 3 to 5 percent require admission to the intensive care unit (ICU), and an estimated 0.56 to 9.38 percent (average of about 2 percent) of people die with the infection.[950,951] Although the numbers range wildly from thousandths of a percent to higher, the general consensus among experts is that the actual mortality rate of COVID-19 is less than 1 percent. The US CDC estimates the infection fatality rate—an estimate of the number of deaths among all infected individuals, both diagnosed and undiagnosed—at a mere 0.0065 percent.[952] These percentages of hospitalizations, ICU admissions, and deaths are likely higher than actual figures because such a high percentage of people who get infected with SARS-CoV-2 are asymptomatic. Knowing this, many people have likely had COVID-19 and never even knew it, which would raise the number of people who did not require any medical treatment and survived without any medical intervention.

The risk of mortality increases the older a person is, with people over age 60 at the greatest risk of dying.[953] The vast majority of deaths after SARS-CoV infection occurred in people aged 55 and older. However, even older individuals have a very low risk of dying. One study determined that chances of hospitalization among people aged 50 to 64 years was 0.057 percent, and the same researchers estimated the case fatality rate (the number of deaths compared to the total number of people diagnosed with the infection) of the same age group to be 0.006 percent.[954] Those over 65 years risk hospitalization and death after a SARS-CoV-2 infection just 0.1 percent and 0.032 percent of the time, respectively. The risks of a SARS-CoV-2 infection seem exaggerated and are likely far lower than many people think.

Research shows that individuals with preexisting health conditions have an increased risk of dying compared to those with no other known health conditions.[955] Illness severity also increases in people with certain underlying medical conditions, particularly those with obesity, cancer, serious heart conditions, type 2 diabetes, chronic kidney disease, chronic obstructive pulmonary disease, a compromised immune system, and sickle cell disease.[956] Other conditions that may increase illness severity include asthma, cerebrovascular disease, cystic fibrosis, high blood pressure, neurological conditions (e.g., dementia), liver disease, pregnancy, pulmonary fibrosis, smoking, blood disorders (e.g., thalassemia), and type 1 diabetes. Many of the conditions that increase the risk of death or severity of illness are lifestyle diseases: obesity (largely caused by diet and inactivity), type 2 diabetes (diet and inactivity are primarily responsible for type 2 diabetes), chronic obstructive pulmonary diseases (smoking is the leading cause of COPD), chronic kidney disease (most often caused by diabetes and high blood pressure), and cancer (strongly linked to diet, physical activity, environmental exposures, and smoking). An important distinction is that people almost always die *with* the infection and not directly *from* it. Instead, COVID-19 acts as a catalyst that makes an already unhealthy person worse. While COVID-19 isn't the direct cause of death, it can contribute to death by decreasing the person's ability to manage a preexisting condition. An Italian study found that the preponderance of people who died with a confirmed COVID-19 infection—99.2 percent—had at least one other health condition.[957] And nearly half of those who died had three preexisting conditions. The US CDC stated that COVID-19 was the only cause of death mentioned for just 6 percent of deaths, but the other 94 percent of people that died with COVID-19 had an average of 2.6 additional health conditions or contributing causes per death.[958] Somehow, COVID-19 is involved in the disruption of the body's ability to manage other health conditions. The existing data suggests that SARS-CoV-2 is almost exclusively dangerous to those with very poor health or advanced age.

In reality, this is not different from other viral illnesses. People with diabetes, obesity, cancer, asthma, heart disease, kidney and liver disorders, chronic neurological conditions, HIV, and who are over age 65 are also considered high-risk groups for flu complications and death.[959] A letter to the US Department of Health and Human Services acknowledges that data provided by the US CDC for flu deaths is "false and misleading," stating that the CDC "acknowledges a difference between flu death and flu-associated death yet uses the terms interchangeably."[960] Like COVID-19, influenza has the potential to initiate a train of events that leads to severe medical complications and death. So the flu is associated with the death, but not the direct cause of death. Here again, we have to make the distinction between dying *from* the flu and dying *with* the flu. Secondary bacterial pneumonia is more frequently the direct cause of death after influenza infection because the opportunistic bacteria thrive in the already weakened human host.[961] Adenoviruses cause a range of illnesses, including the common cold, bronchitis, pneumonia, and conjunctivitis. These viruses usually don't kill a person, but occasionally, they do trigger a cascade of events resulting in death.[962] Whether this cascade of events begins typically has more to do with what preexisting medical conditions that the infected person has rather than other factors.[963] Most coxsackievirus infections only cause mild symptoms and resolve in about a week. However, they can cause serious infections of the heart or brain that result in death in infants and people with a compromised immune system.[964] Even something as common and simple as herpes simplex virus-1 (HSV-1) infection could cause death given the right set of circumstances, such as direct infection of the nervous system in an already unhealthy person.[965] Serious infections, complications, and death after a viral infection tend to occur in people with preexisting conditions or at the extremes of life (very young or very old). Perhaps COVID-19 death totals are better categorized as COVID-19-associated deaths since the virus was only one of the contributing factors that lead to death. What all this information tells us is that we should each be doing everything in our power—eating right, being physically active, managing stress and mood, and limiting exposure to chemicals—to maintain our health and reduce the risk of lifestyle diseases that place us in high-risk categories for complications and death after a viral illness.

Young children and teens rarely have severe COVID-19 or experience complications. They are even less likely to die from COVID-19 when compared to adults. Interestingly, multisystem inflammatory syndrome (MIS-C) has been observed in a small number of children infected with or exposed to COVID-19.[966] MIS-C is a rare but serious condition characterized by inflammation of multiple organs, including the heart, lungs, kidneys, brain, skin, eyes, or gastrointestinal organs. This condition is serious and life-threatening, even in previously healthy children and adolescents, so emergency medical care should be sought if symptoms are noticed. The most common early symptoms include fever, abdominal pain, vomiting, diarrhea, neck pain, rash, bloodshot eyes, and fatigue. Advanced symptoms may include difficulty breathing, confusion, blue lips or face, inability to remain awake, severe abdominal pain, and pain, pressure, or tightness in the chest. MIS-C typically occurs about two to four weeks after the onset of COVID-19 symptoms in children or adolescents. The most common underlying condition among children with MIS-C was obesity followed by chronic lung disease.[967] The medical community is still trying to understand what causes MIS-C, its relationship with COVID-19, and why it seems to only affect children.

While most people who are infected with SARS-CoV-2 fully recover, some people may experience persistent neurological, musculoskeletal, or cardiopulmonary symptoms after a full recovery. When this occurs the condition is called postviral syndrome. It is typically characterized by fatigue, unexplained muscle or joint pain, headache, cognitive problems, sore throat, or swollen lymph nodes. COVID-19 isn't the only virus that may cause lingering symptoms after recovery. It can even develop after simple bouts of a common cold or a mild flu. The exact cause of postviral syndrome is unknown, but experts hypothesize that it may be due to the body's continued attempt to clear remaining virus or the stress and inflammation that occurred in the body as the immune system attacked the virus. Fatigue, racing heartbeat, shortness of breath, foggy thinking, psychiatric symptoms, persistent loss of smell, myocarditis, achy muscles or joints, and damage to the heart or lungs may occur.[968,969,970,971] Why some people have lingering symptoms after recovery is not fully understood.

Description

As of this writing, roughly 200 SARS-CoV-2 vaccines were in various stages of development and testing globally.[972] Although most vaccines take years to develop—the chickenpox vaccine took thirty-four years, and the mumps virus is considered the fastest at just four years—and follow a step-by-step process from laboratory to animals and finally to several human stages, development of coronavirus vaccines is moving at breakneck speed. The steps are overlapping, and in some cases, human testing began before proper animal testing was completed. Progress in vaccine science and technology has led researchers to try new tools in the development of a SARS-CoV-2 vaccine, some of which have never been tested in humans before. Below is a brief explanation of the various approaches scientists are taking to teach the body's immune system to recognize and manage SARS-CoV-2.

Nucleic Acid Vaccines (DNA and mRNA)
Nucleic acid vaccines deliver the instructions (genetic material) for making the viral proteins that cause disease (called a nucleotide sequence) inside human cells. Once the instructions have infiltrated a host cell, the vaccine-derived virus creates proteins that mimic antigens produced when naturally infected by a virus. The hope is that these proteins will act as antigens that the immune system will recognize and mount an immune response to and therefore confer protection against SARS-CoV-2. Nucleic acid vaccines can trigger both antibody production and T-cell responses. The primary idea behind these types of vaccines is that they may mimic a natural infection more closely and elicit a more authentic immune response without allowing the disease to spread. Nucleic acid vaccines can be quickly designed and manufactured and typically cost less to produce.

Although DNA vaccines have been used in preliminary experiments for about three decades, no approved DNA vaccine exists. The primary challenge associated with DNA vaccines is that the DNA must penetrate the cell nucleus—cross not one but two membranes—and then be transcribed in the nucleus into mRNA. If transcription occurs, the mRNA produced moves to the cytoplasm of the cell to stimulate the production of antigens. Another challenge is the fact that DNA vaccines usually require larger doses and often painful delivery methods, like electric shocks, to be effective. DNA vaccines have the potential risk of altering DNA. Once inside a cell's nucleus, DNA vaccines may permanently change your DNA.[973] We have a lot to learn in this rapidly evolving field of vaccination before a DNA vaccine can be used in humans successfully despite their cost-effectiveness and ease of manufacturing.

Contrary to DNA vaccines, mRNA vaccines do not need to be delivered directly to the cell's nucleus. Instead, they deliver a strip of genetic material enclosed in a fat bubble inside the cell. The mRNA creates a protein found on the surface of the virus, which triggers an immune response—usually antibody and T-cell responses. Manufacturers of mRNA vaccines claim they mimic a natural infection with SARS-CoV-2 and stimulate immune protection without the risks of a real infection. The key is they must produce sufficient neutralizing antibodies (an antibody capable of defending a cell against a pathogen or infectious particles by counteracting the biological effects of the virus) to be effective. Like DNA vaccines, no mRNA vaccine has ever been approved for use, and they will likely require at least two doses to be effective.

Companies developing nucleic acid vaccines: Moderna, U.S. National Institutes of Health, Pfizer, BioNTech, Fosun Pharma, AnGes, Osaka University, Takara Bio, Arcturus Therapeutics, Duke-NUS, RNAImmune Inc., Greenlight Biosciences, Fudan University/Shanghai Jiaotong University/RNACure Biopharma, Sanofi Pasteur/Translate Bio, Biocad

Viral-Vectored Vaccines
Viral-vectored vaccines combine the qualities of DNA vaccines and traditional live, attenuated-virus vaccines. They can be replicating or

nonreplicating. Replicating viral-vectored vaccines insert a gene for a viral protein into a different virus that will not cause illness but can replicate. Nonreplicating viral-vectored vaccines add a viral gene to another virus that can't replicate. Basically, COVID-19 genes are placed inside the other virus as a Trojan horse to gain entry inside a cell. The promise of viral-vectored vaccines is that they trigger a robust immune response without the use of an adjuvant (e.g., aluminum) required with traditional vaccines. These types of vaccines have been studied in animals for several decades, but no approved viral-vectored vaccines exist. Like nucleic acid vaccines, viral-vectored vaccines carry DNA into a cell to produce protein antigens that can be customized to stimulate a range of immune responses. They do so through a genetically engineered, live, attenuated virus. They can also actively invade host cells and replicate, similarly to a live attenuated virus, that serves to activate the immune system like an adjuvant.

Most of the time, viral-vectored vaccines produce a robust immune response on their own. However, they may be combined with other vaccine technologies where one vaccine is given as a primer to the immune system followed by a secondary vaccination as a booster. The aim is to produce a stronger overall immune response. While viral-vectored vaccines can be produced quickly, they do have a drawback that people could develop immunity to the viral vector, making booster shots less effective. The immune system has evolved to protect anything it perceives as a threat. Some viral vectors come from parent viruses that the immune system has already encountered and developed antibodies and possibly memory responses to. If the immune system responds to a viral vector it already has immunity to, it impedes delivery of the COVID-19 virus into cells (therefore reducing vaccine efficacy) and, even worse, can cause severe complications.

Companies developing viral-vectored vaccines: AstraZeneca, University of Oxford, CanSino Biologics, Beijing Institute of Biotechnology, Janssen Pharmaceutical, Gamaleya Research Institute, Reithera/Leukocare, Immunitybio/Nantkwest, Erciyes University, Ankara University, ID

Pharma, Valo Therapeutics Ltd, University of Manitoba, University of Georgia/University of Iowa, Geovax/Bravovax, Vaxart

Subunit Vaccines

Instead of an entire virus, subunit vaccines use a specific piece of the virus that produces a strong immune response to that key part of the virus. Think back to the hepatitis B vaccine and the virus surface antigens it uses. By including only the key part of the virus, such as the spike protein, side effects can be reduced. Most subunit vaccines require an adjuvant to trigger a strong protective immune response because the pieces of the pathogen are insufficient to produce adequate long-term immunity. Approved subunit vaccines include those developed for hepatitis B, influenza, pertussis (acellular), HPV, and anthrax. A purported advantage of subunit vaccines is that they can be used in people with weakened immune systems and long-term health problems whereas other vaccines may be prohibited in these individuals due to potential complications.

Companies developing subunit vaccines: Anhui Zhifei Longcom, Chinese Academy of Sciences, Instituto Finlay de Vacunas, Novavax, CSL, Sichuan 'Clover' Biopharmaceuticals, Vaxine and Medytox, University of Queensland, Federal Budgetary Research Institution of Science The State Research Center of Virology and Biotechnology, Farmacologicos Veterinarios Sac/Universidad Peruana Cayetano Heredia, Sorrento Therapeutics, Heat Biologics/University of Miami/Waisman Biomanufacturing, Sanofi Pasteur/GSK, Kentucky Bioprocessing (British American Tobacco), Mynvax, Innomedica, Vabiotech, Vaxil Bio, St. Petersburg Scientific Research Institute of Vaccines and Serums, Lakepharma Inc, Oncogen, Epivax, AJ Vaccines

Live Attenuated or Inactivated Vaccines

More conventional vaccines like those with live-attenuated or inactivated virus are also being developed. The virus is killed or weakened (attenuated) and then administered to a person. Once inside the person's cells, the virus grows and replicates, which stimulates an immune response. Even though the virus replicates, it usually does so without causing symptoms of the actual infection. Severe or fatal reactions can occur if the attenuated or inactivated virus replicates in an uncontrolled manner. This typically occurs in people with a compromised immune system, such as a person with leukemia, human immunodeficiency virus (HIV) infection, or taking an immunosuppressive drug. Except for those administered orally, these vaccines usually only require a single dose for long-term protection. They typically take longer to manufacture and will likely be among the last vaccines fully developed for COVID-19.

Companies developing live-attenuated or inactivated vaccines: Beijing Institute of Biological Products, Codagenix/Serum Institute of India, Indian Immunologicals Ltd/Griffith University, Mehmet Ali Aydinlar University/Acibadem Labmed Health Services A.S., Meissa Vaccines, Sinopharm, Sinovac, Bharat Biotech

Vaccine Manufacturing Process

The vaccine manufacturing process is unknown right now as vaccine inserts are not available for vaccines still in development and the manufacturers have not publicly released this information. It can be expected that subunit and live or attenuated vaccines will be produced similarly to other vaccines manufactured in a similar manner.

Ingredients

Currently unknown.

Controversial ingredients

➢ Currently unknown.

Package insert adverse reactions

Not available at the time of this writing.

Parent or healthcare provider adverse events reported through VAERS

Not available at the time of this writing.

Before we discuss the published literature documenting adverse reactions to various COVID-19 vaccines, the sheer speed at which COVID-19 vaccines have been moved through testing phases and approvals may expose individuals to unnecessary risks and dangers alone. In their rush to produce a vaccine answer to SARS-CoV-2, governments and manufacturers have accepted certain risks by skipping animal testing in some cases and combining trial phases in others. Aside from the safety and efficacy questions that surround any vaccine, these fast-tracked timelines provide reasons to be especially cautious with a COVID-19 vaccine.

Another concern about some of the intramuscular COVID-19 vaccines is their storage requirements. Some require storage at -80 °C (-112 °F) storage to remain viable making transportation and storage of the vaccines problematic.

Some vaccines make an infection worse rather than protect against it. Called antibody-dependent enhancement (ADE), this adverse effect occurs when vaccine-generated viral antibodies bind to the virus without neutralizing it. When this occurs, the non-neutralizing antibodies accelerate viral entry into host cells and make the illness more severe. Scientists and vaccine manufacturers alike acknowledge this risk.[974,975,976] In fact, this phenomenon was observed in mice when scientists attempted to create a vaccine for SARS-CoV-1.[977,978] Moreover, mice that were vaccinated and then naturally infected by the virus experienced severe pneumonia, suggesting that coronavirus vaccines may increase the severity of natural exposure to coronaviruses.[979] Non-neutralizing antibodies have been identified in people infected with coronaviruses, but whether this will increase illness severity or not has yet to be determined.[980] Based on this, it is no wonder that public support and trust in a COVID-19 vaccine is low.

A very small trial of Pfizer's BNT162b1 SARS-CoV-2 modified mRNA vaccine compared three dosage strengths—10 mcg, 30 mcg, and 100 mcg—in twenty-four healthy subjects. Fifty percent of the subjects who received the 10 or 30 mcg dose and 58.3 percent of those who received the 100 mcg dose reported adverse events within one week of vaccination.[981] Only 11.1 percent of participants in the placebo group reported an adverse reaction. The most commonly reported adverse events were fever, moderate fatigue, and headache. Additionally, chills, muscle pain, and joint pain were reported. Two of the participants who received the 30 mcg dose experienced a severe adverse event, which was an extreme fever and sleep disturbance. A higher percentage (58.3%) reported adverse events within one week of receiving a single dose of the high dose (100 mcg) vaccine. And these adverse reactions were seen in healthy individuals because the trial excluded people with compromised immune systems, other viral infections (HIV, Hep C, Hep B), and those with increased risk of severe COVID-19 illness or a history of autoimmune disease.

Moderna has released a preliminary report of a dose-escalation, open-label trial of its mRNA-1273 mRNA vaccine. The trial included forty-five healthy adults who received two vaccinations, twenty-eight days apart, in either a 25 mcg, 100 mcg, or 250 mcg dose. There were fifteen participants in each dosage strength group. No serious adverse events were reported during the trial, but one participant withdrew because of hives related to receipt of the first vaccination.[982] Moreover, systemic adverse events (like fatigue, chills, headache, and muscle pain) were reported in 33 percent, 67 percent, and 53 percent of the 25 mcg, 100 mcg, and 250 mcg groups, respectively, after the first vaccination. These adverse events increased in frequency after a second vaccination dose was received, occurring 54 percent, 100 percent, and 100 percent of the time. Fevers were commonly reported in the 100 mcg (40%) and 250 mcg (57%) group, with one in the 250 mcg group being rated as severe.

Oxford/AstraZeneca's ChAdOx1 nCoV-19 viral-vectored vaccine was assessed in a phase 1/2, single-blind, randomized controlled trial that included 1,077 healthy adults aged 18 to 55. The participants were randomized to receive ChAdOx1 or the MenACWY vaccine. Fifty-six of the subjects received prophylactic paracetamol prior to the shot in order to reduce pain after vaccination. Of the 487 participants who received ChAdOx1 and did not receive paracetamol, 328 (67%) reported mild to moderate pain; while only 180 (38%) of 477 participants who received the MenACWY vaccine and no paracetamol reported pain.[983] Fatigue (70%) and headache were the most commonly reported systemic reactions among those who received ChAdOx1 (68%) and no paracetamol. For comparison, the MenACWY group without paracetamol reported significantly less fatigue (41%) and headaches (37%). Muscle aches (60%), malaise (61%), chills (56%), and feeling feverish (51%) were other common systemic adverse reactions in the ChAdOx1 without paracetamol group. Temporary hematological (relating to blood or blood-forming organs) changes were observed in 46 percent of the ChAdOx1 group compared to only 7 percent in the MenACWY group.

Additionally, AstraZeneca voluntarily halted their large-scale human trials of the ChAdOx1 vaccine in September of 2020 after one participant suffered a serious adverse reaction.[984] Oxford University confirmed in a statement that this was the second time the trial was forced into a mandatory stoppage due to adverse reactions. The adverse reaction that halted the trial was transverse myelitis (TM), a serious inflammatory condition characterized by inflammation of both sides of the spinal cord.[985] Viral infections may cause TM, with the disorder usually appearing after recovery from the infection. TM often damages the protective covering of the nerves (myelin) and interrupts messages sent from the spinal cord throughout the body. Symptoms include pain, muscle weakness, abnormal sensations, bladder or bowel problems, sexual dysfunction, and paralysis. Although, some people recover within months or years of a single bout of TM without any lasting problems, others suffer permanent damage that disrupts their ability to perform ordinary tasks of daily living. After a brief pause—basically a few days—and investigations by independent committees and international regulators, AstraZeneca was permitted to resume the trial in the U.K. Two compulsory pauses in the trials, especially when halted by a devastating condition like TM, certainly creates great concern and doubts about the safety of the vaccine.

Russia approved a COVID-19 vaccine for public use in August of 2020 before important Phase 3 trials were complete. Gam-COVID-Vac, dubbed "Sputnik-V," is a viral-vectored vaccine consisting of a recombinant adenovirus type 26 vector and a recombinant adenovirus type 5 vector, both carrying the gene for the SARS-CoV-2 spike protein. The Phase 1 and Phase 2 trials were combined and included seventy-six health men and women aged 18 to 60. The most common systemic adverse events were fever (50%), headache (42%), fatigue/weakness (28%), and muscle or joint pain (24%).[986] No serious adverse events were reported during the study and the systemic adverse events were considered mild.

A Chinese-manufactured (Beijing Institute of Biotechnology and CanSino Biologics) viral-vectored COVID-19 vaccine in a recombinant adenovirus type 5 vector was tested in a randomized, double-blind, placebo-controlled, phase 2 trial of 603 healthy volunteers. The participants were divided into three groups: two different doses of viral particles (1×10^{11} viral particles per mL or 5×10^{10} viral particles per mL) and a placebo group. Adverse reactions were reported by 72 percent (1×10^{11}) and 74 percent (5×10^{10}) of the vaccine groups, compared to only 37 percent of the placebo group. Additionally, 24 percent (1×10^{11}) and 1 percent (5×10^{10}) of the vaccine groups reported severe adverse reactions.[987] The most common systemic reactions were fatigue (34%–42%), fever (16%–32%), and headache (28%–29%), and the most common localized reaction was injection site pain (56%–57%). A previous study of the same vaccine reported that 81% of participants reported at least one adverse reaction across three tested doses (low, medium, and high).[988] Fever (46%), fatigue (44%), headache (39%), and muscle pain (17%) were the most common systemic reactions in this trial. Six to 14% of participants experienced a severe fever, one reported a severe fever with significant fatigue, muscle pain, and shortness of breath, and a third person reported severe fever accompanied with severe joint pain and fatigue.

The long-term effects of these vaccines are largely unknown because insufficient time has elapsed to determine risk. Another concern is that the vaccines have only been tested in healthy people under the age of 61, which does not satisfactorily represent true populations. Nearly half of all Americans suffer from at least one chronic disease, and 39 and 13 percent of the global population is overweight and obese, respectively.[989,990] Vaccines are known to be less effective in obese adults when compared to people with a lower body mass index.[991,992] This may be because the immune system triggers inflammation on and off as needed, but overweight and obese individuals tend to maintain a constant state of mild inflammation. Vaccines are designed to leverage the immune system's inflammatory response to protect against a pathogen. Hence, the process that vaccines leverage is interfered with in overweight and obese individuals who are under constant inflammation, impairing the immune response to vaccination. The vaccines may also be less effective in people at greatest need of protection, people over the age of 60. The older a person is, the poorer his or her ability to respond to vaccines and generate sufficient antibodies to protect against infections.[993,994] Adverse reactions to vaccines are likely to be greater in those with poor health and possibly less effective in overweight or obese individuals.

INFECTION RISKS	VACCINE RISKS
Death (very rare)	Largely unknown
Postviral syndrome	Transverse myelitis
Multisystem inflammatory syndrome (very rare)	

References

[1] World Health Organization. The power of vaccines: still not fully utilized. Available at: https://www.who.int/publications/10-year-review/vaccines/en/ [Accessed November 2, 2019].

[2] Kim SS, Frimpong JA, Rivers PA, et al. Effects of maternal and provider characteristics on up-to-date immunization status of children aged 19 to 35 months. *Am J Public Health*. 2007 Feb;97(2):259-66.

[3] Gullion JS, Henry L, Gullion G. Deciding to opt out of childhood vaccination mandates. *Public Helath Nurs*. 2008 Sep-Oct;25(5):401-8.

[4] Aharon AA, Nehama H, et al. Reasons why parents do not comply with recommended pediatric vaccines. 5th International Jerusalem Conference on Health Policy, ICC Jerusalem Convention Center. 2013 June 3-5.

[5] O'Leary ST, Nelson C, Duran J. Maternal charactewristics and hospital policies are risk factors for nonreceipt of hepatitis B vaccine in the newborn nursery. *Pediatr Infect Dis J*. 2012 Jan;31(1):1-4.

[6] Pearce A, Law C, Elliman D, et al. Factors Associated With Uptake of Measles, Mumps, and Rubella Vaccine (MMR) and Use of Single Antigen Vaccines in a Contemporary UK Cohort: Prospective Cohort Study. *BMJ*. 2008 Apr 5;336(7647):754-7.

[7] Ogilvie G, Andeson M, Marra F, et al. A Population-Based Evaluation of a Publicly Funded, School-Based HPV Vaccine Program in British Columbia, Canada: Parental Factors Associated With HPV Vaccine Receipt. *PLoS Med*. 2010 May 4;7(5):e1000270.

[8] Martin M, Badalyan V. Vaccination practices among physicians and their children. *Open J Pediatrics*. 2012;2:228-35.

[9] Psfay-Barbe KM, Heininger U, Aebi C, et al. How Do Physicians Immunize Their Own Children? Differences Among Pediatricians and Nonpediatricians. *Pediatrics*. 2005 Nov;116(5):e623-33.

[10] Diesner SA, Peutberger S, Voitl P, et al. Vaccination status of resident pediatricians and the potential risk for their patients - a cross-sectional questionnaire study in pediatric practices in Vienna. *BMC Pediatr*. 2019;19:153.

[11] Association of American Physicians and Surgeons. Statement on Federal Vaccine Mandates. Available at: https://aapsonline.org/measles-outbreak-and-federal-vaccine-mandates/ [Accessed March 7, 2020].

[12] PC Magazine. Facebook, YouTube To Suppress Anti-Vaxxer Content. Available at: https://www.pcmag.com/news/facebook-youtube-to-suppress-anti-vaxxer-content [Accessed November 2, 2019].

[13] CBS News. Tech's fight against anti-vaccine content prompts free speech debate. https://www.cbsnews.com/news/tech-companies-fight-against-vaccine-misinformation-prompts-free-speech-debate/ [Accessed November 2, 2019].

[14] Zhou X, Coiera E, Tsafnat G, et al. Using Social Connection Information to Improve Opinion Mining: Identifying Negative Sentiment About HPV Vaccines on Twitter. *Stud Health Technol Inform*. 2015;216:761-5.

[15] Salathe M, Khandelwal S. Assessing Vaccination Sentiments With Online Social Media: Implications for Infectious Disease Dynamics and Control. *PLoS Comput Biol*. 2011 Oct;7(10):e1002199.

[16] Dunn AG, Leask J, Zhou X, et al. Associations Between Exposure to and Expression of Negative Opinions About Human Papillomavirus Vaccines on Social Media: An Observational Study. *J Med Internet Res*. 2015 Jun 10;17(6)e144.

[17] Du J, Xu J, Song HY, et al. Leveraging Machine Learning-Based Approaches to Assess Human Papillomavirus Vaccination Sentiment Trends With Twitter Data. *BMC Med Inform Decis Mak*. 2017 Jul 15;17(Suppl 2):69.

[18] Nelon JL Moscarelli M, Stupka P, et al. Does Scientific Publication Inform Public Discourse? A Case Study Observing Social Media Engagement Around Vaccinations. *Health Promot Pract*. 2020 Feb 1. [Online ahead of print]

[19] Martin B. On the Suppression of Vaccination Dissent. *Sci Eng Ethics*. 2015 Feb;21(1):143-57.

[20] United States Centers for Disease Control and Prevention. 2019 Recommended Vaccinations for Children (7-18 Years Old) Parent-Friendly Format. Available at: https://www.cdc.gov/vaccines/schedules/easy-to-read/child-easyread.html and https://www.cdc.gov/vaccines/schedules/easy-to-read/adolescent-easyread.html [Accessed January 22, 2020].

[21] Deisher TA, Doan NV, Koyama K, et al. Epidemiologic and Molecular Relationship Between Vaccine Manufacture and Autism Spectrum Disorder Prevalence. *Issues Law Med*. 2015 Spring;30(1):47-70.

[22] Deisher TA, Doan NV, Omalye A, et al. Impact of environmental factors on the prevalence of autistic disorder after 1979. *J Public Health Epidemiology*. 2014 Sep;6(9):271-86.

[23] Hosseini AM, Majidi J, Baradaran B, et al. Toll-Like Receptors in the Pathogenesis of Autoimmune Diseases. *Adv Pharm Bull*. 2015 Dec;5(Suppl 1):605–614.

[24] Chen CY, Shih YC, Hung YF, et al. Beyond defense: regulation of neuronal morphogenesis and brain functions via Toll-like receptors. *J Biomed Sci*. 2019;26:90.

[25] Ratajczak HV. Theoretical Aspects of Autism: Causes--A Review. J Immunotoxicol. 2011 Jan-Mar;8(1):68-79.

[26] Deisher TA, Doan NV, Koyama K, et al. Epidemiologic and Molecular Relationship Between Vaccine Manufacture and Autism Spectrum Disorder Prevalence. *Issues Law Med*. 2015 Spring;30(1):47-70.

[27] Vilchez RA, Butel JS. Emergent Human Pathogen Simian Virus 40 and Its Role in Cancer. *Clin Microbiol Rev*. 2004 Jul; 17(3): 495–508.

[28] Fisher SG, Weber L, Carbone M. Cancer Risk Associated With Simian Virus 40 Contaminated Polio Vaccine. *Anticancer Res*. 1999 May-Jun;19(3B):2173-80.

[29] Carbone M, Pass HI, Miele L, et al. New Developments About the Association of SV40 With Human Mesothelioma. *Oncogene*. 2003 Aug 11;22(33):5173-80.

[30] Hirvonen A, Mattson K, Karjalainen A, et al. Simian Virus 40 (SV40)-like DNA Sequences Not Detectable in Finnish Mesothelioma Patients Not Exposed to SV40-contaminated Polio Vaccines. *Mol Carcinog*. 1999 Oct;26(2):93-9.

[31] Poulin DL, DeCaprio JA. Is There a Role for SV40 in Human Cancer? *J Clin Oncol*. 2006 Sep 10;24(26):4356-65.

[32] Olin P, Giesecke J. Potential Exposure to SV40 in Polio Vaccines Used in Sweden During 1957: No Impact on Cancer Incidence Rates 1960 to 1993. Dev Biol Stand. 1998;94:227-33.

[33] Strickler HD, Rosenberg PS, Devesa SS, et al. Contamination of Poliovirus Vaccines With Simian Virus 40 (1955-1963) and Subsequent Cancer Rates. JAMA. 1998 Jan 28;279(4):292-5.

[34] Richmond JE, Parry JV, Gardner SD. Characterisation of a polyomavirus in two foetal rhesus monkey kidney cell lines used for the growth of hepatitis A virus. *Arch Virol*. 1984;80(2-3):131-46.

[35] United States Centers for Disease Control and Prevention. Rotavirus VIS. Available at: https://www.cdc.gov/vaccines/hcp/vis/vis-statements/rotavirus.html [Accessed January 22, 2020].

[36] Hattermann K, Roedner C, Schmitt C, et al. Infection Studies on Human Cell Lines With Porcine Circovirus Type 1 and Porcine Circovirus Type 2. *Xenotransplantation*. 2004 Mat;11(3):284-94.

[37] Liu X, Ouyang T, Ouyang H, et al. Human cells are permissive for the productive infection of porcine circovirus type 2 in vitro. *Sci Rep*. 2019 Apr;9(5638):1-8.

[38] Kahn AS, USFDA. Investigating Viruses in Cells Used to Make Vaccines; and Evaluating the Potential Threat Posed by Transmission of Viruses to Humans. Available at: https://www.fda.gov/vaccines-blood-biologics/biologics-research-projects/investigating-viruses-cells-used-make-vaccines-and-evaluating-potential-threat-posed-transmission [Accessed January 22, 2020].

[39] Lu HY, Chen YH, Liu HJ. Baculovirus as a vaccine vector. *Bioengineered*. 2012 Sep 1;3(5):271–274.

[40] European commission Health & Consumer Protective Directorate-General. Guidance Document on the assessment of new isolates of baculovirus species already included in Annex I of Council Directive 91/414/EEC. Available at: https://ec.europa.eu/food/sites/food/files/plant/docs/pesticides_aas_guidance_baculovirus.pdf [Accessed January 25, 2020].

[41] Kern JK, Geier DA, Homme KG, et al. Examining the Evidence That Ethylmercury Crosses the Blood-Brain Barrier. *Environ Toxicol Pharmacol*. 2020 Feb;74:103312.

[42] Barrett JR. Thimerosal and Animal Brains: New Data for Assessing Human Ethylmercury Risk. *Environ Health Perspect*. 2005 Aug;113(8):A543–A544.

[43] Dorea JG, Farina M, Rocha JBT. Toxicity of Ethylmercury (And Thimerosal): A Comparison With Methylmercury. *J Appl Toxicol*. 2013 Aug;33(8):700-1.

[44] United States Centers for Disease Control and Prevention. Frequently Asked Questions about Thimerosal. Available at: https://www.cdc.gov/vaccinesafety/concerns/thimerosal/faqs.html?CDC_AA_refVal=https%3A%2F%2F www.cdc.gov%2Fvaccinesafety%2Fconcerns%2Fthimerosal%2Fthimerosal_faqs.html [Accessed November 2, 2019].

[45] Matyja E, Albrecht J. Ultrastructural evidence that mercuric chloride lowers the threshold for glutamate neurotoxicity in an organotypic culture of rat cerebellum. *Neurosci Lett.* 1993;158:155-158.

[46] Albrecht J, Matyja E. Glutamate: a potential mediator of inorganic mercury neurotoxicity. *Metab Brain Dis.* 1996; 11: 175-184.

[47] Rodriguez JI, Kern JK. Evidence of microglial activation in autism and its possible role in brain underconnectivity. *Neuron Glia Biol.* 2011 May;7(2-4):205–213.

[48] Kim JW, Hong JY, Bae SM. Microglia and Autism Spectrum Disorder: Overview of Current Evidence and Novel Immunomodulatory Treatment Options. *Clin Psychopharmacol Neurosci.* 2018 Aug;16(3):246–252.

[49] Teixeira FB, de Oliveira ACA, Leao LKR, et al. Exposure to Inorganic Mercury Causes Oxidative Stress, Cell Death, and Functional Deficits in the Motor Cortex. *Front Mol Neurosci.* 2018 May 15;11(125):1-11.

[50] Geier DA, Sykes LK, Geierr MR, et al. A Review of Thimerosal (Merthiolate) and its Ethylmercury Breakdown Product: Specific Historical Considerations Regarding Safety and Effectiveness. *J Toxicol Environ Health Part B.* 2007 Nov 28;10(8):575-96.

[51] Hooker B, Kern J, Geier D, et al. Methodological Issues and Evidence of Malfeasance in Research Purporting to Show Thimerosal in Vaccines Is Safe. *Biomed Res Int.* 2014;2014:247218. *N Am J Med Sci.* 2014 Oct;6(10):519-31.

[52] Geier DA, King PG, Hooker BS, et al. Thimerosal: clinical, epidemiologica and biochemical studies. *Clin Chim Acta.* 2015 Apr;444:212-20.

[53] Geier DA, Kern JK, Homme KG, et al. The Risk of Neurodevelopmental Disorders Following Thimerosal-containing Hib Vaccine in Comparison to Thimerosal-free Hib Vaccine Administered From 1995 to 1999 in the United States. *Int J Hyg Environ Health.* 2018 May;221(4):677-83.

[54] Geier DA, Kern JK, Homme KG, et al. A Cross-Sectional Study of the Relationship Between Infant Thimerosal-containing Hepatitis B Vaccine Exposure and Attention-Deficit/Hyperactivity Disorder. *J Trace Elem Med Biol.* 2018 Mar;46:1-9.

[55] Geier DA, Kern JK, Homme KG, et al. Thimerosal Exposure and Disturbance of Emotions Specific to Childhood and Adolescence: A Case-Control Study in the Vaccine Safety Datalink (VSD) Database. *Brain Inj.* 2017;31(2):272-278.

[56] Dorea JG. Low-dose Thimerosal in Pediatric Vaccines: Adverse Effects in Perspective. *Environ Res.* 2017 Jan;152:280-293.

[57] Dorea JG, Marques RC, Isejima C. Neurodevelopment of Amazonian infants : antenatal exposure and postnatal exposiure to methyl- an ethylmercury. *J Biomed Biotechnol.* 2012;2012:132876.

[58] Oken E, Bellinger BC. Fish consumption, methylmercury and child neurodevelopment. *Curr Opin Pediatr.* 2008 Apr;20(2):178–183.

[59] Bose-O'Reilly S, McCarty KM, Steckling N, et al. Mercury Exposure and Children's Health. *Curr Probl Pediatr Adolesc Health Care.* 2010 Sep;40(8):186–215.

[60] Geier DA, Kern JK, Hooker BS, et al. Thimerosal-containing Hepatitis B Vaccination and the Risk for Diagnosed Specific Delays in Development in the United States: A Case-Control Study in the Vaccine Safety Datalink.

[61] Mrozeh-Budzyn D, Majewska R, Kieltyka A, et al. Neonatal Exposure to Thimerosal From Vaccines and Child Development in the First 3 Years of Life. *Neurotoxicol Teratol.* 2012 Nov-Dec;34(6):592-7.

[62] Gallagher C, Goodman M. Hepatitis B triple series vaccine and developmental disability in US children aged 1–9 years. *J Toxicol Environ Chem.* 2008 Sep;90(5):997-1008.

[63] Geier DA, Hooker BS, Kern JK, et al. A two-phase study evaluating the relationship between Thimerosal-containing vaccine administration and the risk for an autism spectrum disorder diagnosis in the United States. *Transl Neurodegener.* 2013;2:25.

[64] Geier DA, Geier MR, A comparative evaluation of the effects of MMR immunization and mercury doses from thimerosal-containing childhood vaccines on the population prevalence of autism. *Med Sci Monit.* 2004 Mar;10(3):PI33-9.

[65] Geier DA, Geier MR. A case series of children with apparent mercurytoxic encephalopathies manifesting with clinical symptooms of regressive autistic disorders. *J Toxicol Environ Health A*. 2007 May;70(10):837-51.

[66] Geier DA, Geier MR. A prospective study of thimerosal-containing Rho(D)-immune globulin administration as a risk factor for autistic disorders. *J Matern Fetal Neonatal Med*. 2007 May;20(5):385-90.

[67] Verstraeten TM, Davies R, Gu D, et al. Increased risk of developmental neurologic impairment after high exposure to thimerosal-containing vaccine in first month of life. *Proceedings of the Epidemic Intelligence Service Annual Conference*. 2000 Apr;49.

[68] Geier DA, Hooker BS, Kern JK, et al. A Dose-Response Relationship Between Organic Mercury Exposure From Thimerosal-Containing Vaccines and Neurodevelopmental Disorders. *Int J Environ Res Public Health*. 2014 Sep 5;11(9):9156-70.

[69] Gallagher CM, Goodman MS. Hepatitis B vaccination of male neonates and autism diagnosis, NHIS 1997-2002. *J Toxicol Environ Health A*. 2010;73(24):1665-77.

[70] Jafari T, Rostampour N, Fallah AA, et al. The Association Between Mercury Levels and Autism Spectrum Disorders: A Systematic Review and Meta-Analysis. *J Trace Elem Med Biol*. 2017 Dec;44:289-297.

[71] Geier DA, Kern JK, Geier MR. Increased Risk for an Atypical Autism Diagnosis Following Thimerosal-containing Vaccine Exposure in the United States: A Prospective Longitudinal Case-Control Study in the Vaccine Safety Datalink. *J Trace Elem Med Biol*. 2017 Jul;42:18-24.

[72] Geier DA, Kern JK, Homme KG, et al. Abnormal Brain Connectivity Spectrum Disorders Following Thimerosal Administration: A Prospective Longitudinal Case-Control Assessment of Medical Records in the Vaccine Safety Datalink. *Dose Response*. 2017 Mar 16;15(1):1559325817690849.

[73] Taylor LE, Swerdfeger AL, Eslick GD. Vaccines Are Not Associated With Autism: An Evidence-Based Meta-Analysis of Case-Control and Cohort Studies. *Vaccine*. 2014 Jun 17;32(29):3623-9.

[74] Hurley AM, Tadrous M, Miller ES. Thimerosal-Containing Vaccines and Autism: A Review of Recent Epidemiologic Studies. *J Pediatr Pharmacol Ther*. 2010 Jul-Sep;15(3):173–181.

[75] Cunha GKD, Matos MBD, Trettim JP, et al. Thimerosal-containing Vaccines and Deficit in Child Development: Population-based Study in Southern Brazil. *Vaccine*. 2020 Jan 31 [Epub ahed of print].

[76] Geier D, Geier MR. Neurodevelopmental disorders following thimerosal-containing childhood immunizations: a follow up analysis. *Int J toxicol*. 2004 Nov-Dec;23(6):369-76.

[77] Geier DA, Geier MR. A meta-analysis epidemiological assessment of neurodevelopmental disorders following vaccines administered from 1994 through 2000 in the United States. *Neuro Endocrinol Lett*. 2006 Aug;27(4):401-13.

[78] Geier DA, Geier MR. A two-phased population epidemiological study of the safety of thimerosal-contianing vaccines: a follow-up analysis. *Med Sci Monit*. 2005 Apr;11(4):CR160-70.

[79] Young HA, Geier DA, Geier MR. Thimerosal exposure in infants and neurodevelopmental disorders: an assessment of computerized medical records in the Vaccine Safety Datalink. *J Neurol Sci*. 2008 Aug;271(1-2):110-18.

[80] Geier DA, Geier MR. An Assessment of the Impact of Thimerosal on Childhood Neurodevelopmental Disorders. *Pediatr Rehabil*. 2003 Apr-Jun;6(2):97-102.

[81] Geier D, Geier MR. Neurodevelopmental disorders after thimerosal-containing vaccines: A brief communication. *Exp Biol Med (Maywood)*. 2003 Jun;228(6):660-64.

[82] Geier DA, Kern JK, King PG, et al. The risk of neurodevelopmental disorders following a Thimerosal-preserved DTaP formulation in comparison to its Thimerosal- reduced formulation in the vaccine adverse event reporting system (VAERS). 2014 Jun;2(2):1-10.

[83] Dorea JG. Multiple Low-Level Exposures: Hg Interactions With Co-Occurring Neurotoxic Substances in Early Life. Biochim Biophys Acta Gen Subj. 2019 Dec;1863(12):129243.

[84] Geier DA, Young HA, Geier MR. Thimerosal exposure and increasing trends of premature puberty in the vaccine safety datalink. *Indian J Med Res*. 2010 Apr;131:500-7.

[85] Geier DA, Kern JK, Geier MR. Premature Puberty and Thimerosal-Containing Hepatitis B Vaccination: A Case-Control Study in the Vaccine Safety Datalink. *Toxics*. 2018 Nov 15;6(4).

[86] Bodicoat DH, Schoemaker MJ, Jones ME, et al. Timing of pubertal stages and breast cancer risk: the Breakthrough Generations Study. *Breast Cancer Res*. 2014; 16(1): R18.

[87] Biro FM, Greenspan LC, Glavez MP, et al. Onset of Breast Development in a Longitudinal Cohort. Pediatrics. 2013 Dec;132(6):1019-27.

[88] Shaw CA, Petrik MSJ. Aluminum hydroxide injections lead to motor deficits and motor neuron degeneration. *J Inorg Biochem*. 2009;103:1555–1562.

[89] Shaw CA, Li D, Tomljenovic. Are there negative CNS impacts of aluminum adjuvants used in vaccines and immunotherapy? *Immunotherapy*. 2014;6(10):1055-71.

[90] Crepeaux G, Eidi H, David MO, et al. Non-linear Dose-Response of Aluminium Hydroxide Adjuvant Particles: Selective Low Dose Neurotoxicity. *Toxicology*. 2017 Jan 15;375:48-57.

[91] Khan Z, Combadiere C, Authier FJ, et al. Slow CCL2-dependent translocation of biopersistent particles from muscle to brain. *BMC Med*. 2013;11(99):1-18.

[92] Gheraradi RK, Eidi H, Crepeaux G, et al. Biopersistence and Brain Translocation of Aluminum Adjuvants of Vaccines. *Front Neurol*. 2015;6:4.

[93] Khan Z, Combadiere C, Authier FJ, et al. Slow CCL2-dependent translocation of biopersistent particles from muscle to brain. *BMC Medicine*. 2013;11(99):1-18.

[94] Lu F, Hogenesch H. Kinetics of the inflammatory response following intramuscular injection of aluminum adjuvant. *Vaccine*. 2013 Aug 20; 31(37):3979-86.

[95] Morefield GL, Sokolovska A, Jiang D, et al. Role of aluminum-containing adjuvants in antigen internalization by dendritic cells in vitro. *Vaccine*. 2005 Feb 18;23(13):1588-95.

[96] Perricone C, Colafrancesco S, Maxor RD, et al. Autoimmune/inflammatory syndrome induced by adjuvants (ASIA) 2013: Unveiling the pathogenic, clinical and diagnostic aspects. *J Autoimmun*. 2013 Dec;47:1-16.

[97] Soriano A, Nesher G, Shoelfeld Y. Predicting post-vaccination autoimmunity: Who might be at risk? *Pharmacol Res*. 2015 Feb;92:18-22.

[98] McFarland G, Joie EL, Thomas P, et al. Acute Exposure and Chronic Retention of Aluminum in Three Vaccine Schedules and Effects of Genetic and Environmental Variation. *J Trace Elem Med Biol*. 2020 Mar;58:126444.

[99] Shaw CA, Li D, Tomljenovic L. Are there negative CNS impacts of aluminum adjuvants used in vaccines and immunotherapy? *Immunother*. 2014 Nov 27;6(10:1055-71.

[100] Bai D, Yip BHK, Windham GC, et al. Association of Genetic and Environmental Factors With Autism in a 5-Country Cohort. *JAMA Psychiatry*. 2019;76(10):1035-1043.

[101] Shaw CA, Sheth S, Li D, et al. Etiology of autism spectrum disorders: Genes, environment, or both? *OA Autism*. 2014 Jun;10(2):11.

[102] Tomljenovic L, Shaw CA. Mechanisms of Aluminum Adjuvant Toxicity and Autoimmunity in Pediatric Populations. *Lupus*. 2012 Feb;21(2):223-30.

[103] Shaw CA, Tomljenovic L. Aluminum in the Central Nervous System (CNS): Toxicity in Humans and Animals, Vaccine Adjuvants, and Autoimmunity. *Immunol Res*. 2013 Jul;56(2-3):304-16.

[104] Tomljenovic L, Shaw CA. Do aluminum vaccine adjuvants contribute to the rising prevalence of autism? *J Inorg Biochem*. 2011 Nov;105(11):1489-99.

[105] Shaw CA, Seneff S, Kette SD, et al. Aluminum-induced Entropy in Biological Systems: Implications for Neurological Disease. *J Toxicol*. 2014;2014:491316.

[106] Couette M, Boisse MF, Maison P, et al. Long-term Persistence of Vaccine-Derived Aluminum Hydroxide Is Associated With Chronic Cognitive Dysfunction. *J Inorg Biochem*. 2009 Nov;103(11):15171-8.

[107] Rigolet M, Aouizerate J, Couette M, et al. Clinical Features in Patients with Long-Lasting Macrophagic Myofasciitis. *Front Neurol*. 2014;5:230.

[108] Lach B, Cupler EJ. Macrophagic Myofasciitis in Children Is a Localized Reaction to Vaccination. *J Child Neurol*. 2008 Jul;23(6):614-9.

[109] Chkheidze R, Burns DK, White CL, et al. Morin Stain Detects Aluminum-Containing Macrophages in Macrophagic Myofasciitis and Vaccination Granuloma With High Sensitivity and Specificity. J Neuropathol Exp Neurol. 2017 Apr 1;76(4):323-331.

[110] Gherardi RK, Coquet M, Cherin P, et al. Macrophagic Myofasciitis Lesions Assess Long-Term Persistence of Vaccine-Derived Aluminium Hydroxide in Muscle. *Brain*. 2001 Sep;124(Pt 9):1821-31.

[111] Sebaiti MA, Abrivard M, Blanc-Durand P, et al. Macrophagic Myofasciitis-Associated Dysfunctioning: An Update of Neuropsychological and Neuroimaging Features. Best Pract Res Clin Rheumatol. 2018 Oct;32(5)640-650.

[112] Gherardi RK, Crepeaux G, Authier FJ. Myalgia and Chronic Fatigue Syndrome Following Immunization: Macrophagic Myofasciitis and Animal Studies Support Linkage to Aluminum Adjuvant Persistency and Diffusion in the Immune System. Autoimmun Rev. 2019 Jul;8(7):691-705.

[113] Israeli E, Agmon-Levin N, Blank M, et al. Macrophagic Myofaciitis a Vaccine (Alum) Autoimmune-Related Disease. *Clin Rev Allergy Immunol*. 2011 Oct;41(2):163-8.

[114] Gherard RK, Authier FJ. Macrophagic Myofasciitis: Characterization and Pathophysiology. *Lupus*. 2012 Feb;21(2):184-9.

[115] Authier FJ, Cherin P, Creange A, et al. Central Nervous System Disease in Patients With Macrophagic Myofasciitis. *Brain*. 2001 May;124(Pt 5):974-83.

[116] Gherardi RK. Lessons from macrophagic myofasciitis: towards definition of a vaccine adjuvant-related syndrome. *Rev Neurol (Paris)*. 2003 feb;159(2):162-4.

[117] Gherardi RK. Lessons from macrophagic myofasciitis: towards definition of a vaccine adjuvant-related syndrome. *Rev Neurol (Paris)*. 2003 feb;159(2):162-4.

[118] Exley C, Swarbrick L, Gherardi RK, et al. A Role for the Body Burden of Aluminium in Vaccine-Associated Macrophagic Myofasciitis and Chronic Fatigue Syndrome. Med Hypotheses. 2009 Feb;72(2):135-9.

[119] Shaw CA, Petrik MSJ. Aluminum hydroxide injections lead to motor deficits and motor neuron degeneration. *J Inorg Biochem.* 2009;103:1555–1562.

[120] Petrik MS, Wong MC, Tabata RC, et al. Aluminum Adjuvant Linked to Gulf War Illness Induces Motor Neuron Death in Mice. *Neuromolecular Med.* 2007;9(1):83-100.

[121] Gherardi RK. Lessons from macrophagic myofasciitis: towards definition of a vaccine adjuvant-related syndrome. *Rev Neurol (Paris)*. 2003 feb;159(2):162-4.

[122] Goulle J-P, Grangeot-Keros L. Aluminum and Vaccines: Current State of Knowledge. Med Mal Infect. 2020 Feb;50(1):16-21.

[123] Golos A, Lutynska. ALUMINIUM-ADJUVANTED VACCINES – A REVIEW OF THE CURRENT STATE OF KNOWLEDGE. *Przegl Epidemiol.* 2015;69:731-4.

[124] Ameratunga R, Gillis D, Gold M, et al. Evidence Refuting the Existence of Autoimmune/Autoinflammatory Syndrome Induced by Adjuvants (ASIA). *J Allergy Clin Immunol Prac.* 2017 Nov-Dec;5(6):1551-5.

[125] Tomljenovic L, Shaw CA. Aluminum Vaccine Adjuvants: Are They Safe? *Curr Med Chem.* 2011;18(17):2630-7.

[126] Petrovsky N. Freeing vaccine adjuvants from dangerous immunological dogma. *Expert Rev Vaccines.* 2008 Feb;7(1):7-10.

[127] Petrovsky N, Aguilar JC. Vaccine adjuvants: current state and future trends. *Immunol Cell Biol.* 2004 Oct;82(5):488-96.

[128] Petrovsky N, Aguilar JC. Vaccine adjuvants: current state and future trends. *Immunol Cell Biol.* 2004 Oct;82(5):488-96.

[129] Powell BS, Andrianov AK, Fusco PC. Polyionic vaccine adjuvants: another look at aluminum salts and polyelectrolytes. *Clin Exp Vaccine Res.* 2015 Jan;4(1):23-45.

[130] Vera-Lastra O, Medina G, Cruz-Dominguez Mdel P, et al. Autoimmune/inflammatory syndrome induced by adjuvants (Shoenfeld's syndrome): clinical and immunological spectrum. *Expert Rev Clin Immunol.* 2013 Apr;9(4):361-73.

[131] Nohynek H, Jokinen J, Partinen M, et al. AS03 adjuvanted AH1N1 vaccine associated with an abrupt increase in the incidence of childhood narcolepsy in Finland. *PLoS One.* 2012;7(3):e33536.

[132] Petrovsky N. Comparative safety of vaccine adjuvants: a summary of current evidence and future needs. *Drug Saf.* 2015 Nov;38(11):1059–1074.

[133] European Medicines Agency. The European Agency for the Evaluation of Medicinal Products: Note for Guidance on Plasma-Derived Medicinal Products. 2001. Available at http://www.ema.europa.eu/docs/en_GB/document_library/Scientific_guideline/2009/09/WC500003613.pdf [Accessed October 26, 2019].

[134] Geier DA, Jordan SK, Geier MR. The Relative Toxicity of Compounds Used as Preservatives in Vaccines and Biologics. *Med Sci Monit.* 2010 May;16(5):SR21-7.

[135] Abu-Elnaga HI, Rizk SA, Daoud HM, et al. Studies on the using of 2-Phenoxyethanol as an Alternative to Thiomersal as a Preservative in Foot-and-Mouth Disease Vaccine. *Global J Med Res Vet Sci and Vet Med.* 2019;I(I).

[136] Melin VE, Potineni H, Hunt P, et al. Exposure to common quaternary ammonium disinfectants decreases fertility in mice. *Reprod Toxicol.* 2014 Dec;50:163-70.

[137] Swenberg JA, Moeller BC, Lu K, et al. Formaldehyde Carcinogenicity Research: 30 Years and Counting for Mode of Action, Epidemiology, and Cancer Risk Assessment. *Toxicol Pathol.* 2013 Feb;41(2):181–189.

[138] American Cancer Society, Formaldehyde: What is formaldehyde? Available at: https://www.cancer.org/cancer/cancer-causes/formaldehyde.html [Accessed January 25, 20202].

[139] Eells JT, McMartin KE, Black K, et al. Formaldehyde Poisoning: Rapid Metabolism to Formic Acid. *JAMA.* 1981;246(11):1237-1238.

[140] National Research Council (US) Committee on Toxicology. Formaldehyde - An Assessment of Its Health Effects. *National Acad Press (US).* 1980.

[141] Mitkus RJ, Hess MA, Schwartz SL. Assessing the Safety of Residual Formaldehyde in Infant Vaccines. Vaccine. 2013 Jun 7;31(25):2738-43.

[142] American Chemistry Council. Formaldehyde occurs naturally and is all around us. Available at: https://formaldehyde.americanchemistry.com/Formaldehyde-Occurs-Naturally-and-Is-All-Around-Us.pdf [Accessed January 25, 2020].

[143] Shaffer MP, Belsito DV. Allergic Contact Dermatitis From Glutaraldehyde in Health-Care Workers. Contact Dermatitis. 2000 Sep;43(3):150-6.

[144] United States Centers for Disease Control and Prevention. Glutaraldehyde - Occupational Hazards in Hospitals. Available at: https://www.cdc.gov/niosh/docs/2001-115/default.html [Accessed January 25, 2020].

[145] Hanson JM, Plusa SM, Bennett MK, et al. Glutaraldehyde as a Possible Cause of Diarrhoea After Sigmoidoscopy. Br J Surg. 1998 Oct;85(10):1385-7.

[146] Ahishali E, Uygur-Bayramicli O, Dolapcioglu C, et al. Chemical Colitis Due to Glutaraldehyde: Case Series and Review of the Literature. Dig Dis Sci. 2009 Dec;54(12):2541-5.

[147] Marshall TM, Dardia GP, Colvin KL, et al. Neurotoxicity Associated With Traumatic Brain Injury, Blast, Chemical, Heavy Metal and Quinoline Drug Exposure. Altern Ther Health Med. 2019 Jan;25(1):28-34.

[148] Xiong JS, Branigan D, Li M, et al. Deciphering the MSG controversy. Int J Clin Exp Med. 2009;2(4):329–336.

[149] Yang WH, Drouin MA, Herbert M, et al. The monosodium glutamate symptom complex: assessment in a double-blind, placebo-controlled, randomized study. J Allergy Clin Immunol. 1997 Jun;99(6 Pt 1):757-62.

[150] Schaumburg HH, Byck R, Gerstl R, et al. Monosodium L-glutamate: its pharmacology and role in the Chinese restaurant syndrome. Science. 1969 Feb 21;163(3869):826-8.

[151] United States Environmental Protection Agency. Fact Sheet: Nonylphenols and Nonylphenol Ethoxylates. Available at: https://www.epa.gov/assessing-and-managing-chemicals-under-tsca/fact-sheet-nonylphenols-and-nonylphenol-ethoxylates [Accessed January 25, 2020].

[152] World Health Organization. INTEGRATED RISK ASSESSMENT: NONYLPHENOL CASE STUDY. Available at: https://www.who.int/ipcs/methods/Nonylphenol.pdf [Accessed January 25, 2020].

[153] United States Environmental Protection Agency. Technical Fact Sheet – 1,4-Dioxane, November 2017. Available at: https://www.epa.gov/sites/production/files/2014-03/documents/ffrro_factsheet_contaminant_14-dioxane_january2014_final.pdf [Accessed January 25, 2020].

[154] Oser BL, Oser M. Nutritional studies on rats of diets containing high levels of partial ester emulsifiers. II. Reproduction and lactation. J Nutr. 1956 Dec 10; 60(4):489-505.

[155] Sun W, Xie C, Wang H, et al. Specific Role of Polysorbate 80 Coating on the Targeting of Nanoparticles to the Brain. Biomaterials. 2004 Jul;25(15):3065-71.

[156] Gulyaev AE, Gelperina SE, Skidan IN, et al. Significant Transport of Doxorubicin Into the Brain With Polysorbate 80-coated Nanoparticles. Pharm Res. 1999 Oct;16(10):1564-9.

[157] Pardridge WM. The Blood-Brain Barrier: Bottleneck in Brain Drug Development. NeuroRx. 2005 Jan; 2(1): 3–14.

[158] Gajdová M, Jakubovsky J, Války J. Delayed effects of neonatal exposure to Tween 80 on female reproductive organs in rats. Food Chem Toxicol. 1993 Mar; 31(3):183-90.

[159] Little DT, Ward HRG. Adolescent Premature Ovarian Insufficiency Following Human Papillomavirus Vaccination: A Case Series Seen in General Practice. J Investig Med High Impact Case Rep. 2014 Oct-Dec;2(4):2324709614556129.

[160] Coors EA, Seybold H, Merk HF, et al. Polysorbate 80 in Medical Products and Nonimmunologic Anaphylactoid Reactions. Ann Allergy Asthma Immunol. 2005 Dec;95(6):593-9.

[161] Environmental Working Group. Polysorbate 20. Available at: https://www.ewg.org/skindeep/ingredients/705137-POLYSORBATE20/ [Accessed October 23, 2009].

[162] Greenwood J, Adu J, Davey AJ, et al. The Effect of Bile Salts on the Permeability and Ultrastructure of the Perfused, Energy-Depleted, Rat Blood-Brain Barrier. J Cereb Blood Flow Metab. 1991 Jul;11(4):644-54.

[163] Tomkins O, Friedman O, Ivens S, et al. Blood-brain Barrier Disruption Results in Delayed Functional and Structural Alterations in the Rat Neocortex. Neurobiol Dis. 2007 Feb;25(2)367-77.

[164] Kesarwani K, Gupta R, Mukerjee A. Bioavailability enhancers of herbal origin: an overview. Asian Pac J Trop Biomed. 2013 Apr;3(4):253-66.

[165] United States Centers for Disease Control and Prevention. Hepatitis B. Available at: https://www.cdc.gov/hepatitis/hbv/index.htm [Accessed January 22, 2020].

[166] Fattovich G, Bortolotti F, Donato F. Natural history of chronic hepatitis B: special emphasis on disease progression and prognostic factors. J Hepatol. 2008;48(2):335-52.

[167] United States Centers for Disease Control and Prevention. What is viral hepatitis? Available at: https://www.cdc.gov/hepatitis/abc/index.htm [Accessed January 22, 2020].

[168] Hatami H, Salehi M, Sanei E, et al. Intra-familial Transmission of Hepatitis B virus Infection in Zahedan. Iran Red Crescent Med J. 2013 Jan; 15(1): 4–8.

[169] Salkic NN, Zerem E, Zildzic M, et al. Risk factors for intrafamilial spread of hepatitis B in northeastern Bosnia and Herzegovina. Ann Saudi Med. 2009 Jan-Feb; 29(1): 41–45.

[170] United States Centers for Disease Control and Prevention. Hepatitis B in an extended family -- Alabama. Available at: https://www.cdc.gov/mmwr/preview/mmwrhtml/00001001.htm [Accessed January 23, 2020].

[171] Zervou EK, Gatselis NK, Xanthi E, et al. Intrafamilial Spread of Hepatitis B Virus Infection in Greece. *Eur J Gastroenterol Hepatol.* 2005 Sep;17(9):911-5.

[172] World Health Organization. Hepatitis B. Available at: https://www.who.int/news-room/fact-sheets/detail/hepatitis-b [Accessed January 22, 2022].

[173] Ringehan M, McKeating JA, Protzer U. Viral hepatitis and liver cancer. *Philos Trans R Soc Lond B Biol Sci.* 2017 Oct 19;372(1732):20160274.

[174] Beasley RP. Hepatitis B virus. The major etiology of hepatocellular carcinoma. *Cancer.* 1988;61(10):1942-56.

[175] McMahon BJ. The natural history of chronic hepatitis B virus infection. *Hepatology.* 2009;49(5 Suppl):S45-55.

[176] Ringehan M, McKeating JA, Protzer U. Viral hepatitis and liver cancer. *Philos Trans R Soc Lond B Biol Sci.* 2017 Oct 19;372(1732):20160274.

[177] American Cancer Society. Chronic viral hepatitis. Available at: https://www.cancer.org/cancer/liver-cancer/causes-risks-prevention/risk-factors.html [Accessed Jannuary 23, 2020].

[178] Fattovich G, Bortolotti F, Donato F. Natural history of chronic hepatitis B: special emphasis on disease progression and prognostic factors. *J Hepatol.* 2008 Feb; 48(2):335-52.

[179] World Health Organization. Hepatitis B. Available at: https://www.who.int/news-room/fact-sheets/detail/hepatitis-b [Accessed January 22, 2022].

[180] Bianconi E, Piovesan A, Facchin F, et al. An estimation of the number of cells in the human body. *Ann Hum Biol.* 2013 Nov-Dec;40(6):463-71.

[181] Ron Sender, Shai Fuchs, Ron Milo. Revised Estimates for the Number of Human and Bacteria Cells in the Body. *PLoS Biol.* 2016 Aug;14(8):e1002533.

[182] Wylie KM, Weinstock GM, Storch GA. Emerging view of the human virome. *Transl Res.* 2012 Oct;160(4):283-90.

[183] Williams SCP. The other microbiome. *PNAS.* 2013 Feb 19;10(8):2682-84.

[184] Wilke CO, Sawyer SL. At the mercy of viruses. *eLife.* 2016;5:e16758.

[185] David Enard, Le Cai, Carina Gwennap, Dmitri A Petrov. Viruses are a dominant driver of protein adaptation in mammals. *eLife.* 2016 May 17;5:e12469.

[186] Raviram R, Rocha PP, Luo VM, et al. Analysis of 3D genomic interactions identifies candidate host genes that transposable elements potentially regulate. *Genome Biol.* 2018 Dec 13;19(1):216.

[187] Her M, Kavanaugh A. Alterations in immune function with biologic therapies for autoimmune disease. *J Allergy Clin Immunol.* 2016 Jan;137(1):19-27.

[188] O'Shea DO, Hogan AE. Dysregulation of Natural Killer Cells in Obesity. *Cancers.* 2019;11(4):573.

[189] Lazzerini PE, Hamilton RM, Boutjdir M. Editorial: Cardioimmunology: Inflammation and Immunity in Cardiovascular Disease. *Front Cardiovasc Med.* 2019;6: 181.

[190] Graves DT, Kayal RA. Diabetic complications and dysregulated innate immunity. *Front Biosci.* 2008 Jan 1;13:1227–1239.

[191] Marsland BJ, Konigshoff M, Saglani S, et al. Immune system dysregulation in chronic lung disease. *Eur Respiratory J.* 2011 Jan;38:500-01.

[192] Elia RV, Harrison K, Oyston PC, et al. Targeting the "Cytokine Storm" for Therapeutic Benefit. *Clin Vaccine Immunol.* 2013 Mar;20(3):319–327.

[193] Zhang Y, Li J, Zhan Y, et al. Analysis of serum cytokines in patients with severe acute respiratory syndrome. Infect Immun. 2004;72:4410–4415.

[194] United States Food and Drug Administration. Package Insert – Recombivax HB. Available at: https://www.fda.gov/files/vaccines%2C%20blood%20%26%20biologics/published/package-insert-recombivax-hb.pdf [Accessed January 23, 2020].

[195] United States Food and Drug Administration. Package Insert – Energix-B. Available at: https://www.fda.gov/media/119403/download [Accessed January 23, 2020].

[196] United States Food and Drug Administration. HEPLISAV-B [Hepatitis B Vaccine (Recombinant), Adjuvanted]. Available at: https://www.fda.gov/media/108745/download [Accessed January 23, 2020].

[197] Miller H, Cendrowski W, Schapira K. Multiple sclerosis and vaccination. *Br Med J.* 1967;2:210-13.

[198] Stovicek J. [Effect of Vaccination and Therapeutic Sera on the Appearance and Course of Multiple Sclerosis]. *Cesk Neurol.* 1959 Jul;22:343-8.

[199] Palffy G, Merei FT. The Possible Role of Vaccines and Sera in the Pathogenesis of Multiple Sclerosis. *World Neurol.* 1961 feb;2:167-72.

[200] McAlpine, D, et al. Multiple Sclerosis – A Reappraisal. E & S Livingstone Ltd (1965).

[201] Zipp F, Weil JG, Einhäupl KM. No increase in demyelinating diseases after hepatitis B vaccination. *Nat Med.* 1999 Sep;5(9):964-5.

[202] Sadovnick AD, Scheifele DW. School-based hepatitis B vaccination programme and adolescent multiple sclerosis. *Lancet.* 2000;355(9203):549-50.

[203] Ascherio A, Zhang SM, Hernan MA, et al. Hepatitis B vaccination and the risk of multiple sclerosis. *N Engl J Med.* 2001;344(5):327-32.

[204] DeStephano F, Verstraeten T, Jackson LA, et al. Vaccinations and risk of central nervous system demyelinating diseases in adults. *Arch Neurol.* 2003;60(4):504-9.

[205] Ramagopalan SV, Valdar W, Dyment DA, et al. Canadian Collaborative Study Group. Association of infectious mononucleosis with multiple sclerosis. A population-based study. Neuroepidemiology. 2009 Apr;32(4):257-62.

[206] Touze E, Fourrier A, Rue-Fenouche C, et al. Hepatitis B vaccination and first central nervous system demyelinating event: a case–control study. *Neuroepidemiology.* 2002 Jul-Aug;21(4):180-6.

[207] Sturkenboom MCJM, Abenhaim L, Wolfson C, et al. Vaccinations, demyelination and multiple sclerosis study, a population-based study (VDAMS): a population-based study in the UK. *Pharmacoepidemiol Drug Saf.* 1999;8:S170–S171.

[208] Fourrier A, Begaud B, Alperovitch A, et al. Hepatitis B vaccine and first episodes of central nervous system demyelinating disorders: a comparison between reported and expected number of cases. *Br J Clin Pharmacol.* 2001 May;51(5):489-90.

[209] ANSM. Vaccination anti-Hépatite B, mise à jour des données et des études de pharmacovigilance. Février 2000 (in French). Available at: http://ansm.sante.fr/var/ansm_site/storage/original/application/b460abed4a9a61d8dad78d4364033354.pdf. [Accessed February 15, 2020].

[210] Hernan MA, Jock SS, Olek MJ, et al. Recombinant Hepatitis B Vaccine and the Risk of Multiple Sclerosis: A Prospective Study. Neurology. 2004 Sep 14;63(5):838-42.

[211] Geier DA, geier MR. A case-control study of serious autoimmune adverse events following hepatitis B immunization. *Autoimmunity.* 2005 Jun;38(4):295-301.

[212] Mikaeloff Y, Caridabe G, Suissa S, et al. Hepatitis B Vaccine and the Risk of CNS Inflammatory Demyelination in Childhood. *Neurology.* 2009 Mar 10;72(10):873-80.

[213] Houezec DL. Evolution of multiple sclerosis in France since the beginning of hepatitis B vaccination. *Immunol Res.* 2014;60(2-3):219–225.

[214] Caporale CM, Papola F, Fiorini MA, et al. Susceptibility to Guillain-Barré Syndrome Is Associated to Polymorphisms of CD1 Genes. *J Neuroimmunol.* 2006 Aug;177(1-2):112-8.

[215] Souayah N, Nasar A, Suri MF, et al. Guillain-Barré Syndrome After Vaccination in United States: Data From the Centers for Disease Control and Prevention/Food and Drug Administration Vaccine Adverse Event Reporting System (1990-2005). *J Clin Neuromuscul Dis.* 2009 Sep;11(1):1-6.

[216] Gallagher C, Goodman M. Hepatitis B triple series vaccine and developmental disability in US children aged 1–9 years. *Toxicol Environ Chem.* 2008;90(5):997-1008.

[217] Geier DA, Kern JK, Homme KG, et al. A Cross-Sectional Study of the Association between Infant Hepatitis B Vaccine Exposure in Boys and the Risk of Adverse Effects as Measured by Receipt of Special Education Services. *Int J Environ Res Public Health.* 2018 Jan;15(1):123.

[218] Geier DA, Kern JK, Hooker BS, et al. A longitudinal cohort study of the relationship between Thimerosal-containing hepatitis B vaccination and specific delays in development in the United States: Assessment of attributable risk and lifetime care costs. *J Epidemiology Global Health.* 2016 Jun;6(2):105-18.

[219] Kern JK, Geier D, Sykes LK, et al. The Relationship Between Mercury and Autism: A Comprehensive Review and Discussion. *J Trace Elem Med Biol.* 2016 Sep;37:8-24.

[220] Gallagher CM, Goodman MS. Hepatitis B Vaccination of Male Neonates and Autism Diagnosis, NHIS 1997–2002. *J Toxicol Environ Health Pt A.* 2010;73(24):1665-77.

[221] Rogers TD, McKimm E, Dickson PE, et al. Is autism a disease of the cerebellum? An integration of clinical and pre-clinical research. *Front Syst Neurosci.* 2013;7:15.

[222] Wang SSH, Kloth AD, Badura A. The Cerebellum, Sensitive Periods, and Autism. *Neuron.* 2014 Aug 6;83(3):518–532.

[223] Bruchhage MMK, Bucc MP, Becker EBE. Cerebellar Involvement in Autism and ADHD. *Handb Clin Neurol.* 2018;155:61-72.

[224] Institute of Medicine (US) Immunization Safety Review Committee; Stratton K, Almario D, McCormick MC, editors. Immunization Safety Review: Hepatitis B Vaccine and Demyelinating Neurological Disorders. *National Academies Press (US);* 2002.

[225] Geier DA, Geier MR. A One Year Followup of Chronic Arthritis Following Rubella and Hepatitis B Vaccination Based Upon Analysis of the Vaccine Adverse Events Reporting System (VAERS) Database. *Clin Exp Rheumatol*. 2002 Nov-Dec;20(6):767-71.

[226] Pope JE, Stevens A, Howson W, et al. The Development of Rheumatoid Arthritis After Recombinant Hepatitis B Vaccination. *J Rheumatol*. 1998 Sep;25(9):1687-93.

[227] Tanjena V, David CS. Association of MHC and rheumatoid arthritis: Regulatory role of HLA class II molecules in animal models of RA - studies on transgenic/knockout mice. *Arthritis Res*. 2000;2(3):205–207.

[228] Kampstra ASB, Toes REM. HLA class II and rheumatoid arthritis: the bumpy road of revelation. *Immunogenetics*. 2017;69(8):597–603.

[229] Attia AM, Attalla SM, Shaat RM, et al. Study of The Role of Mercury Poisoning in Rheumatoid Arthritis Patients and Its Relation with Zinc and Copper Levels. *Mansoura J Forensic Med Clin Toxicol*. 2012 Summer-Autumn;20(2):49-64.

[230] Pamphlett R, Jew SK. Mercury Is Taken Up Selectively by Cells Involved in Joint, Bone, and Connective Tissue Disorders. *Front Med (Lausanne)*. 2019 Jul 19;6:168.

[231] Troeger C, Khalil IA, Rao PC. Rotavirus Vaccination and the Global Burden of Rotavirus Diarrhea Among Children Younger Than 5 Years. *JAMA Pediatr*. 2018 Oct;172(1):958-65.

[232] Dennehy PH. Rotavirus Vaccines: an Overview. *Clin Microbiol Rev*. 2008 Jan;21(1):198–208.

[233] United States Centers for Disease Control and Prevention. Rotavirus. Available at: https://www.cdc.gov/vaccines/pubs/pinkbook/downloads/rota.pdf [Accessed January 24, 2020].

[234] World Health Organization. Estimated rotavirus deaths for children under five years of age: 2013, 215 000. Available at: https://www.who.int/immunization/monitoring_surveillance/burden/estimates/rotavirus/en/ [Accessed January 24, 2020].

[235] Troeger C, Khalil IA, Rao PC. Rotavirus Vaccination and the Global Burden of Rotavirus Diarrhea Among Children Younger Than 5 Years. *JAMA Pediatr*. 2018 Oct;172(1):958-65.

[236] Bruijning-Verhagen P, Nipshagen MD, Graaf HD, et al. Rotavirus Disease Course Among Immunocompromised Patients; 5-year Observations From a Tertiary Care Medical Centre. *J Infect*. 2017 Nov;75(5):448-454.

[237] United States Centers for Disease Control and Prevention. Questions & Answers about Intussusception and Rotavirus Vaccine. Available at: https://www.cdc.gov/vaccines/vpd/rotavirus/about-intussusception.html [Accessed January 24, 2020].

[238] Bucardo F, Reyes Y, Ronnelid Y, et al. Histo-blood group antigens and rotavirus vaccine shedding in Nicaraguan infants. *Sci Rep*. 2019 Jul 24;9(1):10764.

[239] Ye S, Whiley DM, Ware RS, et al. Multivalent Rotavirus Vaccine and Wild-type Rotavirus Strain Shedding in Australian Infants: A Birth Cohort Study. Clin Infect Dis. 2018 Apr 17;66(9):1411-1418.

[240] Anderson EJ. Rotavirus Vaccines: Viral Shedding and Risk of Transmission. *Lancet Infect Dis*. 2008 Oct;8(10):642-9.

[241] United States Food and Drug Administration. Rotateq® Package Insert - 2/23/2017. Available at: https://www.fda.gov/media/75718/download [Accessed January 24, 2020].

[242] United States Food and Drug Administration. Package Insert and Patient Information-Rotarix. Available at: https://www.fda.gov/media/75726/download [Accessed January 24, 2020].

[243] Bakare N, Menschik D, Tiernan R, et al. Severe Combined Immunodeficiency (SCID) and Rotavirus Vaccination: Reports to the Vaccine Adverse Events Reporting System (VAERS). *Vaccine*. 2010 Sep 14;28(40):6609-12.

[244] United States Food and Drug Administration. Rotateq® Package Insert - 2/23/2017. Available at: https://www.fda.gov/media/75718/download [Accessed January 24, 2020].

[245] United States Food and Drug Administration. Package Insert and Patient Information-Rotarix. Available at: https://www.fda.gov/media/75726/download [Accessed January 24, 2020].

[246] Geier DA, King PG, Sykes LK, et al. The Temporal Relationship Between RotaTeq Immunization and Intussusception Adverse Events in the Vaccine Adverse Event Reporting System (VAERS). Med Sci Monit. 2012 Feb;18(2):PH12-17.

[247] Geier DA, King PG, Sykes LK, et al. RotaTeq Vaccine Adverse Events and Policy Considerations. Med Sci Monit. 2008 Mar;14(3)PH9-16.

[248] Koch J, Harder T, von Kried R, et al. Risk of Intussusception After Rotavirus Vaccination: A Systematic Literature Review and Meta-Analysis. *Dtsch Arztebl Int*. 2017 Apr;114(15):255–262.

[249] Buettcher M, Baer G, Bonhoeffer J, et al. Three-year surveillance of intussusception in children in Switzerland. *Pediatrics*. 2007;120(3):473-80

[250] Clark AD, Hasso-Agopsowicz M, Kraus MW, et al. Update on the global epidemiology of intussusception: a systematic review of incidence rates, age distributions and case-fatality ratios among children aged <5 years, before the introduction of rotavirus vaccination. *In J Epidemiol*. 2019 Aug;48(4):1316-26.

[251] Kramer A, Schwebke I, Kampf G. How long do nosocomial pathogens persist on inanimate surfaces? A systematic review. *BMC Infect Dis*. 2006 Aug 16;6:130.

[252] Clarke KEN, MacNeil A, Hadler S, et al. Global Epidemiology of Diphtheria, 2000–2017. *Synopsis*. 2019 Oct;25(10):1834-42.

[253] Clarke KEN, MacNeil A, Hadler S, et al. Global Epidemiology of Diphtheria, 2000–2017. *Synopsis*. 2019 Oct;25(10):1834-42.

[254] Clarke KEN, MacNeil A, Hadler S, et al. Global Epidemiology of Diphtheria, 2000–2017. *Synopsis*. 2019 Oct;25(10):1834-42.

[255] The immunization Advisory Centre. Tetanus. Available at: https://www.immune.org.nz/diseases/tetanus [Accessed January 25, 2020].

[256] The immunization Advisory Centre. Tetanus. Available at: https://www.immune.org.nz/diseases/tetanus [Accessed January 25, 2020].

[257] Pascual FB, McGinley EL, Zanardi LR, et al. Tetanus surveillance--United States, 1998—2000. *MMWR Surveill Summ*. 2003;52(3):1-8.

[258] World Health Organization. Pertussis. Available at: https://www.who.int/immunization/monitoring_surveillance/burden/vpd/surveillance_type/passive/pertussis/en/ [Accessed January 25, 2020].

[259] Yeung KHT, Duclos P, Nelson EAS, et al. An Update of the Global Burden of Pertussis in Children Younger Than 5 Years: A Modelling Study. *Lancet Infect Dis*. 2017 Sep;17(9):974-80.

[260] United States Centers for Disease Control and Prevention. Diphtheria. Available at: https://www.cdc.gov/diphtheria/clinicians.html [Accessed January 25, 2020].

[261] United States Centers for Disease Control and Prevention. Tetanus. Available at: https://www.cdc.gov/vaccines/pubs/pinkbook/tetanus.html [Accessed January 25, 2020].

[262] Our World in Data. Tetanus. Available at: https://ourworldindata.org/tetanus [Accessed January 25, 2020].

[263] World Health Organization. Immunization, Vaccines and Biologicals. Available at: https://www.who.int/immunization/diseases/tetanus/en/ [Accessed January 25, 2020].

[264] United States Centers for Disease Control and Prevention. Pertussis. Available at: https://www.cdc.gov/pertussis/about/complications.html [Accessed January 25, 2020].

[265] United States Centers for Disease Control and Prevention. Pertussis. Available at: https://www.cdc.gov/pertussis/about/complications.html [Accessed January 25, 2020].

[266] United States Centers for Disease Control and Prevention. Pertussis frequently asked questions. Available at: https://www.cdc.gov/pertussis/about/faqs.html [Accessed January 25, 2020].

[267] United States Food and Drug Administration. Sanofi Pasteur 253 – Daptacel. Available at: https://www.fda.gov/files/vaccines%2C%20blood%20%26%20biologics/published/Package-Insert---DAPTACEL.pdf [Accessed January 25, 2020].

[268] United States Food and Drug Administration. Infanrix. Available at: https://www.fda.gov/media/75157/download [Accessed January 25, 2020].

[269] United States Food and Drug Administration. Highlights of Prescribing Information, Kinrix. Available at: https://www.fda.gov/media/80128/download [Accessed January 25, 2020].

[270] United States Food and Drug Administration. Highlights of Prescribing Information, Pediarix. Available at: https://www.gsksource.com/pharma/content/dam/GlaxoSmithKline/US/en/Prescribing_Information/Pediarix/pdf/PEDIARIX.PDF [Accessed January 25, 2020].

[271] United States Food and Drug Administration. Sanofi Pasteur 242 – Pentacel. Available at: https://www.fda.gov/media/74385/download [Accessed January 25, 2020].

[272] United States Food and Drug Administration. Sanofi Pasteur 243 – Quadracel. Available at: https://www.fda.gov/media/91640/download [Accessed January 25, 2020].

[273] United States Food and Drug Administration. Sanofi Pasteur 306 – Adacel. Available at: https://www.fda.gov/files/vaccines%2C%20blood%20%26%20biologics/published/Package-Insert---Adacel.pdf [Accessed January 25, 2020].

[274] United States Food and Drug Administration. Highlights of prescribing information, Boostrix. Available at: https://gsksource.com/pharma/content/dam/GlaxoSmithKline/US/en/Prescribing_Information/Boostrix/pdf/BOOSTRIX.PDF [Accessed January 25, 2020].

[275] United States Food and Drug Administration. Sanofi Pasteur Full Prescribing Information, 426 – Diphtheria and Tetanus Toxoids Adsorbed. Available at: https://www.fda.gov/media/75962/download [Accessed January 25, 2020].

[276] United States Food and Drug Administration. HIGHLIGHTS OF PRESCRIBING INFORMATION, TENIVAC. Available at: https://www.fda.gov/media/76610/download [Accessed January 25, 2020].

[277] United States Food and Drug Administration. Package Insert - TDVAX (NDC 14362-0111). Available at: https://www.fda.gov/media/76430/download [Accessed January 25, 2020].

[278] Vaccineshoppe.com. Tetanus Toxin Adsorbed. Available at: https://www.vaccineshoppe.com/image.cfm?doc_id=5976&image_type=product_pdf [Accessed January 25, 2020].

[279] Bart MJ, Harris SR, Advani A, et al. Global Population Structure and Evolution of Bordetella pertussis and Their Relationship with Vaccination. *mBio*. 2014 Apr 22;5(2):e01074.

[280] Moori FR, van Loo IHM, van Gent M, et al. Bordetella pertussis Strains with Increased Toxin Production Associated with Pertussis Resurgence. *Emerg Infect Dis*. 2009 Aug;15(8):1206–1213.

[281] Schmidtke AJ, Boney KO, Martin SW, et al. Population Diversity Among Bordetella Pertussis Isolates, United States, 1935-2009. *Emerg Infect Dis*. 2012 Aug;18(8):248-55.

[282] Mooi FR, van Der Maas NAT, de Melker HE. Pertussis resurgence: waning immunity and pathogen adaptation – two sides of the same coin. 2014 Apr;142(4):685-94.

[283] Cherry JD. Why do pertussis vaccine fail? *Pediatrics*. 2012 May 1;129(5):968-70.

[284] Cherry JD. Epidemic pertussis in 2012 — the resurgence of a vaccine-preventable disease. *N Engl J Med*. 2012 Aug;367(9):785-87.

[285] Cherry JD. Pertussis: Challenges today and for the future. *PLoS Pathog*. 2013;9(7):e1003418.

[286] Queenan AM, Cassiday PK, Evangelista A. Pertactin-negative variants of Bordetella pertussis in the United States. *N Engl J Med*. 2013 Feb 7;368(6):5843-4.

[287] Otsuka N, Han HJ, Toyoizumi-Ajisaka H, et al. *PLoS One*. 2012;7(2):e31985.

[288] Stefanelli P, Faxio C, Fedele G, et al. A Natural Pertactin Deficient Strain of Bordetella Pertussis Shows Improved Entry in Human Monocyte-Derived Dendritic Cells. New Microbiol. 2009 Apr;32(2)159-66.

[289] Barkoff AM, Mertsola J, Pierard D, et al. Pertactin-deficient Bordetella pertussis isolates: evidence of increased circulation in Europe, 1998 to 2015. *Euro Surveill*. 2019 Feb 14;24(7):1700832.

[290] Octavia S, Sintchenko V, Gilbert GL, et al. Newly Emerging Clones of Bordetella Pertussis Carrying prn2 and ptxP3 Alleles Implicated in Australian Pertussis Epidemic in 2008-2010. J Infect Dis. 2012 Apr 5;205(8):1220-4.

[291] van Boven M, Mooi FR, Schellekens JFP, et al. Pathogen Adaptation Under Imperfect Vaccination: Implications for Pertussis. Proc Biol Sci. 2005 Aug 7;272(1572):1617-24.

[292] Cherry JD, Seaton BL. Patterns of Bordetella parapertussis respiratory illnesses: 2008-2010. *Clin Infect Dis*. 2012 Feb15;54(4):534-7.

[293] Guiso N. Bordetella pertussis and pertussis vaccines. *Clin Infect Dis*. 2009 Nov 15;49(10):1565-69.

[294] Liese JG, Renner C, Stojanov S, et al. Clinical and Epidemiological Picture of B Pertussis and B Parapertussis Infections After Introduction of Acellular Pertussis Vaccines. Arch Dis Child. 2003 Aug;88(8):684-7.

[295] Kamiya H, Otsuka N, Ando Y, et al. Transmission of Bordetella holmesii during Pertussis Outbreak, Japan. *Emerg Infect Dis*. 2012 Jul;18(7):1166–1169.

[296] Long GH, Karanikas AT, Harvill ET, et al. Acellular Pertussis Vaccination Facilitates Bordetella Parapertussis Infection in a Rodent Model of Bordetellosis. *Proc Biol Sci*. 2010 Jul 7;277(1690):2017-25.

[297] Zhang X, Weyrich LS, Lavine JS, et al. Lack of Cross-protection against Bordetella holmesii after Pertussis Vaccination. *Emerg Infect Dis*. 2012 Nov;18(11):1771–1779.

[298] Pittet LF, Emonet S, Schrenzel J, et al. Bordetella Holmesii: An Under-Recognised Bordetella Species. Lancet Infect Dis. 2014 Jun;14(6):510-9.

[299] Hergele N, Paris AS, Brun D, et al. Evolution of French Bordetella Pertussis and Bordetella Parapertussis Isolates: Increase of Bordetellae Not Expressing Pertactin. Clin Microbiol Infect. 2012 Sep;18(9):E340-6.

[300] Zerbo O, Bartlett J, Goddard K, et al. Acellular Pertussis Vaccine Effectiveness Over Time. *Pediatrics*. 2019 Jul;144(1):e20183466.

[301] Tartof SY, Lewis M, Kenyon C, et al. Waning Immunity to Pertussis Following 5 Doses of DTaP. Pediatrics. 2013 Apr;131(4):e1047-52.

[302] Barkoff AM, Mertsola J, Guillot S, et al. Appearance of Bordetella Pertussis Strains Not Expressing the Vaccine Antigen Pertactin in Finland. *Clin Vaccine Immunol*. 2012 Oct;19(10):1703-4.

300

[303] Acosta AM, DeBolt C, Tasslimi A, et al. Tdap Vaccine Effectiveness in Adolescents During the 2012 Washington State Pertussis Epidemic. *Pediatrics*. 2015 Jun;135(6):981-9.

[304] Althouse BM, Scarpino SV. Asymptomatic transmission and the resurgence of Bordetella pertussis. *BMC Medicine*. 2015;13(1):146.

[305] Lam C, Octavia S, icafort L, et al. Rapid Increase in Pertactin-deficient Bordetella pertussis Isolates, Australia. *Emerg Infect Dis*. 2014 May;20(4):626-33.

[306] Munoz FM. Safer Pertussis Vaccines for Children: Trading Efficacy for Safety. *Pediatrics*. 2018 Jul;142(1):e20181036.

[307] Sun Y, Christnense J, Hviid A, et al. Risk of Febrile Seizures and Epilepsy After Vaccination With Diphtheria, Tetanus, Acellular Pertussis, Inactivated Poliovirus, and Haemophilus Influenzae Type B. *JAMA*. 2012 Feb 22;307(8):823-31.

[308] Barloe WE, Davis RL, Glasser JW, et al. The Risk of Seizures After Receipt of Whole-Cell Pertussis or Measles, Mumps, and Rubella Vaccine. *N Engl J Med*. 2001 Aug 30;345(9):656-61.

[309] Pruna D, Balestri P, Zamponi N, et al. Epilepsy and Vaccinations: Italian Guidelines. *Epilepsia*. 2013 Oct;54(Suppl 7):13-22.

[310] Tartof SY, Tseng HF, Liu AL, et al. Exploring the Risk Factors for Vaccine-Associated and Non-Vaccine Associated Febrile Seizures in a Large Pediatric Cohort. *Vaccine*. 2014 May 7;32(22):2574-81.

[311] Principi N, Esposito S. Vaccines and Febrile Seizures. *Expert Rev Vaccines*. 2013 Aug;12(8):885-92.

[312] Gold M, Dugdale S, Woodman RJ, et al. Use of the Australian Childhood Immunisation Register for Vaccine Safety Data Linkage. *Vaccine*. 2010 Jun 11;28(26):4308-11.

[313] Miller E, Andrews N, Stowe J, et al. Risks of Convulsion and Aseptic Meningitis Following Measles-Mumps-Rubella Vaccination in the United Kingdom. *Am J Epidemiol*. 2007 Mar 15;165(6):704-9.

[314] Feenstra B, Pasternak B, Geller F, et al. Common Variants Associated With General and MMR Vaccine-Related Febrile Seizures. *Nat Genet*. 2014 Dec;46(12):1274-82.

[315] Feenstra B, Pasternak B, Geller F, et al. Common Variants Associated With General and MMR Vaccine-Related Febrile Seizures. *Nat Genet*. 2014 Dec;46(12):1274-82.

[316] Klein NP, Fireman B, Yih WK, et al. Measles-mumps-rubella-varicella Combination Vaccine and the Risk of Febrile Seizures. *Pediatrics*. 2010 Jul;126(1):e1-8.

[317] O'Leary ST, Suh CA, Marin M, et al. Febrile Seizures and Measles-Mumps-Rubella-Varicella (MMRV) Vaccine: What Do Primary Care Physicians Think? *Vaccine*. 2012 Nov 6;30(48):6731-3.

[318] MacDonald SE, Dover DC, Simmonds KA, et al. Risk of Febrile Seizures After First Dose of Measles-Mumps-Rubella-Varicella Vaccine: A Population-Based Cohort Study. *CMAJ*. 2014 Aug 5;186(11):824-9.

[319] Schink T, Holstiege J, Garbe E. Risk of Febrile Convulsions After MMRV Vaccination in Comparison to MMR or MMR+V Vaccination. *Vaccine*. 2013 Feb;32(6):645-50.

[320] Schink T, Holstiege J, Garbe E. Risk of Febrile Convulsions After MMRV Vaccination in Comparison to MMR or MMR+V Vaccination. *Vaccine*. 2013 Feb;32(6):645-50.

[321] Ma SJ, Xiong YQ, Jiang LN, et al. Risk of Febrile Seizure After Measles-Mumps-Rubella-Varicella Vaccine: A Systematic Review and Meta-Analysis. *Vaccine*. 2015 Jul 17;33(31):3636-49.

[322] Vestergaard M, HviiD A, Madsen KM, et al. MMR Vaccination and Febrile Seizures: Evaluation of Susceptible Subgroups and Long-Term Prognosis. *JAMA*. 2014 Jul 21;292(3):351-7.

[323] Li X, Yao G, Wang, Y. The Influence of Vaccine on Febrile Seizure. *Curr Neuropharmacol*. 2018;16(1):59-65.

[324] Ma SJ, Xiong YQ, Jiang LN, et al. Risk of Febrile Seizure After Measles-Mumps-Rubella-Varicella Vaccine: A Systematic Review and Meta-Analysis. *Vaccine*. 2015 Jul 17;33(31):3636-49.

[325] von Spiczak S, Helbig I, Drechsel-Baeuerle U, et al. A Retrospective Population-Based Study on Seizures Related to Childhood Vaccination. *Epilepsia*. 2011 Aug;52(8):1506-12.

[326] Hurwitz EL, Morgenstern H. Effects of diphtheria-tetanus-pertussis or tetanus vaccination on allergies and allergy-related respiratory symptoms among children and adolescents in the United States. *J Manipulative physiol Therap*. 2000 Feb;23(2):81-90.

[327] Odent MR, Culpin EE, Kimmel T. Pertussis vaccination and asthma: Is there a link? *JAMA*. 1994;272(8):592-3.

[328] Bernsen RMD, Nagelkerke NJD, Thijs C, et al. Reported Pertussis Infection and Risk of Atopy in 8- To 12-yr-old Vaccinated and Non-Vaccinated Children. *Pediatr Allergy Immunol*. 2008 Feb;19(1):46-52.

[329] Kemp T, Pearce N, Fitzharris P, et al. Is Infant Immunization a Risk Factor for Childhood Asthma or Allergy? *Epidemiology*. 1997 Nov;8(6):678-80.

[330] McDonald KL, Huq SI, Lix LM, et al. Delay in Diphtheria, Pertussis, Tetanus Vaccination Is Associated With a Reduced Risk of Childhood Asthma. *J Allergy Clin Immunol*. 2008 Mar;121(3):626-31.

[331] Bremner SSA, Carey IM, DeWilde S, et al. Timing of Routine Immunisations and Subsequent Hay Fever Risk. *Arch Dis Child*. 2005 Jun;90(6):567-73.

[332] Bernsen RM, Nagelkerke NJ, Thijs C, et al. Reported Pertussis Infection and Risk of Atopy in 8- To 12-yr-old Vaccinated and Non-Vaccinated Children. *Pediatr Allergy Immunol*. 2008 Feb;19(1):46-52.

[333] L Nilsson, N-IM Kjellman, J Storsaeter, et al. Lack of association between pertussis vaccination and symptoms of asthma and allergy [letter]. *JAMA*. 1996;275:760.

[334] J Henderson, K North, M Griffiths, et al. Pertussis vaccination and wheezing illnesses in young children: prospective cohort study. *BMJ*. 1999;318:1173-1176

[335] Mogensen SW, Andersen A, Rodrigues A, et al. The Introduction of Diphtheria-Tetanus-Pertussis and Oral Polio Vaccine Among Young Infants in an Urban African Community: A Natural Experiment. *EBioMedicine*. 2017 Mar;17:192-198.

[336] Aaby P, Mogensen SW, Rodrigues A, et al. Evidence of Increase in Mortality After the Introduction of Diphtheria-Tetanus-Pertussis Vaccine to Children Aged 6-35 Months in Guinea-Bissau: A Time for Reflection? *Front Public Health*. 2018 Mar 19;6:79.

[337] Higgins JP, Soares-Weiser K, López-López JA, et al. Association of BCG, DTP, and measles containing vaccines with childhood mortality: systematic review. *BMJ*. 2016 Oct 13;355:i5170.

[338] United States Food and Drug Administration. Package Insert – VAXELIS. Available at: https://www.fda.gov/media/119465/download [Accessed February 22, 2020].

[339] Filiano JJ, Kinney HC. Arcuate Nucleus Hypoplasia in the Sudden Infant Death Syndrome. *J Neuropathol Exp Neurol*. 1992 Jul;51(4):394-403.

[340] von Kries R, Tosche AM, Strassburger K, et al. Sudden and Unexpected Deaths After the Administration of Hexavalent Vaccines (Diphtheria, Tetanus, Pertussis, Poliomyelitis, Hepatitis B, Haemophilius Influenzae Type B): Is There a Signal? *Eur J Pediatr*. 2005 Feb;164(2):61-9.

[341] Traversa G, Spila-Alegiani S, Bianchi C, et al. Sudden Unexpected Deaths and Vaccinations during the First Two Years of Life in Italy: A Case Series Study. *PLoS One*. 2011 Jan;6(1):e16363.

[342] Kuhnert R, Hecker H, Pothko-Muller C, et al. A Modified Self-Controlled Case Series Method to Examine Association Between Multidose Vaccinations and Death. *Stat Med*. 2011 Mar 15;30(6):666-77.

[343] GlaxoSmithKilne. Bridging clinical safety and pharmacovigilance confidential report to regulatory authorities on Infanrix hexa (combined diphtheria, tetanus, and acellular pertussis, hepatitis B, inactivated poliomyelitis, and Haemophilus influenzae type B vaccine), October 23, 2009 to October 22, 2011. *GSK Confidential Summary Bridging Report*. 2011 Dec 16:246-9.

[344] Puliyel J, Sathyamala C. Comment: Infanrix hexa and sudden death: a review of the periodic safety update reports submitted to the European Medicines Agency. *Indian J Med Ethics*. 2018;3(1).

[345] Zinka B, Rauch E, Buettner A, et al. Unexplained cases of sudden infant death shortly after hexavalent vaccination. *Vaccine*. 2006 Jul 26;24(31-32):5779-80.

[346] D'Errico S, Neri M, Riezzo I, et al. β-Tryptase and quantitative mast-cell increase in a sudden infant death following hexavalent immunization. *Forensic Sci Int*. 2008 Aug 6;179(2-3):e25-e29.

[347] Ottaviani G, Lavezzi AM, Matturri L. Sudden Infant Death Syndrome (SIDS) Shortly After Hexavalent Vaccination: Another Pathology in Suspected SIDS? *Virchows Arch*. 2006 Jan;448(1):100-4.

[348] Matturri L, Corno GD, Lavezzi AM. Sudden Infant Death Following Hexavalent Vaccination: A Neuropathologic Study. *Curr Med Chem*. 2014 Mar;21(7):941-6.

[349] Baldo V, Bonanni P, Castro M, et al. Combined Hexavalent Diphtheria-Tetanus-Acellular Pertussis-Hepatitis B-inactivated poliovirus-Haemophilus Influenzae Type B Vaccine; Infanrix™ Hexa: Twelve Years of Experience in Italy. *Hum Vaccin Immunother*. 2014;10(1):129-37.

[350] Orsi A, Azzari C, Bozzola E, et al. Hexavalent vaccines: characteristics of available products and practical considerations from a panel of Italian experts. *J Prev Med Hyg*. 2018 Jun;59(2):E107–E119.

[351] Omenenaca F, Vazquez L, Garcia-Corbeira P, et al. Immunization of Preterm Infants With GSK's Hexavalent Combined Diphtheria-Tetanus-Acellular Pertussis-Hepatitis B-inactivated poliovirus-Haemophilus Influenzae Type B Conjugate Vaccine: A Review of Safety and Immunogenicity. *Vaccine*. 2018 Feb 8;36(7):986-996.

[352] Osawa M, Nagao R, Kakimoto Y, et al. Sudden Infant Death After Vaccination Survey of Forensic Autopsy Files. *Am J Forensic Med Pathol*. 2019 Sep;40(3):232-7.

[353] Moro PL, Perez-Vilar S, Lewis P, et al. Safety Surveillance of Diphtheria and Tetanus Toxoids and Acellular Pertussis (DTaP) Vaccines. *Pediatrics*. 2018;142(1):e20174171.

[354] Moro PL, Arana J, Cano M, et al. Deaths Reported to the Vaccine Adverse Event Reporting System, United States, 1997-2013. *Clin Infect Dis*. 2015;61(6):980-7.

[355] Eriksen EM, Perlman JA, Miller A, et al. Lack of association between hepatitis B birth immunization and neonatal death: a population-based study from the vaccine safety datalink project. *Pediatr Infect Dis J.* 2004;23(7):656-62.

[356] Griffin MR, Ray WA, Livengood JR, et al. Risk of sudden infant death syndrome after immunization with diphtheria-tetanus-pertussis vaccine. *N Engl J Med.* 1988 Sep 8;319(10):618-23.

[357] Institute of Medicine (US) Immunization Safety Review Committee. Immunization Safety Review: Vaccinations and Sudden Unexpected Death in Infancy. Washington, DC: National Academies Press, 2003.

[358] Institute of Medicine (US) Vaccine Safety Committee: Stratton KR, Howe CJ, Johnston Jr RB. Adverse Events Associated With Childhood Vaccines: Evidence Bearing on Causality. Washington (DC): National Academies Press (US); 1994. The National Academies Collection: Reports funded by National Institutes of Health.

[359] General recommendations on immunization --- recommendations of the Advisory Committee on Immunization Practices (ACIP). *MMWR Recomm Rep.* 2011;60(RR-2):1-64.

[360] Gruslin A, Steben M, Halperin S, et al. Immunization in pregnancy: No. 220, December 2008. *Int J Gynaecol Obstet.* 2009;105:187-91.

[361] American Academy of Pediatrics Committee on Infectious Diseases, Kimberlin DW, Brady MT et al. Red Book: 2015 Report of the Committee on Infectious Diseases. 30th ed. Elk Grove Village, IL: American Academy of Pediatrics. 2015.

[362] World Health Organization. WHO Position Paper on Haemophilus infl uenzae type b conjugate vaccines. *Wkly Epidemiol Rec.* 2006; 81: 445–52.

[363] Watt JP, Wolfson LJ, O'Brien KL, et al. Burden of disease caused by Haemophilus influenzae type b in children younger than 5 years: global estimates. *Lancet.* 2009 Sep;374:903-11.

[364] Watt JP, Wolfson LJ, O'Brien KL, et al. Burden of disease caused by Haemophilus influenzae type b in children younger than 5 years: global estimates. *Lancet.* 2009 Sep;374:903-11.

[365] Snedeker JD, Kaplan SL, Dodge PR, et al. Subdural Effusion and Its Relationship With Neurologic Sequelae of Bacterial Meningitis in Infancy: A Prospective Study. *Pediatrics.* 1990 Aug;86(2):163-70.

[366] World Health Organization. Haemophilus influenza type B. Available at: http://www.emro.who.int/health-topics/haemophilus-influenzae-type-b/disease-burden.html [Accessed February 1, 2020].

[367] United States Centers for Disease Control and Prevention. ABCs Report: Haemophilus influenzae, 2013. https://www.cdc.gov/abcs/reports-findings/survreports/hib13.html Available at: {Accessed February 1, 2020].

[368] Soeters HM, Blain A, Pondo T, et al. Current Epidemiology and Trends in Invasive Haemophilus influenzae Disease—United States, 2009–2015. *Clin Infect Dis.* 2018 Sep 15;67(6):881-9.

[369] United States Food and Drug Administration. Sanofi Pasteur 095 – ActHIB. Available at: https://www.fda.gov/media/74395/download [Accessed February 1, 2020].

[370] United States Food and Drug Administration. HIGHLIGHTS OF PRESCRIBING INFORMATION. HIBERIX. Available at: https://www.fda.gov/media/77017/download [Accessed February 1, 2020].

[371] United States Food and Drug Administration. Liquid PedvaxHIB. Available at: https://www.fda.gov/media/80438/download [Accessed February 1, 2020].

[372] Merck & Co., Inc. Comvax. Available at: https://id-ea.org/wp-content/uploads/2012/05/COMVAX-Package-Insert.pdf [Accessed February 1, 2020].

[373] Adam HJ, Richardsom SE, Jamieson FB, et al. Changing Epidemiology of Invasive Haemophilus Influenzae in Ontario, Canada: Evidence for Herd Effects and Strain Replacement Due to Hib Vaccination. Vaccine. 2010 May 28;28(24):4073-8.

[374] Sadeghi-Aval P, Tsang RS, Jamieson FB, et al. Emergence of Non-Serotype B Encapsulated Haemophilus Influenzae as a Cause of Pediatric Meningitis in Northwestern Ontario. *Can J Infect Dis Med Microbiol.* 2013 Spring;24(1):13-6.

[375] Cerqueira A, Byce S, Tsang RSW, et al. Continuing Surveillance of Invasive Haemophilus influenzae Disease in Northwestern Ontario Emphasizes the Importance of Serotype a and Non-Typeable Strains as Causes of Serious Disease: A Canadian Immunization Research Network (CIRN) Study. Can J Microbiol. 2019 Nov;65(11):805-813.

[376] Tsang RSW, Ulanova M. The Changing Epidemiology of Invasive Haemophilus Influenzae Disease: Emergence and Global Presence of Serotype a Strains That May Require a New Vaccine for Control. *Vaccine.* 2017 Jul 24;35(33):4270-4275.

[377] Rubach MP, Bender JM, Mottice S, et al. Increasing Incidence of Invasive Haemophilus Influenzae Disease in Adults, Utah, USA. *Emerg Infect Dis.* 2011 Sep;17(9):1645-50.

[378] Blain A, MacNeil J, Wang X, et al. Invasive Haemophilus influenzae Disease in Adults ≥65 Years, United States, 2011. 2014 Summer;1(2):ofu044.

303

[379] Shuel M, HoangL, Law DKS, et al. Invasive Haemophilus Influenzae in British Columbia: non-Hib and Non-Typeable Strains Causing Disease in Children and Adults. *Int J Infect Dis*. 2011 Mar;15(3):e167-73.

[380] Langereis JD, Jonge MID. Invasive Disease Caused by Nontypeable Haemophilus influenza. *Emerg Infect Dis*. 2015 Oct;21(10):1711–1718.

[381] Dworkin MS, Park L, Borchardt SM. The Changing Epidemiology of Invasive Haemophilus Influenzae Disease, Especially in Persons > or = 65 Years Old. *Clin Infect Dis*. 2007 Mar 15;44(6):810-6.

[382] Zanella RC, Bokermann S, Lucia A, et al. Changes in Serotype Distribution of Haemophilus Influenzae Meningitis Isolates Identified Through Laboratory-Based Surveillance Following Routine Childhood Vaccination Against H. Influenzae Type B in Brazil. *Vaccine*. 2011 Nov 8;29(48):8937-42.

[383] Ribeiro GS, Reis JN, Cordeiro SM, et al. Prevention of Haemophilus Influenzae Type B (Hib) Meningitis and Emergence of Serotype Replacement With Type a Strains After Introduction of Hib Immunization in Brazil. *J Infect Dis*. 2003 Jan 1;187(1):109-16.

[384] Bruce MG, ZulZ T, DeByle C, et al. Haemophilus influenzae Serotype a Invasive Disease, Alaska, USA, 1983–2011. *Emerg Infect Dis*. 2013 Jun;19(6):932–937.

[385] Filippi CM, von Herrath MG. Viral Trigger for Type 1 Diabetes: Pros and Cons. *Diabetes*. 2008 Nov;57(11):2863–2871.

[386] Stene LC, Oikarinen S, Hyoty H, et al. Enterovirus Infection and Progression From Islet Autoimmunity to Type 1 Diabetes: The Diabetes and Autoimmunity Study in the Young (DAISY). *Diabetes*. 2010 Dec;59(12):3174-80.

[387] Kimpimäki T, Kupila A, Hämäläinen AM, et al. The first signs of beta-cell autoimmunity appear in infancy in genetically susceptible children from the general population: the Finnish Type 1 Diabetes Prediction and Prevention Study. *J Clin Endocrinol Metab*. 2001 Oct;86(10):4782-8.

[388] Lönnrot M, Korpela K, Knip M, et al. Enterovirus infection as a risk factor for beta-cell autoimmunity in a prospectively observed birth cohort: the Finnish Diabetes Prediction and Prevention Study. *Diabetes*. 2000 Aug;49(8):1314-8.

[389] Richardson SJ, Morgan NG. Enteroviral infections in the pathogenesis of type 1 diabetes: new insights for therapeutic intervention. *Curr Opin Pharmacol*. 2018 Dec;43:11–19.

[390] Classen JB, Classen DC. Clustering of cases of insulin dependent diabetes (IDDM) occurring three years after Hemophilus influenza B (HiB) immunization support causal relationship between immunization and IDDM. *Autoimmunity*. 2002;35:247-53.

[391] Classen JB, Classen DC. Clustering of cases of IDDM occurring 2-4 years after vaccination is consistent with clustering after infections and progression to IDDM in autoantibody positive individuals. *JPEM*. 2003;16:495-508.

[392] Classen JB, Classen DC. Association between type 1 diabets and Hib vaccine: causal relation is likely. *BMJ*. 199 Oct 23;319(7217):1133.

[393] Classen DC, Classen JB. The timing of pediatric immunization and the risk of insulin-dependent diabetes mellitus. *Infect Dis Clin Pract*. 1997 Oct 22;6(7):449-54.

[394] Classen JB, Classen DC. Vaccines and the risk of insulin-dependent diabetes (IDDM): potential mechanism of action. *Med Hypoth*. 2001;57(5):532-8.

[395] Wahlberg J, Fredriksson J, Vaarala O, et al. Vaccinations may induce diabetes related autoantibodies in one year old children. *Ann N Y Acad Sci*. 2003;1005:404-8.

[396] Cheng BW, Lo FS, Wang AM, et al. Autoantibodies against islet cell antigens in children with type 1 diabetes mellitus. *Oncotarget*. 2018 Mar 27;9(23):16275–16283.

[397] Classen JB, Classen DC. Vaccines and the risk of insulin-dependent diabetes (IDDM): potential mechanism of action. *Med Hypoth*. 2001;57(5):532-8.

[398] Wahlberg J, Fredriksson J, Vaarala O, et al. Vaccinations may induce diabetes related autoantibodies in one year old children. *Ann N Y Acad Sci*. 2003;1005:404-8.

[399] Karjalainen J, Vahasalo P, Knip M, et al. Islet cell autoimmunity and progression to insulin dependent diabetes mellitus in genetically high and low siblings of diabetic children. *Eur J Clin Invest*. 1996;26:640-9.

[400] Kulmala P, Savola K, Reijonen H, et al. Genetic markers, humoral autoimmunity, and prediction of type 1 diabetes in siblings of affected children. *Diabetes*. 2000;49:48-58

[401] Karjalainen J, Vahasalo P, Knip M, et al. Islet cell autoimmunity and progression to insulin dependent diabetes mellitus in genetically high and low siblings of diabetic children. *Eur J Clin Invest*. 1996;26:640-9.

[402] Zeigler AG, Hummel M, Schenker M, et al. Autoantibody appearance and risk for development of childhood diabetes in offspring of parents with type I diabetes: the 2 year analysis of the German BABYDIAB study. *Diabetes*. 1999;48:460-8.

[403] Clasen JB. Prevalence of Autism is Positively Associated with the Incidence of Type 1 Diabetes, but Negatively Associated with the Incidence of Type 2 Diabetes, Implication for the Etiology of the Autism Epidemic. *Open Acces Sci Rep*. 2013;2(3):679.

[404] Imai Y, Dobrian AD, Weaver JR, et al. Interaction between cytokines and inflammatory cells in islet dysfunction, insulin resistance, and vascular disease. *Diabetes Obes Metab*. 2013 Sep;15(0 3):117–129.

[405] Wang C, Guan Y, Yang J. Cytokines in the Progression of Pancreatic β-Cell Dysfunction. *Int J Endocrinol*. 2010;2010:515136.

[406] Newby BN, Mathews CE. Type I Interferon Is a Catastrophic Feature of the Diabetic Islet Microenvironment. *Front Endocrinol (Lausanne)*. 2017;8:232.

[407] Lombardi A, Tsomos E, Hammerstad SS, et al. INTERFERON ALPHA: THE KEY TRIGGER OF TYPE 1 DIABETES. *J Autoimmun*. 2018 Nov;94:7–15.

[408] Classen JB. Review of Evidence That Epidemics of Type 1 Diabetes and Type 2 Diabetes/Metabolic Syndrome Are Polar Opposite Responses to Iatrogenic Inflammation. *Curr Diabetes Rev*. 2012 Nov;8(6):413-8.

[409] Classed JB. Italian Pediatric Data Support Hypothesis That Simultaneous Epidemics of Type 1 Diabetes and Type 2 Diabetes/Metabolic Syndrome/Obesity Are Polar Opposite Responses (i.e., Symptoms) to a Primary Inflammatory Condition. *J Pediatr Endocrinol Metab*. 2011;24(7-8):455-6.

[410] Classen JB. Review of Vaccine Induced Immune Overload and the Resulting Epidemics of Type 1 Diabetes and Metabolic Syndrome, Emphasis on Explaining the Recent Accelerations in the Risk of Prediabetes and other Immune Mediated Diseases. *J Mol Genet Med*. 2014;S1:025.

[411] Classen JB. Risk of Vaccine Induced Diabetes in Children with a Family History of Type 1 Diabetes. *Open Ped Med J*. 2008;2:7-10.

[412] Classen JB, Classen DC. Clustering of cases of IDDM occurring 2-4 years after vaccination is consistent with clustering after infections and progression to IDDM in autoantibody positive individuals. *JPEM*. 2003;16:495-508.

[413] Classen JB, Classen DC. Public should be told that vaccines may have long term adverse effects. *BMJ*. 1999 Jan 16;318(7177):193.

[414] Classen JB. Diabetes epidemic follows hepatitis B immunization program. *N Z Med J*. 1996 May 24;109(1022):195.

[415] Classen JB, Classen DC. Clustering of cases of insulin dependent diabetes (IDDM) occurring three years after Hemophilus influenza B (HiB) immunization support causal relationship between immunization and IDDM. *Autoimmunity*. 2002;35:247-53.

[416] Hyoty H, Hiltunen M, Reunanen A, et al. Decline of Mumps Antibodies in Type 1 (Insulin-Dependent) Diabetic Children and a Plateau in the Rising Incidence of Type 1 Diabetes After Introduction of the Mumps-Measles-Rubella Vaccine in Finland. Childhood Diabetes in Finland Study Group. *Diabetologia*. 1993 Dec;36(12):1303-8.

[417] Otten A, Helmke K, Stief T, et al. Mumps, Mumps Vaccination, Islet Cell Antibodies and the First Manifestation of Diabetes Mellitus Type I. *Behring Inst Mitt*. 1984 Jul;(75)83-8.

[418] Sinaniotis CA, Daskalopoulou E, Lapatsanis P, et al. Letter: Diabetes mellitus after mumps vaccination. *Arch Dis Child*. 1975 Sep;50(9):749–750.

[419] Arumugham V. Bioinformatics analysis links type 1 diabetes to vaccines contaminated with animal proteins and autoreactive T cells express skin homing receptors consistent with injected vaccines as causal agent. *Zenodo*. 2017:1034775.

[420] Hviid A, Stellfeld M, Wohlfahrt J, et al. Childhood Vaccination and Type 1 Diabetes. *N Engl J Med*. 2004;350:1398-1404.

[421] Patterson CC. Infections and vaccinations as risk factors for childhood type I diabetes mellitus: a multicenter case-control investigation. *Diabetologia*. 2000;43:47-53.

[422] DeStefano F, Mullooly JP, Okoro CA, et al. Childhood vaccinations, vaccination timing, and risk of type 1 diabetes mellitus. *Pediatrics*. 2001;108:e112.

[423] Geno KA, Gilbert GL, Song JY, et al. Pneumococcal Capsules and Their Types: Past, Present, and Future. *Clin Microbiol Rev*. 2015 Jul;28(3):871-99.

[424] Gray BM, Converse GM 3rd, Dillon HC Jr. Epidemiologic studies of Streptococcus pneumoniae in infants: acquisition, carriage, and infection during the first 24 months of life. *J Infect Dis*. 1980 Dec; 142(6):923-33.

[425] Cho EY, Kang HM, Lee J, et al. Changes in serotype distribution and antibiotic resistance of nasopharyngeal isolates of Streptococcus pneumoniae from children in Korea, after optional use of the 7-valent conjugate vaccine. *J Korean Med Sci*. 2012 Jul; 27(7):716-22.

305

[426] Kim KH, Hong JY, Lee H, et al. Nasopharyngeal pneumococcal carriage of children attending day care centers in Korea: comparison between children immunized with 7-valent pneumococcal conjugate vaccine and non-immunized. *J Korean Med Sci*. 2011 Feb; 26(2):184-90.

[427] Sleeman KL, Griffiths D, Shackley F, et al. Capsular serotype-specific attack rates and duration of carriage of Streptococcus pneumoniae in a population of children. *J Infect Dis*. 2006 Sep 1; 194(5):682-8.

[428] United States Centers for Disease Control and Prevention. Pneumococcal Disease. Available at: https://www.cdc.gov/vaccines/pubs/pinkbook/pneumo.html [Accessed February 8, 2020].

[429] Wahl B, O'Brian KL, Greenbaum A, et al. Burden of Streptococcus pneumoniae and Haemophilus influenzae type b disease in children in the era of conjugate vaccines: global, regional, and national estimates for 2000–15. *Lancet Global Health*. 2018 Jul;6(7):PE744-57.

[430] Bogaert D, De Groot R, Hermans PW. Streptococcus pneumoniae colonisation: the key to pneumococcal disease. *Lancet Infect Dis*. 2004 Mar; 4(3):144-54.

[431] Ferreira DM, Jambo KC, Gordon SB. Experimental human pneumococcal carriage models for vaccine research. *Trends Microbiol*. 2011 Sep; 19(9):464-70.

[432] European Centre for Disease Prevention and Control. Invasive pneumococcal disease - Annual Epidemiological Report 2016 [2014 data]. Available at: https://www.ecdc.europa.eu/en/publications-data/invasive-pneumococcal-disease-annual-epidemiological-report-2016-2014-data [Accessed February 29, 2020].

[433] Backhaus E, Berg S, Andersson R, et al. Epidemiology of invasive pneumococcal infections: manifestations, incidence and case fatality rate correlated to age, gender and risk factors. *BMC Infect Dis*. 2016;16:367.

[434] Maimaiti N, Ahmed Z, Isa Z, et al. Clinical Burden of Invasive Pneumococcal Disease in Selected Developing Countries. *Value Health Reg Issues*. 2013 Sep-Oct;2(2):259-63.

[435] GBD 2016 Lower Respiratory Infections Collaborators. Estimates of the global, regional, and national morbidity, mortality, and aetiologies of lower respiratory infections in 195 countries, 1990-2016: A systematic analysis for the Global Burden of Disease Study 2016External. *Lancet Infect Dis*. 2018 Sep 19. pii: S1473-3099(18)30310-4.

[436] United States Centers for Disease Control and Prevention. Global Pneumococcal Disease and Vaccine. Available at: https://www.cdc.gov/pneumococcal/global.html [Accessed February 8, 2020].

[437] Backhaus E, Berg S, Andersson R, et al. Epidemiology of invasive pneumococcal infections: manifestations, incidence and case fatality rate correlated to age, gender and risk factors. *BMC Infect Dis*. 2016;16:367.

[438] O'Brien K, Wolfson LJ, Watt JP, et al. Burden of Disease Caused by Streptococcus Pneumoniae in Children Younger Than 5 Years: Global Estimates. *Lancet*. 2009 Sep 12;374(9693):893-902.

[439] Maimaiti N, Ahmed Z, Isa Z, et al. Clinical Burden of Invasive Pneumococcal Disease in Selected Developing Countries. *Value Health Reg Issues*. 2013 Sep-Oct;2(2):259-63.

[440] Meningitisnow.org. Pneumococcal. Available at: https://www.meningitisnow.org/meningitis-explained/what-is-meningitis/types-and-causes/pneumococcal/ [Accessed February 8, 2020].

[441] United States Centers for Disease Control and Prevention. Pneumococcal Disease. Available at: https://www.cdc.gov/vaccines/pubs/pinkbook/pneumo.html [Accessed February 8, 2020].

[442] United States Food and Drug Administration. Package Insert – Prevnar 13. Available at: https://www.fda.gov/files/vaccines%2C%20blood%20%26%20biologics/published/Package-Insert------Prevnar-13.pdf [Accessed February 8, 2020].

[443] European Medicines Agency. Synflorix, Summary of Produce Characteristics. Available at: https://www.ema.europa.eu/en/documents/product-information/synflorix-epar-product-information_en.pdf [Accessed February 8, 2020].

[444] United States Food and Drug Administration. Package Insert - Pneumovax 23. Available at: https://www.fda.gov/media/80547/download [Accessed February 8, 2020].

[445] Tan TQ. Serious and invasive pediatric pneumococcal disease epidemiology and vaccine impact in the USA. *Expert Rev Anti Infect Ther*. 2010 Feb;8(2):117-25.

[446] Oikawa J, Ishiwada N, Takahashi Y, et al. Changes in Nasopharyngeal Carriage of Streptococcus Pneumoniae, Haemophilus Influenzae and Moraxella Catarrhalis Among Healthy Children Attending a Day-Care Centre Before and After Official Financial Support for the 7-valent Pneumococcal Conjugate Vaccine and H. Influenzae Type B Vaccine in Japan. *J Infect Chemother*. 2014 Feb;20(2):146-9.

[447] Alexandre C, Dubos F, Courouble C, et al. Rebound in the Incidence of Pneumococcal Meningitis in Northern France: Effect of Serotype Replacement. *Acta Paediatr*. 2010 Nov;99(11):1686-90.

[448] Huang SS, Hinrichsen VL, Stevenson AE, et al. Continued Impact of Pneumococcal Conjugate Vaccine on Carriage in Young Children. *Pediatrics*. 2009 Jul;124(1):e1-11.

[449] Melegaro A, Choi YH, George R, et al. Dynamic models of pneumococcal carriage and the impact of the Heptavalent Pneumococcal Conjugate Vaccine on invasive pneumococcal disease. *BMC Infect Dis*. 2010 Apr 8;10:90.

[450] Dagan R. Serotype replacement in perspective. *Vaccine*. 2009 Aug 21;27(Sup 3):C22-24.

[451] Sahni V, Naus M, Hoang L, et al. The Epidemiology of Invasive Pneumococcal Disease in British Columbia Following Implementation of an Infant Immunization Program: Increases in Herd Immunity and Replacement Disease. *Can J Public Health*. 2012 Jan-Feb;103(1):29-33.

[452] Norton NB, Stanek RJ, Mufsom MA. Routine Pneumococcal Vaccination of Children Provokes New Patterns of Serotypes Causing Invasive Pneumococcal Disease in Adults and Children. Am J Med Sci. 2013 Feb;345(2):112-20.

[453] Mehtala J, Antonio M, Kaltoft MS, et al. Competition Between Streptococcus Pneumoniae Strains: Implications for Vaccine-Induced Replacement in Colonization and Disease. *Epidemiology*. 2013 Jul;24(4):522-9.

[454] Lee GM, Kleinman K, Pelton SI, et al. Impact of 13-Valent Pneumococcal Conjugate Vaccination on Streptococcus Pneumoniae Carriage in Young Children in Massachusetts. *J Pediatric Infect Dis Soc*. 2014 Mar;3(1):23-32.

[455] Asner SA, Agyeman PKA, Gradoux E, et al. Burden of Streptococcus pneumoniae Sepsis in Children After Introduction of Pneumococcal Conjugate Vaccines: A Prospective Population-based Cohort Study. *Clin Infect Dis*. 2019 Nov;69(9):1574-80.

[456] Vadlamudi NK, Chen A, Marra F. Impact of the 13-Valent Pneumococcal Conjugate Vaccine Among Adults: A Systematic Review and Meta-analysis. *Clin Infect Dis*. 2019 Jun 18;69(1):34-49.

[457] Ricketson LJ, Wood ML, Vanderkooi OG, et al. Trends in Asymptomatic Nasopharyngeal Colonization With Streptococcus Pneumoniae After Introduction of the 13-valent Pneumococcal Conjugate Vaccine in Calgary, Canada. *Pediatr Infect Dis J*. 2014 Jul;33(7):724-30.

[458] Flasche S, Edmunds WJ, Miller E, et al. The Impact of Specific and Non-Specific Immunity on the Ecology of Streptococcus Pneumoniae and the Implications for Vaccination. Proc Biol Sci. 2013 Oct 2;280(1771):20131939.

[459] United States Centers for Disease Control and Prevention. Poliomyelitis. Available at: https://www.cdc.gov/vaccines/pubs/pinkbook/polio.html [Accessed February 8, 2020].

[460] European Centre for Disease Prevention and Control. Disease factsheet about poliomyelitis. Available at: https://www.ecdc.europa.eu/en/poliomyelitis/facts [Accessed March 6, 2020].

[461] Jobra J, Diop OM, Iber J, et al. Update on Vaccine-Derived Poliovirus Outbreaks — Worldwide, January 2018–June 2019. *Weekly*. 2019 Nov 15;68(45):1024-8.

[462] Jobra J, Diop OM, Iber J, et al. Update on Vaccine-Derived Poliovirus Outbreaks — Worldwide, January 2018–June 2019. *Weekly*. 2019 Nov 15;68(45):1024-8.

[463] University of Minnesota. Center for Infectious Disease Research and Policy. World Polio Day: Wild poliovirus type 3 declared eradicated. Available at: http://www.cidrap.umn.edu/news-perspective/2019/10/world-polio-day-wild-poliovirus-type-3-declared-eradicated [Accessed February 8, 2020].

[464] Polio Global Eradication Initiative. Available at: http://polioeradication.org/polio-today/polio-now/this-week/ [Accessed February 8, 2020].

[465] World Health Organization. Poliomyelitis. Available at: https://www.who.int/news-room/fact-sheets/detail/poliomyelitis [Accessed February 8, 2020].

[466] United States Centers for Disease Control and Prevention. What is Polio? Available at: https://www.cdc.gov/polio/what-is-polio/index.htm [Accessed February 8, 2020].

[467] World Health Organization. Model Insert Oral Polio Vaccine for Children. Available at: https://www.who.int/immunization_standards/vaccine_quality/insert_opv_2002.pdf [Accessed February 8, 2020].

[468] United States Food and Drug Administration. Sanofi Pasteur 059 IPOL. Poliovirus Vaccine Inactivated IPOL. Available at: https://www.fda.gov/files/vaccines%2C%20blood%20%26%20biologics/published/Package-Insert---IPOL.pdf [Accessed February 8, 2020].

[469] World Health Organization. Model Insert Oral Polio Vaccine for Children. Available at: https://www.who.int/immunization_standards/vaccine_quality/insert_opv_2002.pdf [Accessed February 8, 2020].

[470] World Health Organization. Information Sheet Observed Rate of Vaccine Reactions Polio Vaccines. Available at: https://www.who.int/vaccine_safety/initiative/tools/polio_vaccine_rates_information_sheet.pdf [Accessed February 8, 2020].

[471] Mudur G. Doctors question India's polio strategy after surge in number of cases. *BMJ*. 2006 Sep 16; 333(7568): 568.

[472] Vashisht N, Puliyel J. Polio Programme: Let Us Declare Victory and Move On. *Indian J Med Ethics.* 2012 Apr-Jun;9(2)114-7.

[473] Dhiman R, Prkash SC, Sreenivas V, et al. Correlation between Non-Polio Acute Flaccid Paralysis Rates with Pulse Polio Frequency in India. *Int J Environ Res Public Health.* 2018 Aug;15(8):1755.

[474] Vashisht N, Puliyel J, Sreenivas V. Trends in Nonpolio Acute Flaccid Paralysis Incidence in India 2000 to 2013. *Pediatrics.* 2015 Feb;135(Sup 1):S16-S17.

[475] Maan HS, Dhole TN, Chowdhary R. Identification and characterization of nonpolio enterovirus associated with nonpolio-acute flaccid paralysis in polio endemic state of Uttar Pradesh, Northern India. *PLoS One.* 2019 Jan;14(1):e0208902.

[476] Faleye TOC, Adewumi MO, Japhet MO, et al. Non-polio Enteroviruses in Faeces of Children Diagnosed With Acute Flaccid Paralysis in Nigeria. *Virol J.* 2017 Sep 12;14(1)175.

[477] Suresh S, Forgie S, Robinson J. Non-polio Enterovirus Detection With Acute Flaccid Paralysis: A Systematic Review. *J Med Virol.* 2018 Jan;90(1)3-7.

[478] Prussin AJ, Garcia EB, Marr LC. Total Concentrations of Virus and Bacteria in Indoor and Outdoor Air. *Environ Sci Technol Lett.* 2015;2(4):84-88.

[479] Yan J, Grantham M, Pantelic J, et al. Infectious virus in exhaled breath of symptomatic seasonal influenza cases from a college community. 2018 Jan 30;115(5):1081-86.

[480] Leitmeyer K, Adlhoch C. Influenza Transmission on Aircraft A Systematic Literature Review. *Epidemiology.* 2016 Sep;27(5):743-51.

[481] World Health Organization. Influenza (Seasonal). Available at: https://www.who.int/news-room/fact-sheets/detail/influenza-(seasonal) [Accessed February 8, 2020].

[482] Czaja CA, Miller L, Alden N, et al. Age-Related Differences in Hospitalization Rates, Clinical Presentation, and Outcomes Among Older Adults Hospitalized With Influenza—U.S. Influenza Hospitalization Surveillance Network (FluSurv-NET). *Open Forum Infect Dis.* 2019 Jul;6(7):1-8.

[483] United States Centers for Disease Control and Prevention. Children & Influenza (Flu). Available at: https://www.cdc.gov/flu/highrisk/children.htm [Accessed February 8, 2020].

[484] United States Centers for Disease Control and Prevention. Live Attenuated Influenza Vaccine [LAIV] (The Nasal Spray Flu Vaccine). Available at: https://www.cdc.gov/flu/prevent/nasalspray.htm#anchor_1528460157435 [Accessed February 8, 2020].

[485] United States Food and Drug Administration. Seqirus, Influenza Vaccine STN BL 1254. Available at: https://www.fda.gov/media/99883/download [Accessed February 8, 2020].

[486] United States Food and Drug Administration. Package Insert - Fluad. Available at: https://www.fda.gov/media/94583/download [Accessed February 8, 2020].

[487] United States Food and Drug Administration. Package Insert - FLUARIX QUADRIVALENT. Available at: https://www.fda.gov/media/115744/download [Accessed February 8, 2020].

[488] United States Food and Drug Administration. Package Insert - Flublok Quadrivalent. Available at: https://www.fda.gov/media/123144/download [Accessed February 8, 2020].

[489] United States Food and Drug Administration. Package Insert - Flucelvax Quadrivalent. Available at: https://www.fda.gov/media/115862/download [Accessed February 8, 2020].

[490] European Medicines Agency. Fluenz Tetra, INN-influenza vaccine (live attenuated, nasal). Available at: https://www.ema.europa.eu/en/documents/product-information/fluenz-tetra-epar-product-information_en.pdf [Accessed February 8, 2020].

[491] United States Food and Drug Administration. Package Insert - FLULAVAL QUADRIVALENT. Available at: https://www.fda.gov/media/115785/download [Accessed February 8, 2020].

[492] United States Food and Drug Administration. Package Insert - FluMist Quadrivalent. Available at: https://www.fda.gov/media/83072/download [Accessed February 8, 2020].

[493] United States Food and Drug Administration. Package Insert - Fluvirin. Available at: https://www.fda.gov/media/75156/download [Accessed February 8, 2020].

[494] United States Food and Drug Administration. Package Insert - Fluzone Quadrivalent. Available at: https://www.fda.gov/media/119856/download [Accessed February 8, 2020].

[495] United States Food and Drug Administration. Package Insert - Fluzone Quadrivalent. Available at: https://www.fda.gov/media/119856/download [Accessed February 8, 2020].

[496] United States Food and Drug Administration. Package Insert - Fluzone High-Dose. Available at: https://www.fda.gov/media/119870/download [Accessed February 8, 2020].

[497] Jefferson T, Rivetti A, Pietrantonj CD, et al. Vaccines for Preventing Influenza in Healthy Children. *Cochrane Database Syst Rev.* 2012 Aug 15;2012(8):CD004879.

[498] Jefferson T, Rivetti A, Pietrantonj CD, et al. Vaccines for Preventing Influenza in Healthy Children. *Cochrane Database Syst Rev.* 2018 Feb 1;2(2):CD004879.

[499] Lewnard JA, Cobey S. Immune History and Influenza Vaccine Effectiveness. *Vaccines (Basel)*. 2018 Jun;6(2):28.

[500] Kissling E, Rose A, Emborg HD, et al. Interim 2018/19 influenza vaccine effectiveness: six European studies, October 2018 to January 2019. *Euro Surveill*. 2019 Feb 21;24(8):1900121.

[501] United States Centers for Disease Control and Prevention. US Flu VE Data from 2018–2019. Available at: https://www.cdc.gov/flu/vaccines-work/2018-2019.html [Accessed February 19, 2020].

[502] United States Centers for Disease Control and Prevention. Past Seasons Vaccine Effectiveness Estimates. Available at: https://www.cdc.gov/flu/vaccines-work/past-seasons-estimates.html [Accessed February 19, 2020].

[503] Simonsen L, Reichert TA, Viboud C, et al. Impact of Influenza Vaccination on Seasonal Mortality in the US Elderly Population. *Arch Intern Med*. 2005 Feb 14;165(3):265-72.

[504] Reichert T, Chowell G, McCullers JA. The age distribution of mortality due to influenza: pandemic and peri-pandemic. *BMC Med*. 2012 Dec 12;10:162.

[505] Fireman B, Lee J, Lewis N, et al. Influenza Vaccination and Mortality: Differentiating Vaccine Effects From Bias. *Am J Epidemiology*. 2009 Sep 1;170(5):650-6.

[506] Poudel S, Shehadeh F, Zacharioudakis IM, et al. The Effect of Influenza Vaccination on Mortality and Risk of Hospitalization in Patients With Heart Failure: A Systematic Review and Meta-analysis. *Open Forum Infect Dis*. 2019 Apr;6(4):ofz159.

[507] Groenwold RHH, Hoes AW, Hak E. Impact of influenza vaccination on mortality risk among the elderly. 2009;34(1):56-62.

[508] Bodewes R, Kreijtz JHCM, Rimmelzwaan GF. Yearly Influenza Vaccinations: A Double-Edged Sword? *Lancet Infect Dis*. 2009 Dec;9(12):784-8.

[509] Skowronski DM, Serres GD, Crowcroft NS, et al. Association Between the 2008-09 Seasonal Influenza Vaccine and Pandemic H1N1 Illness During Spring-Summer 2009: Four Observational Studies From Canada. *PLoS Med*. 2010 Apr 6;7(4):e1000258.

[510] Crum-Cianflone NF, Blair PJ, Faix D, et al. Clinical and Epidemiologic Characteristics of an Outbreak of Novel H1N1 (Swine Origin) Influenza A Virus among United States Military Beneficiaries. *Clin Infect Dis*. 2009 Dec 15;49(12):1801–1810.

[511] Bodewes R, Fraaij PLA, Kreijtz JHKCM, et al. Annual Influenza Vaccination Affects the Development of Heterosubtypic Immunity. *Vaccine*. 2012 Dec 7;30(51):7407-10.

[512] Kreijtz JHCM, Bodewes R, van den Brand JMA, et al. Infection of Mice With a Human Influenza A/H3N2 Virus Induces Protective Immunity Against Lethal Infection With Influenza A/H5N1 Virus. *Vaccine*. 2009 Aug 6;27(36):4983–9.

[513] Kreijtz JHCM, Bodewes R, van Amerongen G, et al. Primary Influenza A Virus Infection Induces Cross-Protective Immunity Against a Lethal Infection With a Heterosubtypic Virus Strain in Mice. *Vaccine*. 2007 Jan 8;25(4):612-20.

[514] Groves HT, McDonald JU, Langat P, et al. Mouse Models of Influenza Infection with Circulating Strains to Test Seasonal Vaccine Efficacy. *Front Immunol*. 2018;9:126.

[515] Bodewes R, Kreijtz JHCM, Baas C, et al. Vaccination Against Human Influenza A/H3N2 Virus Prevents the Induction of Heterosubtypic Immunity Against Lethal Infection With Avian Influenza A/H5N1 Virus. *PLoS One*. 2009;4(5):e5538.

[516] Bodewes R, Kreijtz JHCM, Geelhoed-Mieras MM, et al. Vaccination Against Seasonal Influenza A/H3N2 Virus Reduces the Induction of Heterosubtypic Immunity Against Influenza A/H5N1 Virus Infection in Ferrets. *J Virol*. 2011 Mar;85(6):695-702.

[517] Wolff GG. Influenza Vaccination and Respiratory Virus Interference Among Department of Defense Personnel During the 2017-2018 Influenza Season. Vaccine. 2020 Jan 10;38(2):350-354.

[518] Rudenko L, Kiseleva I, Krutikova E, et al. Rationale for vaccination with trivalent or quadrivalent live attenuated influenza vaccines: Protective vaccine efficacy in the ferret model. *PLoS One*. 2018;13(12):e0208028.

[519] Dong W, Bhide Y, Sicca F, et al. Cross-Protective Immune Responses Induced by Sequential Influenza Virus Infection and by Sequential Vaccination With Inactivated Influenza Vaccines. *Front Immunol*. 2018;9:2312.

[520] Wang Y, Fan G, Horby P, et al. Comparative Outcomes of Adults Hospitalized With Seasonal Influenza A or B Virus Infection: Application of the 7-Category Ordinal Scale. *Open Forum Infect Dis*. 2019 Mar;6(3):1-9.

[521] Ohmit SE, Petrie JG, Malosh RE, et al. Influenza Vaccine Effectiveness in the Community and the Household. *Clin Infect Dis*. 2013 May;56(10):1363-9.

522 Ramsay LC, Buchan SA, Stirling RG, et al. The impact of repeated vaccination on influenza vaccine effectiveness: a systematic review and meta-analysis. *BMC Med*. 2019;17(9):2019.

523 McLean HQ, Capsard H, Griffin MR, et al. Association of Prior Vaccination With Influenza Vaccine Effectiveness in Children Receiving Live Attenuated or Inactivated Vaccine. *JAMA Netw Open*. 2018 Oct 5;1(6):e183742.

524 Jefferson T, Di Pietrantonj C, Debalini MG, et al. Relation of Study Quality, Concordance, Take Home Message, Funding, and Impact in Studies of Influenza Vaccines: Systematic Review. *BMJ*. 2009 Feb 12;338:b354.

525 Doshi P. Are U.S. flu-death figures more PR than science? *BMJ*. 2005 Dec 10;331:1412.

526 Joshi AY, Iyer VN, Hartz MF, et al. Effectiveness of Trivalent Inactivated Influenza Vaccine in Influenza-Related Hospitalization in Children: A Case-Control Study. Allergy Asthma Proc. 2012 Mar-Apr;33(2)e23-7.

527 Vasileiou E, Sheikh A, Butler C, et al. Effectiveness of Influenza Vaccines in Asthma: A Systematic Review and Meta-Analysis. *Clin Infect Dis*. 2017 Oct 15;65(8):1388-95.

528 Ray GT, Lewis N, Goddard K, et al. Asthma exacerbations among asthmatic children receiving live attenuated versus inactivated influenza vaccines. *Vaccine*. 2017 May9;35(20):2668-75.

529 Duffy J, Lewis M, Harrington T, et al. Live attenuated influenza vaccine use and safety in children and adults with asthma. *Ann Allergy Asthma Immunol*. 2017 Apr;118(4):439-444.

530 Cowling BJ, Fang VJ, Nishiura H, et al. Increased Risk of Noninfluenza Respiratory Virus Infections Associated With Receipt of Inactivated Influenza Vaccine. *Clin Infect Dis*. 2012 Jun;54(12):1778-83.

531 Ayoub DM, Yazbak FE, et al. Influenza Vaccination During Pregnancy: A Critical Assessment of the Recommendations of the Advisory Committee on Immunization Practices (ACIP). *J Am Physicians Surgeons*. 2006 Summer;11(2):41-7.

532 Goldman GS. Comparison of VAERS fetal-loss reports during three consecutive influenza seasons. *Hum Exp Toxicol*. 2013 May;32(5):464–475.

533 Thomas RE, Jefferson T, Lasserson TJ. Influenza vaccination for healthcare workers who care for elderly people aged 60 or older living in long-term care institutions. *Cochrane Database Syst Rev.* 2013;7:CD005187.

534 Thomas RE, Jefferson T, Lasserson TJ. Influenza vaccination for healthcare workers who work with the elderly: systemic review. *Vaccine*. 2010 Dec 16;29(2):344-56.

535 Abramson ZH. What, in fact, is the evidence that vaccinating healthcare workers against seasonal influenza protects their patients? A critical review. *Int J Fam Med*. 2012;2012:205464

536 Jefferson T, Mar CD, Dooley L, et al. Physical Interventions to Interrupt or Reduce the Spread of Respiratory Viruses: Systematic Review. *BMJ*. 2009 Sep 21;339:b3675.

537 Jefferson T, Mar CBD, Dooley L, et al. Physical Interventions to Interrupt or Reduce the Spread of Respiratory Viruses. *Cochrane Database Syst Rev*. 2011 Jul 6;2011(7):CD006207.

538 Centers for Disease Control and Prevention (CDC). Updated recommendations for isolation of persons with mumps. *MMWR Morb Mortal Wkly Rep*. 2008 Oct 10;57(40):1103-5.

539 Sane J, Gouma S, Koopmans M, et al. Epidemic of Mumps Among Vaccinated Persons, The Netherlands, 2009-2012. *Emerg Infect Dis*. 2014 Apr;20(4):643-8.

540 World Health Organization. Surveillance Guidelines for Measles, Rubella and Congenital Rubella Syndrome in the WHO European Region. Available at: https://www.ncbi.nlm.nih.gov/books/NBK143257/ [Accessed February 17, 2020].

541 Webster WS. Teratogen update: congenital rubella. Teratology 1998;58(1):13–23.

542 World Health Organization. More than 140,000 die from measles as cases surge worldwide. Available at: https://www.who.int/news-room/detail/05-12-2019-more-than-140-000-die-from-measles-as-cases-surge-worldwide [Accessed February 17, 2020].

543 Beleni AI, Borgmann S. Mumps in the Vaccination Age: Global Epidemiology and the Situation in Germany. *Int J Environ Res Public Health*. 2018 Aug; 15(8): 1618.

544 WHO-Europe-UNICEF. Global and regional immunization profile. Global. WHO-UNICEF 2014 December 1. Available from: http://www.who.int/immunization/monitoring_surveillance/data/gs_gloprofile.pdf?ua=1 [Accessed February 17, 2020].

545 WHO-Europe-UNICEF. Global and regional immunization profile. Global. WHO-UNICEF 2014 December 1. Available from: http://www.who.int/immunization/monitoring_surveillance/data/gs_gloprofile.pdf?ua=1 [Accessed February 17, 2020].

[546] Infectious Disease Advisor, Anne Gershon. Infectious Diseases, Measles Virus (Rubeola). Available at: https://www.infectiousdiseaseadvisor.com/home/decision-support-in-medicine/infectious-diseases/measles-virus-rubeola/ [Accessed February 17, 2020].

[547] World Health Organization. More than 140,000 die from measles as cases surge worldwide. Available at: https://www.who.int/news-room/detail/05-12-2019-more-than-140-000-die-from-measles-as-cases-surge-worldwide [Accessed February 17, 2020].

[548] United States Centers for Disease Control and Prevention. Mumps. Available at: https://www.cdc.gov/vaccines/pubs/pinkbook/mumps.html [Accessed February 17, 2020].

[549] United States Centers for Disease Control and Prevention. Mumps. Available at: https://www.cdc.gov/vaccines/pubs/pinkbook/mumps.html [Accessed February 17, 2020].

[550] Maldonado Y. Mumps. In Behrman RE, Kliegman RM, Jenson HB (eds). Nelson Textbook of Pediatrics. 16.Ed. Philadelphia: WB Saunders, 2000:954-955.

[551] United States Centers for Disease Control and Prevention. Mumps. Available at: https://www.cdc.gov/vaccines/pubs/pinkbook/mumps.html [Accessed February 17, 2020].

[552] United States Centers for Disease Control and Prevention. Mumps. Available at: https://www.cdc.gov/vaccines/pubs/pinkbook/mumps.html [Accessed February 17, 2020].

[553] Cutts FT, Vynnycky E. Modelling the incidence of congenital rubella syndrome in developing countries. *Int J Epidemiol*. 1999;28:1176-84.

[554] World Health Organization. Surveillance Guidelines for Measles, Rubella and Congenital Rubella Syndrome in the WHO European Region. Available at: https://www.ncbi.nlm.nih.gov/books/NBK143257/ [Accessed February 17, 2020].

[555] United States Food and Drug Administration. Package Insert – MMR. Available at: https://www.fda.gov/media/75191/download [Accessed February 17, 2020].

[556] United States Food and Drug Administration. Package Insert - ProQuad Frozen HSA. Available at: https://www.fda.gov/media/75203/download [Accessed February 17, 2020].

[557] GlaskoSmithKline. Priorix-Tetra Product Information. Available at: https://au.gsk.com/media/217228/priorix_tetra_pi_008_approved.pdf [Accessed February 17, 2020].

[558] Lievano F, Galea SA, Thronton M, et al. Measles, Mumps, and Rubella Virus Vaccine (M-M-R™II): A Review of 32 Years of Clinical and Postmarketing Experience. *Vaccine*. 2012 Nov 6;30(48):6918-26.

[559] Lievano F, Galea SA, Thronton M, et al. Measles, Mumps, and Rubella Virus Vaccine (M-M-R™II): A Review of 32 Years of Clinical and Postmarketing Experience. *Vaccine*. 2012 Nov 6;30(48):6918-26.

[560] Kubota Y, Iso H, Tamakoshi A, et al. Association of Measles and Mumps With Cardiovascular Disease: The Japan Collaborative Cohort (JACC) Study. Atherosclerosis. 2015 Aug;241(2):682-6.

[561] Swirski FK, Nahrendorf M. Cardioimmunology: the immune system in cardiac homeostasis and disease. *Nature Rev Immunol*. 2018;18:733-44.

[562] Shaheen SO, AAby P, Hall AJ, et al. Measles and Atopy in Guinea-Bissau. *Lancet*. 1996 Jul 29;347(9018):1792-6.

[563] Roselund H, Bergstrom A, Alm JS, et al. Allergic Disease and Atopic Sensitization in Children in Relation to Measles Vaccination and Measles Infection. *Pediatrics*. 2009 Mar;123(3):771-8.

[564] Kuckosmanoglu E, Cetinkaya F, Akcay F, et al. Frequency of allergic diseases following measles. *Allergologia et Immunopathologia*. 2006 Aug;34(4):146-9.

[565] Kuyucu S, Sarc,r Y, Tuncer A, et al. Determinants of Atopic Sensitization in Turkish School Children: Effects of Pre- And Post-Natal Events and Maternal Atopy. *Pediatr Allergy Immunol*. 2004 Feb;15(1):62-71.

[566] Warner JA, Warner JO. Early life events in allergic sensitization. *Br Med Bull*. 2000;56(4):883-93.

[567] Neeland MR, Koplin JJ, Dang TD, et al. Early life innate immune signatures of persistent food allergy. *J Allergy Clin Immunol*. 2018 Sep;142(3):857-64.

[568] Bremner SSA, Carey IM, DeWilde S, et al. Timing of Routine Immunisations and Subsequent Hay Fever Risk. *Arch Dis Child*. 2005 Jun;90(6):567-73.

[569] Kondo N, Fukutomi O, Ozawa T, et al. Improvement of Food-Sensitive Atopic Dermatitis Accompanied by Reduced Lymphocyte Responses to Food Antigen Following Natural Measles Virus Infection. *Clin Exp Allergy*. 1993 Jan;23(1):44-50.

[570] Alm J, Swartz JS, Lilja G, et al. Atopy in children of families with an anthroposophic lifestyle. *Lancet*. 1999 May 1;353(9163):1485-8.

[571] Floistrup H, Swartz J, Bergstrom A, et al. Allergic Disease and Sensitization in Steiner School Children. *J Allergy Clin Immunol*. 2006 Jan;117(1):59-66.

[572] Koning H, Baert MR, Oranje AP, et al. Development of Immune Functions Related to Allergic Mechanisms in Young Children. *Pediatr Res*. 1996 Sep;40(3):363-75.

[573] Sakaguchi M, Inouye S. IgE sensitization to gelatin: the probable role of gelatin-containing diphtheria-tetanus-acellular pertussis (DTaP) vaccines. *Vaccine*. 2000;18(19):2055-2058.

[574] Nagao M, Fujisawa T, Ihara T, et al. Highly Increased Levels of IgE Antibodies to Vaccine Components in Children With Influenza Vaccine-Associated Anaphylaxis. *J Allergy Clin Immunol*. 2016 Mar;137(3):861-7.

[575] Penaloza-MacMaster P, Barber DL, Wherry EJ, et al. Vaccine-elicited CD4 T cells induce immunopathology after chronic LCMV infection. *Science*. 2015;347(6219): 278.

[576] Cohen J, Hohman P, Fulton R, et al. Kinetics of Serum Cytokines after Primary or Repeat Vaccination with the Smallpox Vaccine. *J Infect Dis*. 2010 Apr 15;201(8):1183–1191.

[577] Talaat KR, Halsey NA, Cox AB, et al. Rapid Changes in Serum Cytokines and Chemokines in Response to Inactivated Influenza Vaccination. *Influenza Other Respir Viruses*. 2018 Mar;12(2):202-210.

[578] Eriksson JC, Cox RJ, Szyszko E, et al. Local and systemic cytokine and chemokine responses after parenteral influenza vaccination. *Influenza Other Respir Viruses*. 2007 Jul;1(4):139-46.

[579] Todryk SM. T Cell Memory to Vaccination. *Vaccines (Basel)*. 2018 Dec;6(4):84.

[580] Grivennikov SI, Greten FR, Karin M. Immunity, Inflammation, and Cancer. *Cell*. 2010 Mar 19;140(6):883–899.

[581] Cann SAH, van Netten JP, van Netten C. Acute Infections as a Means of Cancer Prevention: Opposing Effects to Chronic Infections? *Cancer Detect Prev*. 2006;30(1):83-93.

[582] Kim KC. Role of epithelial mucins during airway infection. *Pulm Pharmacol Ther*. 2012 Dec;25(6):415–419.

[583] Linden SK, Florin THJ, McGuckin MA. Mucin Dynamics in Intestinal Bacterial Infection. *PLoS One*. 2008;3(12):e3952.

[584] Horm TM, Schroeder JA. MUC1 and metastatic cancer: Expression, function and therapeutic targeting. *Cell Adh Migr*. 2013 Mar 1;7(2):187–198.

[585] Cramer DW, Vitonis AF, Pinheiro SP, et al. Mumps and ovarian cancer: modern interpretation of an historic association. *Cancer Causes Control*. 2010 Aug;21(8):193–1201.

[586] von Mensdorff-Pouilly S, Moreno M, Verheijen RHM. Natural and Induced Humoral Responses to MUC1. *Cancers (Basel)*. 2011 Sep;3(3):3073–3103.

[587] Donnelly OG, Errington-Mais F, Steele L, et al. Measles Virus Causes Immunogenic Cell Death in Human Melanoma. *Gene Ther*. 2013 Jan;20(1):7-15.

[588] Russel SJ, Peng KW. Measles Virus for Cancer Therapy. *Curr Top Microbiol Immunol*. 2009;330:213-41.

[589] Bell JC. Taming Measles Virus to Create an Effective Cancer Therapeutic. *Mayo Clinic Proc*. 2014 Jul;89(7):863-5.

[590] Touchefeu Y, Schick U, Harrington KJ. [Measles Virus: A Future Therapeutic Agent in Oncology?] *Med Sci (Paris)*. 2012 Apr;28(4):388-94.

[591] Meyers R, Greiner S, Harvey M, et al. Oncolytic Activities of Approved Mumps and Measles Vaccines for Therapy of Ovarian Cancer. *Cancer Gene Ther*. 2005 Jul;12(7):593-9.

[592] Leske H, Haase R, Restle F, et al. Varicella Zoster Virus Infection of Malignant Glioma Cell Cultures: A New Candidate for Oncolytic Virotherapy? *Anticancer Res*. 2012 Apr;32(4):1137-44.

[593] Cramer DW, Vitonis AF, Pinheiro SP, et al. Mumps and ovarian cancer: modern interpretation of an historic association. *Cancer Causes Control*. 2010 Aug;21(8):193–1201.

[594] Buckley JD, Buckley Cm, Ruccione K, et al. Epidemiological Characteristics of Childhood Acute Lymphocytic Leukemia. Analysis by Immunophenotype. The Childrens Cancer Group. *Leukemia*. 1994 May;8(5):856-64.

[595] Ma X, Does MB, Metayer C, et al. Vaccination history and risk of childhood leukaemia. *Int J Epidemiology*. 2005 Oct;34(5):1100-9.

[596] Innis MD, Immunisation and childhood leukaemia. *Lancet*. 1965 Mar 13;1(7385):605.

[597] Mac Arthur AC, McBride ML, Spinelli JJ, et al. Risk of Childhood Leukemia Associated with Vaccination, Infection, and Medication Use in Childhood: The Cross-Canada Childhood Leukemia Study. *Am J Epidemiology*. 2008;167(5):598-606.

[598] Mallol-Mesnard N, Meneguax F, Auvrignon A, et al. Vaccination and the risk of childhood acute leukaemia: the ESCALE study (SFCE). *Int J Epidemiol*. 2007 Feb;36(1):110–116.

[599] West RO. Epidemiological study of malignancies of the ovaries. *Cancer*. 1966;19:1001-7.

[600] Menczer J, Modan M, et al. Possible role of mumps virus in the etiology of ovarian cancer. *Cancer*. 179 Apr;43(4):1375-9.

[601] Cramer DW, Vitonis AF, Pinheiro SP, et al. Mumps and ovarian cancer: modern interpretation of an historic association. *Cancer Causes Control*. 2010 Aug;21(8):193–1201.

[602] Newhouse ML, Pearson RM, Fullerton, KM, et al. A case control study of carcinoma of the ovary. *Br J Prev Soc Med*. 1977 Sep;31(3):148–153.

[603] Albonico HU, Braker HU, Husler J. Febrile history infectious of cancer childhood diseases in the patients and matched controls. *Med Hypotheses*. 1998;51:315-20.

[604] Wrensch M, Weinberg A, Wiencke J, et al. Does Prior Infection With Varicella-Zoster Virus Influence Risk of Adult Glioma? *Am J Epidemiol*. 1997 Apr 1;145(7):594-7.

[605] Schlehofer B, Blettner M, Preston-Martin S, et al. Role of Medical History in Brain Tumour Development. Results From the International Adult Brain Tumour Study. *Int J Cancer*. 1999 Jul 19;82(2):155-60.

[606] Wrensch M, Weinberg A, Wiencke J, et al. History of Chickenpox and Shingles and Prevalence of Antibodies to Varicella-Zoster Virus and Three Other Herpesviruses among Adults with Glioma and Controls. *AM J Epidemiol*. 2005 May 15;161(1):929-38.

[607] Canniff J, Donson Am, Foreman NK, et al. Cytotoxicity of Glioblastoma Cells Mediated Ex Vivo by Varicella-Zoster Virus-Specific T Cells. *J Neurovirol*. 2011 Oct;17(5):448-54.

[608] Lee ST, Bracci P, Zhou M, et al. Interaction of Allergy History and Antibodies to Specific Varicella-Zoster Virus Proteins on Glioma Risk. *Int J Cancer*. 2014 May 1;134(9):2199-210.

[609] Montella M, Maso LF, Crispo A, et al. Do Childhood Diseases Affect NHL and HL Risk? A Case-Control Study From Northern and Southern Italy. *Leuk Res*. 2006 Aug;30(8):917-22.

[610] Alexander FE, Jarrett RF, Lawrence D, et al. Risk Factors for Hodgkin's Disease by Epstein-Barr Virus (EBV) Status: Prior Infection by EBV and Other Agents. *Br J Cancer*. 2000 Mar;82(5):1117-21.

[611] Glaser SL, Keegan THM, Clarke CA, et al. Exposure to Childhood Infections and Risk of Epstein-Barr Virus--Defined Hodgkin's Lymphoma in Women. *Int J Cancer*. 2005 Jul 1;115(4):599-605.

[612] Gutensohn N, Cole P. Childhood social environment and Hodgkin's disease. *N Engl J Med*. 1981 Jan 15;304:135-40.

[613] Paffernbarger RS Jr., Wing AL, Hyde RT. Characteristics in youth indicative of adult-onset Hodgkin's disease. *J Natl Cancer Inst*. 1977 May;58(5):1489-91.

[614] Chang ET, Zheng T, Weir EG, et al. Childhood Social Environment and Hodgkin's Lymphoma: New Findings from a Population-Based Case-Control Study. *Cancer Epidemiol Biomarkers Prev*. 2004 Aug;13(8):1361-70.

[615] Rudant J, Orsi L, Monnereau A, et al. Childhood hodgkin's lymphoma, non-Hodgkin's lymphoma and factors related to the immune system: the Escale study (SFCE). *Int J Cancer*. 2011;129(9):2236–2247.

[616] Parodi S, Crosignani P, Miligi L, et al. Childhood Infectious Diseases and Risk of Leukaemia in an Adult Population. *Int J Cancer*. 2013 Oct 15;133(8):1892-9.

[617] Van Steensel-Moll HA, Valkenburg HA, van Zanen GE. Childhood Leukemia and Infectious Diseases in the First Year of Life: A Register-Based Case-Control Study. *Am J Epidemiol*. 1986 Oct;124(4):590-4.

[618] Urayama KY, Biffler PA, Gallagher ER, et al. A Meta-Analysis of the Association Between Day-Care Attendance and Childhood Acute Lymphoblastic Leukaemia. *Int J Epidemiol*. 2010 Jun;39(3):718-32.

[619] Gilham C, Roman E, Eden TOB, et al. Day care in infancy and risk of childhood acute lymphoblastic leukaemia: findings from UK case-control study. *BMJ*. 2005;330:1294.

[620] Ma X, Buffler PA, Selvin S, et al. Daycare attendance and risk of childhood acute lymphoblastic leukaemia. *Br J Cancer*. 2002 May 6;86(9):1419–1424.

[621] Maia RDRP, Filho VW. Infection and childhood leukemia: review of evidence. *Rev Saude Publica*. 2013 Dec;47(6):1172–1185.

[622] Jourdan-Da Silva N, Perel Y, Mechinaud F, et al. Infectious Diseases in the First Year of Life, Perinatal Characteristics and Childhood Acute Leukaemia. *Br J Cancer*. 2004 Jan 12;90(1):139-45.

[623] Urayama KY, Ma X, Selvin S, et al. Early Life Exposure to Infections and Risk of Childhood Acute Lymphoblastic Leukemia. *Int J Cancer*. 2011 Apr 1;128(7):1632-43.

[624] Petridou E, Kassimos D, Kalmanti M, et al. Age of Exposure to Infections and Risk of Childhood Leukaemia. *BMJ*. 1993 Sep 25;307(6907):774.

[625] Komel KF, Gefeller B, Haferkamp B. Febrile Infections and Malignant Melanoma: Results of a Case-Control Study. *Melanoma Res*. 1992 Sep;2(3):207-11.

[626] Kolmel KF, Pfahlberg A, Mastrangelo G, et al. Infections and Melanoma Risk: Results of a Multicentre EORTC Case-Control Study. European Organization for Research and Treatment of Cancer. *Melanoma Res*. 1999 Oct;9(5):511-9.

[627] Mastrangelo G, FaddA E, Milan G. Cancer Increased After a Reduction of Infections in the First Half of This Century in Italy: Etiologic and Preventive Implications. *Eur J Epidemiol*. 1998 Dec;14(8):749-54.

[628] Rossinck MJ. Move Over, Bacteria! Viruses Make Their Mark as Mutualistic Microbial Symbionts. *J Virology*. 2015 Jul;89(13):6532-5.

313

[629] Chow J, Lee SM, Shen Y, et al. Host–Bacterial Symbiosis in Health and Disease. *Adv Immunol.* 2010;107:243–274.

[630] Mina M, Kula T, Leng Y, et al. Measles virus infection diminishes preexisting antibodies that offer protection from other pathogens. *Science.* 2019;366(6465):599.

[631] Rosen JB, Rota JS, Hickman CJ, et al. Outbreak of Measles Among Persons With Prior Evidence of Immunity, New York City, 2011. *Clin Infect Dis.* 2014 May;58(9):1205-10.

[632] Nkowane BM, Bart SW, Orenstein WA, et al. Measles outbreak in a vaccinated school population: epidemiology, chains of transmission and the role of vaccine failures. *Am J Public Health.* 1987 April;77(4):434–438.

[633] Chen RT, Goldbaum GM, Wassilak SGF, et al. An explosive point–Source measles outbreak in a highly vaccinated population: Modes of transmission and risk factors for disease. *AM J Epidemiology.* 1989 Jan;129(1):173-82.

[634] Business Insider. A US warship hit hard by the mumps is finally virus-free after being quarantined at sea for months. Available at: https://www.businessinsider.com/mumps-outbreak-on-us-warship-is-over-after-5-months-quarantined-at-sea-2019-5 [Accessed March 7, 2019].

[635] De Serres G, Markowski F, Toth E, et al. Largest Measles Epidemic in North America in a decade--Quebec, Canada, 2011: Contribution of Susceptibility, Serendipity, and Superspreading Events. *J Infect Dis.* 2013 Mar 15;207(6):990-8.

[636] Avramovich E, Indenbaum V, Haber M, et al. Measles Outbreak in a Highly Vaccinated Population — Israel, July–August 2017. *Weekly.* 2018 Oct 26;67(42):1186–1188.

[637] Ma R, Lu L, Zhangzhu J, et al. A Measles Outbreak in a Middle School With High Vaccination Coverage and Evidence of Prior Immunity Among Cases, Beijing, P.R. China. *Vaccine.* 2016 Apr 4;34(15):1853-60.

[638] Kurata T, Kanbayashi D, Egawa K, et al. A Measles Outbreak From an Index Case With Immunologically Confirmed Secondary Vaccine Failure. *Vaccine.* 2020 Feb 5;38(6):1467-1475.

[639] Zhang Z, Chen M, Ma R, et al. Outbreak of Measles Among Persons With Secondary Vaccine Failure, China, 2018. *Hum Vaccin Immunother.* 2019 Sep 5 [Online ahead of print].

[640] Trier H, Ronne T. [Duration of Immunity and Occurrence of Secondary Vaccine Failure Following Vaccination Against Measles, Mumps and Rubella]. *Ugeskr Laeger.* 1992 Jul 13;154(29):2008-13.

[641] Morfin F, Beguin A, Lina B, et al. Detection of Measles Vaccine in the Throat of a Vaccinated Child. *Vaccine.* 2002 Feb 22;20(11-12):1541-3.

[642] Kaic B, Gjenero-Margan I, Aleraj B, et al. Spotlight on Measles 2010: Excretion of Vaccine Strain Measles Virus in Urine and Pharyngeal Secretions of a Child With Vaccine Associated Febrile Rash Illness, Croatia, March 2010. *Euro Surveill.* 2010 Sep 2;15(35).

[643] Nestibo L, Lee BE, Fonesca K, et al. Differentiating the wild from the attenuated during a measles outbreak. *Paediatr Child Health.* 2012 Apr;17(4):e32–e33.

[644] Wilson K, Hawken S, Kwong JC, et al. Adverse Events following 12 and 18 Month Vaccinations: a Population-Based, Self-Controlled Case Series Analysis. *PLoS One.* 2011;6(12):e27897.

[645] Wilson K, Ducharme R, Ward B, et al. Increased Emergency Room Visits or Hospital Admissions in Females After 12-month MMR Vaccination, but No Difference After Vaccinations Given at a Younger Age. *Vaccine.* 2014 Feb 26;32(10):1153-9.

[646] Sorup S, Benn CS, Poulsen A. Live Vaccine Against Measles, Mumps, and Rubella and the Risk of Hospital Admissions for Nontargeted Infections. *JAMA.* 2014;311(8):826-35.

[647] Black C, Kaye JA, Jick H. MMR vaccine and idiopathic thrombocytopaenic purpura. *Br J Clin Pharmacol.* 2003 Jan; 55(1): 107–111.

[648] Miller E. Waight P, Farrington CP, et al. Idiopathic thrombocytopenic purpura and MMR vaccine. *Arch Dis Child.* 2001 Mar;84(3):227-9.

[649] Andrews N, Stowe J, Miller E, et al. A Collaborative Approach to Investigating the Risk of Thrombocytopenic Purpura After Measles-Mumps-Rubella Vaccination in England and Denmark. *Vaccine.* 2012 Apr 9;30(19):3042-6.

[650] Rinaldi M, Perricone C, Ortega-Hernandez O-D, et al. Immune Thrombocytopaenic Purpura: An Autoimmune Cross-Link Between Infections and Vaccines. *Lupus.* 2014 May;23(6):554-67.

[651] Andrews N, Stowe J, Miller E, et al. Post-licensure Safety of the Meningococcal Group C Conjugate Vaccine. *Hum Vaccin.* 2007 Mar-Apr;3(2):59-63.

[652] France EK, Glanz J, Xu S, et al. Risk of Immune Thrombocytopenic Purpura After Measles-Mumps-Rubella Immunization in Children. *Pediatrics.* 12008 Mar;121(3):e687-92

314

[653] Bertouola F, Morando C, Menniti-Ippolito F, et al. Association Between Drug and Vaccine Use and Acute Immune Thrombocytopenia in Childhood: A Case-Control Study in Italy. *Drug Saf.* 2010 Jan 1;33(1):65-72.

[654] Rajante J, Zeller B, Treutiger I, et al. Vaccination associated thrombocytopenic purpura in children. *Vaccine.* 2007 Feb;25(10):1838-40.

[655] Nieminen U, Peltola H, Syrjala MT, et al. Acute thrombocytopenic purpura following measles, mumps and rubella vaccination. A report on 23 patients. *Acta Paediatric.* 1993 Mar;82(3):267-70.

[656] O'Leary ST, Glanz JM, McClure DL, et al. The Risk of Immune Thrombocytopenic Purpura After Vaccination in Children and Adolescents. *Pediatrics.* 2012 Feb;129(2):248-55.

[657] Cecinati V, Principi N, Brescia L, et al. Vaccine administration and the development of immune thrombocytopenic purpura in children. *Human Vaccines Immunother.* 2013;9(5):1158-62.

[658] Hseieh YL, Lin LH. Thrombocytopenic purpura following vaccination in early childhood: Experience of a medical center in the past 2 decades. *J Chin Med Assoc.* 2010 Dec;73(12):634-7.

[659] Ronchi F, Cecchi P, Falconi F, et al. Thrombocytopenic purpura as adverse reaction to recombinant hepatitis B vaccine. *Arch Dis Chil.* 1998;78:273-4.

[660] Nuevo H, Nascimento-Carvalho C, Athayde-Oliveira C, et al. Thrombocytopenic purpura after hepatitis B vaccine: case report and review of the literature. *Ped Infect Dis J.* 2004 Feb;23(2):183-4.

[661] Neau D, Bonnet F, Michaud M, et al. Immune Thrombocytopenic Purpura After Recombinant Hepatitis B Vaccine: Retrospective Study of Seven Cases. *Scand J Infect Dis.* 1998;30(2):115-8.

[662] Shafiee A, Nazari S, Hashemiaghdam A, et al. Idiopathic Thrombocytopenic Purpura Is More Severe in Children with a Recent History of Vaccination. *Arch Ped Infect Dis.* 2013;1(3):113-7.

[663] Cecinati V, Principi N, Brescia L, et al. Vaccine administration and the development of immune thrombocytopenic purpura in children. *Human Vaccines Immunother.* 2013;9(5):1158-62.

[664] Rajante J, Zeller B, Treutiger I, et al. Vaccination associated thrombocytopenic purpura in children. *Vaccine.* 2007 Feb;25(10):1838-40.

[665] Cecinati V, Principi N, Brescia L, et al. Vaccine administration and the development of immune thrombocytopenic purpura in children. *Human Vaccines Immunother.* 2013;9(5):1158-62.

[666] Singh VK, Jensen RL. Elevated Levels of Measles Antibodies in Children With Autism. *Pediatr Neurol.* 2003 Apr;28(4):292-4.

[667] Singh VK, Lin SX, Newell E, et al. Abnormal Measles-Mumps-Rubella Antibodies and CNS Autoimmunity in Children With Autism. *J Biomed Sci.* 2002 Jul-Aug;9(4):359-64.

[668] Deisher TA, Doan NV, Omalye A, et al. Impact of environmental factors on the prevalence of autistic disorder after 1979. *J Public Health Epidemiology.* 2014 Sep;6(9):271-86.

[669] Deisher TA, Doan NV, Koyama K, et al. Epidemiologic and Molecular Relationship Between Vaccine Manufacture and Autism Spectrum Disorder Prevalence. *Issues Law Med.* 2015 Spring;30(1)47-70.

[670] Baird G, Pickles A, Simonoff E, et al. Measles Vaccination and Antibody Response in Autism Spectrum Disorders. *Arch Dis Child.* 2008 Oct;93(10):832-7.

[671] Wutzler P, Bonanni P, Burgess M, et al. Varicella vaccination - the global experience. *Expert Rev Vaccines.* 2017 Aug;16(8):833–843.

[672] Boëlle PY, Hanslik T. Varicella in non-immune persons: incidence, hospitalization and mortality rates. *Epidemiol Infect.* 2002 Dec;129(3):599-606.

[673] United States Centers for Disease Control and Prevention. Varicella Vaccine Effectiveness and Duration of Protection. Available at: https://www.cdc.gov/vaccines/vpd-vac/varicella/hcp-effective-duration.htm [Accessed: February 17, 2020].

[674] United States Food and Drug Administration. Package Insert - Varivax (Refrigerator). Available at: https://www.fda.gov/media/76000/download [Accessed February 8, 2020].

[675] Forbes H, Douglas I, Finn A, et al. Risk of herpes zoster after exposure to varicella to explore the exogenous boosting hypothesis: self controlled case series study using UK electronic healthcare data. *BMJ.* 2020;368.

[676] Goldman GS, King PG. Review of the United States Universal Varicella Vaccination Program: Herpes Zoster Incidence Rates, Cost-Effectiveness, and Vaccine Efficacy Based Primarily on the Antelope Valley Varicella Active Surveillance Project Data. *Vaccine.* 2013 Mar 25;31(13):1680-94.

[677] Wu PY, Wu HDI, Chou TC, et al. Varicella Vaccination Alters the Chronological Trends of Herpes Zoster and Varicella. *PLoS One.* 2003 Oct 30;8(10):e77709.

[678] Goldman GS. Cost-benefit analysis of universal varicella vaccination in the U.S. taking into account the closely related herpes-zoster epidemiology.

[679] Golman GS. The case against universal varicella vaccination. *Int J Toxicol.* 2006 Sep-Oct;25(5):313-7.

680 Goldman GS, King PG. Vaccination to Prevent Varicella: Goldman and King's Response to Myers' Interpretation of Varicella Active Surveillance Project Data. *Hum Exp Toxicol*. 2014 Aug;33(8):886-93.

681 Thomas SL, Wheeler JG, Hall AJ. Contacts with varicella or with children and protection against herpes zoster in adults: a case-control study. *Lancet*. 2002 Aug 31;360(9334):678-82.

682 Jardine A, Conaty SJ, Vally H. Herpes Zoster in Australia: Evidence of Increase in Incidence in Adults Attributable to Varicella Immunization? *Epidemiol Infect*. 2011 May;139(5):658-65.

683 Patel MS, Gebremariam A, Davis MM. Herpes zoster-related hospitalizations and expenditures before and after introduction of the varicella vaccine in the United States. *Infect Control Hosp Epidemiol*. 2008 Dec;29(12):1157-63.

684 Yih WK, Brooks DR, Lett SM, et al. The incidence of varicella and herpes zoster in Massachusetts as measured by the Behavioral Risk Factor Surveillance System (BRFSS) during a period of increasing varicella vaccine coverage, 1998–2003. *BMC Public Health*. 2005;5:68.

685 Kelly HA, Grant KA, Gidding H, et al. Decreased Varicella and Increased Herpes Zoster Incidence at a Sentinel Medical Deputising Service in a Setting of Increasing Varicella Vaccine Coverage in Victoria, Australia, 1998 to 2012. *Euro Surveill*. 2014 Oct 16;19(41).

686 Ogunjimi B, Willem L, Beutels P, et al. Integrating Between-Host Transmission and Within-Host Immunity to Analyze the Impact of Varicella Vaccination on Zoster. *Elife*. 2015 Jul 11;4:e07116.

687 Goldman GS. Universal varicella vaccination: efficacy trends and effect on herpes zoster. *Int J Toxicol*. 2005 Jul-Aug;24(4):205-13.

688 Oh SH, Choi EH, Shin SH, et al. Varicella and Varicella Vaccination in South Korea. *Clin Vaccine Immunol*. 2014 May;21(5):762–768.

689 Michalik DE, Steinberg SP, LaRussa PS, et al. Primary Vaccine Failure after 1 Dose of Varicella Vaccine in Healthy Children. *J Infect Dis*. 2008 Apr 1;197(7):944–949.

690 Bonanni P, Gershon A, Gershon M, et al. *Pediatr Infect Dis J*. 2013 Jul;32(7):e305–e313.

691 Michalik DE, Steinberg SP, LaRussa PS, et al. Primary Vaccine Failure after 1 Dose of Varicella Vaccine in Healthy Children. *J Infect Dis*. 2008 Apr 1;197(7):944–949.

692 Galil K, Fair E, Mountcastle N, et al. Younger Age at Vaccination May Increase Risk of Varicella Vaccine Failure. *J Infect Dis*. 2002 Jul 1;186(1):102-5.

693 Bonanni P, Gershon A, Gershon M, et al. *Pediatr Infect Dis J*. 2013 Jul;32(7):e305–e313.

694 Weinmann S, Chun C, Schmid DS, et al. Incidence and Clinical Characteristics of Herpes Zoster Among Children in the Varicella Vaccine Era, 2005-2009. *J Infect Dis*. 2013 Dec 1;208(11):1859-68.

695 Chun C, Weinmann S, Riedlinger K, et al. Laboratory Characteristics of Suspected Herpes Zoster in Vaccinated Children. *Pediatr Infect Dis J*. 2011 Aug;30(8):719-21.

696 Moodley A, Swanson J, Grose C, et al. Severe Herpes Zoster Following Varicella Vaccination in Immunocompetent Young Children. *J Child Neurol*. 2019 Mar;34(4):184–188.

697 Civen R, Chaves SS, Jumaan A, et al. The Incidence and Clinical Characteristics of Herpes Zoster Among Children and Adolescents After Implementation of Varicella Vaccination. *Pediatr Infect Dis J*. 2009 Nov;28(11):954-9.

698 Brisson M, Gay NJ, Edmunds WJ, et al. Exposure to Varicella Boosts Immunity to Herpes-Zoster: Implications for Mass Vaccination Against Chickenpox. *Vaccine*. 2002 Jun 7;20(19-20):2500-7.

699 Edmunds WJ, Brisson M, Gay NK, et al. Varicella Vaccination: A Double-Edged Sword? *Commun Dis Public Health*. 2002 Sep;5(3):185-6.

700 Marin M, Leung J, Gershon AA. Transmission of Vaccine-Strain Varicella-Zoster Virus: A Systematic Review. *Pediatrics*. 2019 Sep;144(3):e20191305.

701 Rafferty E, McDonald W, Qian W, et al. Evaluation of the effect of chickenpox vaccination on shingles epidemiology using agent-based modeling. *PeerJ*. 2018;6:e5012.

702 Davies EC, Pavan-Langston D, Chodosh J, et al. Herpes Zoster Ophthalmicus: Declining Age at Presentation. *Br J Ophthalmol*. 2016 Mar;100(3):312-4.

703 Leung J, Harpaz R, Molinari NA, et al. Herpes Zoster Incidence Among Insured Persons in the United States, 1993–2006: Evaluation of Impact of Varicella Vaccination. *Clinical Infect Dise*. 2011 Feb;52(3):332-40.

704 Grillo AP, Fraunfelder FW. Keratitis in Association With Herpes Zoster and Varicella Vaccines. 2017 Jul;53(7):393-7.

705 Krall P, Kubal A. Herpes Zoster Stromal Keratitis After Varicella Vaccine Booster in a Pediatric Patient. *Cornea*. 2014 Sep;33(9):988-9.

706 Nagpal A, Vora R, Margolis TP, et al. Interstitial Keratitis Following Varicella Vaccination. *Arch Opthalmol*. 2009 feb;127(2):222-23.

[707] University of Missouri Health. Chickenpox, Shingles Vaccine May Cause Corneal Inflammation in Some Patients. Available at: https://medicine.missouri.edu/news/chickenpox-shingles-vaccine-may-cause-corneal-inflammation-some-patients [Accessed February 19, 2020].

[708] Pesonen E, Andsberg E, Ohlin H, et al. Dual Role of Infections as Risk Factors for Coronary Heart Disease. *Atherosclerosis*. 2007 Jul;192(2):370-5.

[709] Min-Chul Kim, Sung-Cheol Yun, Han-Bin Lee, et al. Herpes Zoster Increases the Risk of Stroke and Myocardial Infarction. Journal of the American College of *Cardiology*. 2017;70(2):295-6.

[710] Silverberg JI, Kleiman E, Silverberg NB, et al. Chickenpox in Childhood Is Associated With Decreased Atopic Disorders, IgE, Allergic Sensitization, and Leukocyte Subsets. *Pediatr Allergy Immunol*. 2012 Feb;23(1):50-8.

[711] Quiros-Tejeira RE, Edwards MS, Rand EB, et al. Overview of hepatitis A virus infection in children. 2019 Nov 26. Available at: https://www.uptodate.com/contents/overview-of-hepatitis-a-virus-infection-in-children. *Vaccine*. 2005 May 9;23(25):3349-55.

[712] Hadler SC, Webster HM, Erben JJ, et al. Hepatitis A in day-care centers. A community-wide assessment. *N Engl J Med*. 1980;302(22):1222-1227.

[713] Lednar WM, Lemon SM, Kirkpatrick JW, et al. Frequency of illness associated with epidemic hepatitis A virus infections in adults. *Am J Epidemiol*. 1985;122(2):226-233.

[714] Tong MJ, el-Farra NS, Grew MI. Clinical manifestations of hepatitis A: recent experience in a community teaching hospital. *J Infect Dis*. 1995;171 Suppl 1:S15-18.

[715] Sjogren MH, Tanno H, Fay O, et al. Hepatitis A virus in stool during clinical relapse. *Ann Int Med*. 1987;106(2):221-226.

[716] Gordon SC, Reddy KR, Schiff L, et al. Prolonged intrahepatic cholestasis secondary to acute hepatitis A. *Ann Int Med*. 1984;101(5):635-637.

[717] World Health Organization. Hepatitis A. Available at: https://www.who.int/immunization/diseases/hepatitisA/en/ [Accessed February 17, 2002].

[718] Jefferies M, Rauff B, Rashid H, et al. Update on global epidemiology of viral hepatitis and preventive strategies. *World J Clin Cases*. 2018 Nov 6;6(13):589–599.

[719] United States Centers for Disease Control and Prevention. Hepatitis A. Available at: https://www.cdc.gov/vaccines/pubs/pinkbook/hepa.html [Accessed February 17, 2020].

[720] Wasley A, Fiore A, Bell BP. Hepatitis A in the era of vaccination. *Epidemiol Rev*. 2006; 28():101-11.

[721] Taylor RM, Davern T, Munoz S, et al. Fulminant hepatitis A virus infection in the United States: Incidence, prognosis, and outcomes. *Hepatology*. 2006 Dec; 44(6):1589-97.

[722] United States Centers for Disease Control and Prevention. Hepatitis A. Available at: https://www.cdc.gov/vaccines/pubs/pinkbook/hepa.html [Accessed February 17, 2020].

[723] United States Food and Drug Administration. Package Insert – HAVRIX. Available at: https://www.fda.gov/files/vaccines%2C%20blood%20%26%20biologics/published/Package-Insert---HAVRIX.pdf [Accessed February 17, 2020].

[724] United States Food and Drug Administration. Package Insert – VAQTA. Available at: https://www.fda.gov/media/74519/download [Accessed February 17, 2020].

[725] United States Food and Drug Administration. Package Insert - TWINRIX Available at: https://www.fda.gov/media/119351/download [Accessed February 17, 2020].

[726] O'Leary ST, Glanz JM, McClure DL, et al. The Risk of Immune Thrombocytopenic Purpura After Vaccination in Children and Adolescents. *Pediatrics*.2012 Feb;129(2):248-55.

[727] Cecinati V, Principi N, Brescia L, et al. Vaccine administration and the development of immune thrombocytopenic purpura in children. *Hum Vaccin Immunother*. 2013 May 1;9(5):1158–1162.

[728] Muñoz N, Bosch FX, de Sanjosé S, et al. Epidemiologic classification of human papillomavirus types associated with cervical cancer. *N Engl J Med*. 2003 Feb 6; 348(6):518-27.

[729] Clifford GM, Smith JS, Aguado T, et al. Comparison of HPV type distribution in high-grade cervical lesions and cervical cancer: a meta-analysis. *Br J Cancer*. 2003 Jul 7;89(1):101-5.

[730] Sellors JW, Karwalajtys TL, Kaczorowski J, et al. Incidence, clearance and predictors of human papillomavirus infection in women. Survey of HPV in Ontario Women Group. *CMAJ*. 2003 Feb 18; 168(4):421-5.

[731] Nyitray A, Nielson CM, Harris RB, et al. Prevalence of and risk factors for anal human papillomavirus infection in heterosexual men. *J Infect Dis*. 2008 Jun 15; 197(12):1676-84.

[732] United States Centers for Disease Control and Prevention. About HPV. Available at: https://www.cdc.gov/hpv/parents/about-hpv.html [Accessed February 17, 2020].

[733] Ho GY, Bierman R, Beardsley L, et al. Natural history of cervicovaginal papillomavirus infection in young women. *N Engl J Med*. 1998 Feb 12; 338(7):423-8.

317

[734] Van Doornum GJ, Prins M, Juffermans LH, et al. Regional distribution and incidence of human papillomavirus infections among heterosexual men and women with multiple sexual partners: a prospective study. *Genitourin Med*. 1994 Aug; 70(4):240-6.

[735] Sanjose SD, Diz M, Castellsague X, et al. Worldwide Prevalence and Genotype Distribution of Cervical Human Papillomavirus DNA in Women With Normal Cytology: A Meta-Analysis. *Lancet Infect Dis*. 2007 Jul;7(7):453-9.

[736] Winer RL, Lee SK, Hughes JP, et al. Genital human papillomavirus infection: incidence and risk factors in a cohort of female university students. *Am J Epidemiol*. 2003 Feb 1; 157(3):218-26.

[737] Centers for Disease Control and Prevention, authors. Genital HPV Infection Fact Sheet. Rockville, MD: CDC National Prevention Information Network; 2004.

[738] Dunne EF, Nielson CM, Stone KM, et al. Prevalence of HPV infection among men: A systematic review of the literature. *J Infect Dis*. 2006 Oct 15; 194(8):1044-57.

[739] Castellsague X, Munoz N. Chapter 3: Cofactors in Human Papillomavirus Carcinogenesis—Role of Parity, Oral Contraceptives, and Tobacco Smoking. *J Nat Cancer Institute Monographs*. 2003;31:20-28.

[740] de Martel C, Plummer M, Vignat J, et al. Worldwide burden of cancer attributable to HPV by site, country and HPV type. *Int J Cancer*. 2017 Aug 15;141(4):664–670.

[741] World Health Organization. Cervical Cancer. Available at: https://www.who.int/cancer/prevention/diagnosis-screening/cervical-cancer/en/ [Accessed February 21, 2020].

[742] Safaeian M, Solomon D. Cervical Cancer Prevention - Cervical Screening: Science in Evolution. *Obstet Gynecol Clin North Am*. 2007 Dec;34(4):739–ix.

[743] United States Food and Drug Administration. Package Insert - GARDASIL 9. Available at: https://www.fda.gov/media/90064/download [Accessed February 17, 2020].

[744] United States Food and Drug Administration. Gardasil Package Insert. Available at: https://www.fda.gov/files/vaccines,%20blood%20&%20biologics/published/Package-Insert---Gardasil.pdf [Accessed February 17, 2020].

[745] United States Food and Drug Administration. Package Insert with Patient Package Information section – cervarix. Available at: https://www.fda.gov/media/79773/download [Accessed February 17, 2020].

[746] Poddighe D, Vadala M, Laurino C, et al. Somatoform and Neurocognitive Syndromes After HPV Immunization Are Not Associated to Cell-Mediated Hypersensitivity to Aluminum. *Toxicol In Vitro*. 2017 Sep;43:58-61.

[747] United States Centers for Disease Control and Prevention. Questions about HPV Vaccine Safety. Available at: https://www.cdc.gov/vaccinesafety/vaccines/hpv/hpv-safety-faqs.html [Accessed February 18, 2020].

[748] Tomljenovic L, Spinosa JP, Shaw CA. Human Papillomavirus (HPV) Vaccines as an Option for Preventing Cervical Malignancies: (How) Effective and Safe? *Curr Pharm Des*. 2013;19(8):1466-87.

[749] Mello MM, Abiola S, Colgrove J. Pharmaceutical Companies' Role in State Vaccination Policymaking: The Case of Human Papillomavirus Vaccination. *Am J Public Health*. 2012 May;102(5):893–898.

[750] Tomljenovic L, Shaw CA. Too Fast or Not Too Fast: The FDA's Approval of Merck's HPV Vaccine Gardasil. *J Law Med Ethics*. 2012 Fall;40(3):673-81.

[751] Tomljenovic L, Shaw CA. No autoimmune safety signal after vaccination with quadrivalent HPV vaccine Gardasil? *J Intern Med*. 2012 Nov;272(5):514-5; author reply 516.

[752] Tomljenovic L, Shaw CA. Who Profits From Uncritical Acceptance of Biased Estimates of Vaccine Efficacy and Safety? *Am J Public Health*. 2012 September;102(9):e13–e14.

[753] Spinosa JP, Riva C, Biollaz J. Letter to the Editor Response to the article of Luisa Lina Villa HPV prophylactic vaccination: The first years and what to expect from now, in press. *Cancer Lett*. 2011 May;304(1):70.

[754] Gerhardus A, Razum O. A long story made too short: surrogate variables and the communication of HPV vaccine trial results. *J Epidemiology Comm Health*. 2010 Apr;64(5):377-8.

[755] Tomljenovic L, Wilyman J, Vanamee E, et al. HPV vaccines and cancer prevention, science versus activism. *Infect Agent Cancer*. 2013;8:6.

[756] Tomljenovic L, Shaw CA, et al. Human Papillomavirus (HPV) Vaccine Policy and Evidence-Based Medicine: Are They at Odds? *Ann Med*. 2013 Mar;45(2):182-93.

[757] Tomljenovic L, Spinosa JP, Shaw CA. Human Papillomavirus (HPV) Vaccines as an Option for Preventing Cervical Malignancies: (How) Effective and Safe? *Curr Pharm Des*. 2013;19(8):1466-87.

[758] Wadman M. Merck settles Vioxx lawsuits for $4.85 billion. *Nature*. 2007.

[759] United States District Court for the Eastern District of Pennsylvania. Available at: https://www.naturalnews.com/gallery/documents/Merck-False-Claims-Act.pdf [Accessed February 21, 2020].

[760] Rees CP, Brhlikova P, Pollock AM. Will HPV vaccination prevent cervical cancer? *J Royal Soc Med.* 2020;113(2):64-78.

[761] Gatto M, Agmon-Levin N, Soriano A, et al. Human Papillomavirus Vaccine and Systemic Lupus Erythematosus. *Clin Rheumatol.* 2013 Sep;32(9):1301-7.

[762] Geier DA, Geier MR. A case–control study of quadrivalent human papillomavirus vaccine-associated autoimmune adverse events. *Clin Rheumatol.* 2015;34(7):1225–1231.

[763] Martinez-Lavin M, Amezcua-Guerra L. Serious Adverse Events After HPV Vaccination: A Critical Review of Randomized Trials and Post-Marketing Case Series. *Clin Rheumatol.* 2017 Oct;36(10):2169-2178.

[764] Tomljenovic L, Shaw CA. Death after Quadrivalent Human Papillomavirus (HPV) Vaccination: Causal or Coincidental? *Pharmaceut Reg Affairs.* 2012;S12:001.

[765] Gomez SM, Glover M, Malone M, et al. Vasculitis following HPV immunization. *Rheumatol.* 2013 Mar;52(3):581-2.

[766] Martinez-Lavin M. Hypothesis: Human Papillomavirus Vaccination Syndrome--Small Fiber Neuropathy and Dysautonomia Could Be Its Underlying Pathogenesis. *Clin Rheumatol.* 2015 Jul;34(7):1165-9.

[767] Yaju Y, Tsubaki H. Safety concerns with human papilloma virus immunization in Japan: Analysis and evaluation of Nagoya City's surveillance data for adverse events. *Jpn J Nurs Sci.* 2019 Oct;16(4):433–449.

[768] Chandler RE. Safety Concerns with HPV Vaccines Continue to Linger: Are Current Vaccine Pharmacovigilance Practices Sufficient? *Drug Saf.* 2017;40(12):1167–1170.

[769] Svetlana B, Brinth L, Hendrickson JE, et al. Autonomic Dysfunction and HPV Immunization: An Overview. *Immunol Res.* 2018 Dec;66(6):744-754.

[770] Palmieri B, Poddghe D, Vadala M, et al. Severe somatoform and dysautonomic syndromes after HPV vaccination: case series and review of literature. *Immunol Res.* 2017;65(1):106–116.

[771] Ozawa K, Hineno A, Kinoshita T, et al. Suspected Adverse Effects After Human Papillomavirus Vaccination: A Temporal Relationship Between Vaccine Administration and the Appearance of Symptoms in Japan. *Drug Saf.* 2017;40(12):1219–1229.

[772] Ikeda SI, Hineno A, Ozawa K, et al. Suspected Adverse Effects After Human Papillomavirus Vaccination: A Temporal Relationship. Immunol Res. 2018 Dec;66(6):723-725.

[773] Ozawa K, Hineno A, Kinoshita T, et al. Suspected Adverse Effects After Human Papillomavirus Vaccination: A Temporal Relationship Between Vaccine Administration and the Appearance of Symptoms in Japan. *Drug Saf.* 2017 Dec;40(12):1219-1229.

[774] Brinth L, Theibel AC, Pors K, et al. Suspected Side Effects to the Quadrivalent Human Papilloma Vaccine. *Dan Med J.* 2015 Apr;62(4):A5064.

[775] Hanley SJB, Pollock KGJ, Cushieri K. Peripheral Sympathetic Nerve Dysfunction in Adolescent Japanese Girls Following Immunization With the Human Papillomavirus Vaccine. *Intern Med.* 2015;54(15):1953.

[776] Brinth L, Pors K, Alexandra A, et al. Is Chronic Fatigue Syndrome/Myalgic Encephalomyelitis a Relevant Diagnosis in Patients with Suspected Side Effects to Human Papilloma Virus Vaccine? *Int J Vaccines Vaccin.* 2015;1(1):00003.

[777] Kinoshita T, Abe RT, Hinero A, et al. Peripheral Sympathetic Nerve Dysfunction in Adolescent Japanese Girls Following Immunization With the Human Papillomavirus Vaccine. *Intern Med.* 2014;53(19):2185-200.

[778] Alvarez-Soria MJ, Hernandez-Gonzalez A, Carrasco-Garcia de Leon S, et al.. [Demyelinating disease and vaccination of the human papillomavirus]. *Rev Neurol.* 2011;52:472–6.

[779] Sutton I, Lahoria R, Tan I, et al. CNS demyelination and quadrivalent HPV vaccination. *Mult Scler.* 2009;15:116–9.10.

[780] Brinth LS, Pors K, Theibel AC, et al. Orthostatic Intolerance and Postural Tachycardia Syndrome as Suspected Adverse Effects of Vaccination Against Human Papilloma Virus. *Vaccine.* 2015 May 21;33(22):2602-5.

[781] Campbell JP, Turner JE. Debunking the Myth of Exercise-Induced Immune Suppression: Redefining the Impact of Exercise on Immunological Health Across the Lifespan. *Front Immunol.* 2018 Apr 16;9:648.

[782] Taneja V. Sex Hormones Determine Immune Response. *Front Immunol.* 2018;9:1931.

[783] Palmieri B, Poddighe D, Vadal M, et al. Severe somatoform and dysautonomic syndromes after HPV vaccination: case series and review of literature. *Immunol Res.* 2017;65(1):106–116.

[784] Souayah N, Michas-Martin PA, Nasar A, et al. Guillain-Barré syndrome after Gardasil vaccination: data from Vaccine Adverse Event Reporting System 2006-2009. *Vaccine.* 2011;29:886–9.

[785] Phillips A, Patel C, Pillsbury A, et al. Safety of Human Papillomavirus Vaccines: An Updated Review. *Drug Saf.* 2018 Apt;41(4):329-346.

[786] Blitshteyn S, Brinth L, Hendrickson JE, et al. Autonomic Dysfunction and HPV Immunization: An Overview. *Immunol Res*. 2018 Dec;66(6):744-754.

[787] Wellons M. Cardiovascular Disease and Primary Ovarian Insufficiency. *Semin Reprod Med*. 2011 Jul;29(4):328–341.

[788] Gruber N, Shoenfeld Y. A Link Between Human Papilloma Virus Vaccination and Primary Ovarian Insufficiency: Current Analysis. *Curr Opin Obstet Gynecol*. 2015 Aug;27(4):265-70.

[789] Little DT, Ward HR. Ongoing inadequacy of quadrivalent HPV vaccine safety studies. *BMJ Evid Based Med*. 2019 Jan 7 [Online ahead of print].

[790] Little DT, Ward HRG. Adolescent Premature Ovarian Insufficiency Following Human Papillomavirus Vaccination: A Case Series Seen in General Practice. *J Investig Med High Impact Case Rep*. 2014 Oct-Dec;2(4):2324709614556129.

[791] Colafrancesco S, Perricone C, Tomljenovic L, et al. Human Papilloma Virus Vaccine and Primary Ovarian Failure: Another Facet of the Autoimmune/Inflammatory Syndrome Induced by Adjuvants. *Am J Reprod Immunol*. 2013 Oct;70(4):309-16.

[792] Little DT, Ward HRG. Premature ovarian failure 3 years after menarche in a 16-year-old girl following human papillomavirus vaccination. *BMJ Case Rep*. 2012;2012:bcr2012006879.

[793] DeLong G. A lowered probability of pregnancy in females in the USA aged 25–29 who received a human papillomavirus vaccine injection. *J Toxicol Environ Health A*. 2018;81(14):661–74.

[794] Naleway AL, Mittendorf KF, Irving SA, et al. Primary Ovarian Insufficiency and Adolescent Vaccination. Pediatrics. 2018 Sep;142(3):1-16.

[795] Christianson MS, Wodi P, Talaat K, et al. Primary ovarian insufficiency and human papilloma virus vaccines: a review of the current evidence. *Am J Obstet Gynecol*.
2019 Aug 31 [Online ahead of print].

[796] Hawkes D, Buttery JP. Human papillomavirus vaccination and primary ovarian insufficiency: An association based on ideology rather than evidence. *Curr Opin Obstet Gynecol*. 2016 Feb;28(1):70-2.

[797] Jafri RZ, Ali A, Messonnier NE, et al. Global epidemiology of invasive meningococcal disease. *Popul Health Metr*. 2013;11:17.

[798] Diermayer M, Hedberg K, Hoesly F, et al. Epidemic serogroup B meningococcal disease in Oregon: the evolving epidemiology of the ET-5 strain. *JAMA*. 1999 Apr 28; 281(16):1493-7.

[799] Baker MG, Martin DR, Kieft CE, et al. A 10-year serogroup B meningococcal disease epidemic in New Zealand: descriptive epidemiology, 1991-2000. *J Paediatr Child Health*. 2001 Oct; 37(5):S13-9.

[800] van Kessel F, van den Ende C, Oordt-Speets AM, et al. Outbreaks of meningococcal meningitis in non-African countries over the last 50 years: a systematic review. *J Glob Health*. 2019 Jun; 9(1): 010411.

[801] Mayer SB, Esposito S. Meningococcal disease in childhood: epidemiology, clinical features and prevention. *J Prev Med Hyg*. 2015 Aug;56(3):E121–E124.

[802] Jafri RZ, Ali A, Messonnier NE, et al. Global epidemiology of invasive meningococcal disease. *Popul Health Metr*. 2013;11:17.

[803] World Health Organization. Menigococcal meningitis. Available at: https://www.who.int/news-room/fact-sheets/detail/meningococcal-meningitis [Accessed February 15, 2020].

[804] United States Centers for Disease Control and Prevention. Meningococcal Disease. Diagnosis, Treatment, and Complications. Available at: https://www.cdc.gov/meningococcal/about/diagnosis-treatment.html [Accessed February 15, 2020].

[805] United States Centers for Disease Control and Prevention. Recommendations for Use of Meningococcal Conjugate Vaccines in HIV-Infected Persons — Advisory Committee on Immunization Practices, 2016 Available at: http://www.cdc.gov/mmwr/volumes/65/wr/pdfs/mm6543a3.pdf [Accessed February 17, 2020].

[806] United States Food and Drug Administration. Package Insert - Menveo. Available at: https://www.fda.gov/media/78514/download [Accessed February 17, 2020].

[807] United States Food and Drug Administration. Package Insert - Menactra. Available at: https://www.fda.gov/files/vaccines,%20blood%20&%20biologics/published/Package-Insert---Menactra.pdf [Accessed February 17, 2020].

[808] United States Food and Drug Administration. Package Insert - BEXSERO. Available at: https://www.fda.gov/media/90996/download [Accessed February 17, 2020].

[809] United States Food and Drug Administration. Package Insert - TRUMENBA. Available at: https://www.fda.gov/files/vaccines,%20blood%20&%20biologics/published/Package-Insert---TRUMENBA.pdf [Accessed February 17, 2020].

[810] Myers TR, McNeil MM, Ng CS, et al. Adverse Events Following Quadrivalent Meningococcal CRM-Conjugate Vaccine (Menveo®) Reported to the Vaccine Adverse Event Reporting System (VAERS), 2010–2015. *Vaccine.* 2017 Mar 27;35(14):1758–1763.

[811] Velentgas P, Amato AA, Bohn RL, et al. Risk of Guillain-Barré Syndrome After Meningococcal Conjugate Vaccination. *Pharmacoepidemiol Drug Saf.* 2012 Dec;21(12):1350-8.

[812] Centers for Disease Control and Prevention. Update: Guillain-Barré Syndrome Among Recipients of Menactra Meningococcal Conjugate vaccine--United States, June 2005-September 2006. *MMWR Morb Mortal Wkly Rep.* 2006 Oct 20;55(41):1120-4.

[813] Cho BH, Clark TA, Messonnier NE, et al. MCV Vaccination in the Presence of Vaccine-Associated Guillain-Barré Syndrome Risk: A Decision Analysis Approach. *Vaccine.* 2010 Jan 8;28(3):817-22.

[814] Tseng HF, Sy LS, Ackerson BK, et al. Safety of Quadrivalent Meningococcal Conjugate Vaccine in 11- to 21-Year-Olds. *Pediatrics.* 2017 Jan;139(1):e20162084.

[815] Rowhani-Rahbar A, Klein NP, Lewis N, et al. Immunization and Bell's Palsy in Children: A Case-Centered Analysis. *Am J Epidemiol.* 2012 May 1;175(9):787-85.

[816] Mayson AR, Ray BD, Bhuiyan AR, et al. Pilot comparative study on the health of vaccinated and unvaccinated 6- to 12- year old U.S. children. *J Translational Sci.* 2017;3(3):1-12.

[817] Zimmerman P, Curtis N. Factors That Influence the Immune Response to Vaccination. *Clin Microbiol Rev.* 2019 Apr;32(2):e00084-18.

[818] Melville JM, Moss TJM. The immune consequences of preterm birth. *Front Neurosci.* 2013;7:79.

[819] Ment LR, Vohr BR. Preterm birth and the developing brain. *Lancet Neurol.* 2008 May;7(5):378–379.

[820] O'Conor AR, Wilson CM, Fielder AR. Ophthalmological problems associated with preterm birth. *Eye.* 2007;21:1254-60.

[821] Collin AA, McEvoy C, Castile RG. Respiratory Morbidity and Lung Function in Preterm Infants of 32 to 36 Weeks' Gestational Age. *Pediatrics.* 2010 Jul;126(1):115–128.

[822] Bhutani V, Wong RJ. Bilirubin Neurotoxicity in Preterm Infants: Risk and Prevention. *J Clin Neonatol.* 2013 Apr-Jun;2(2):61–69.

[823] Bavineni M, Wassemaar TM, Agnihotri K, et al. Mechanisms linking preterm birth to onset of cardiovascular disease later in adulthood. *Eur Heart J.* 2019Apr;40(14):1107-12.

[824] Chu PY, Li JS, Kosinski AS, et al. Congenital Heart Disease in Premature Infants 25-32 Weeks' Gestational Age. *J Pediatr.* 2017 Feb;181:37-41.e1.

[825] Rosen L. Adverse events induced by first immunization in extremely premature Infants. School of Medicine, Örebro University, thesis. Available at: http://www.diva-portal.org/smash/get/diva2:974924/FULLTEXT01.pdf [Accessed February 29, 2020].

[826] D'Angio CT. Active Immunization of Premature and Low Birth-Weight Infants: A Review of Immunogenicity, Efficacy, and Tolerability. *Paediatr Drugs.* 2007;9(1):17-32.

[827] D'Angio CT, Maniscalco WM, Pichichero ME. Immunologic Response of Extremely Premature Infants to Tetanus, Haemophilus Influenzae, and Polio Immunizations. *Pediatrics.* 1995 Jul;96(1 Pt 1):18-22.

[828] Khalak R, Pichichero ME, D-Angio CT. Three-year Follow-Up of Vaccine Response in Extremely Preterm Infants. *Pediatrics.* 1998 Apr;101(4 Pt 1):597-603.

[829] Kuzniewicz MW, Klein NP. Differentiating Sepsis From Adverse Events After Immunization in the Neonatal Intensive Care Unit: How Is a Physician to Know? *JAMA Pediatr.* 2015 Aug;169(8):718-19.

[830] Pourcyros M, Korones SB, Arheart KL, et al. Primary Immunization of Premature Infants With Gestational Age <35 Weeks: Cardiorespiratory Complications and C-reactive Protein Responses Associated With Administration of Single and Multiple Separate Vaccines Simultaneously. *J Pediatr.* 2007 Aug;151(2):167-72.

[831] Celik IH, Demirel G, Canplat FE, et al. Inflammatory responses to hepatitis B virus vaccine in healthy term infants. *Eur J Pediatr.* 2013 Jun;172(6):839-42.

[832] Menius C, Schmalisch G, Hartenstein S, et al. Adverse Cardiorespiratory Events Following Primary Vaccination of Very Low Birth Weight Infants. *J Pediatr (Rio J).* 2012 Mar-Apr; 88(2):137-42.

[833] Mialet-Marty T, Beuchee A, Jmaa WB, et al. Possible Predictors of Cardiorespiratory Events After Immunization in Preterm Neonates. *Neonatology.* 2013;104(2):151-5.

[834] Sen S, Cloete Y, Hassan K, et al. Adverse Events Following Vaccination in Premature Infants. *Acta Paediatr.* 2001 Aug;90(8):916-20.

[835] Lee J, Robinson JL, Spady DW. Frequency of Apnea, Bradycardia, and Desaturations Following First Diphtheria-Tetanus-Pertussis-Inactivated polio-Haemophilus Influenzae Type B Immunization in Hospitalized Preterm Infants. *BMC Pediatr.* 2006 Jun 19;6:20.

[836] Klein NP, Masolo ML, Green J, et al. Risk Factors for Developing Apnea After Immunization in the Neonatal Intensive Care Unit. *Pediatrics.* 2008 Mar;121(3):463-9.

[837] Hacking DF, Davis PG, Wong E, et al. Frequency of Respiratory Deterioration After Immunisation in Preterm Infants. *J Paediatr Child Health*. 2010 Dec;46(12):742-8.

[838] Dangio CT, Hall CB. Timing of Vaccinations in Premature Infants. *BioDrugs*. 2000 May;13(5):335-46.

[839] Buijs SC, Boersma B. [Cardiorespiratory Events After First Immunization in Premature Infants: A Prospective Cohort Study]. *Ned Tijdschr Geneeskd*. 2012;156(3):A3797.

[840] Pourcyrous M, Koronoes SB, Crouse D, et al. Interleukin-6, C-reactive Protein, and Abnormal Cardiorespiratory Responses to Immunization in Premature Infants. *Pediatrics*. 1988 Mar;101(3):E3.

[841] Lee J, Robinson JL, Spady DW. Frequency of Apnea, Bradycardia, and Desaturations Following First Diphtheria-Tetanus-Pertussis-Inactivated polio-Haemophilus Influenzae Type B Immunization in Hospitalized Preterm Infants. *BMC Pediatr*. 2006 Jun 19;6:20.

[842] Schulzke S, Heininger U, Lucking-Famira M, et al. Apnoea and Bradycardia in Preterm Infants Following Immunisation With Pentavalent or Hexavalent Vaccines. *Eur J Pediatr*. 2005 Jul;164(7):432-5.

[843] Flatz-Jequier A, Posfay-Barbe KM, Pfister RE, et al. Recurrence of Cardiorespiratory Events Following Repeat DTaP-based Combined Immunization in Very Low Birth Weight Premature Infants. *J Pediatr*. 2008 Sep;153(3):429-31.

[844] Clifford V, Crawford NW, Royle J, et al. Recurrent Apnoea Post Immunisation: Informing Re-Immunisation Policy. *Vaccine*. 2011 Aug 5;29(34):5681-7.

[845] Sanchez PJ, Laptoo AR, Fisher L, et al. Apnea after immunization of preterm infants.*J Pediatrics*. 1997 May;130(5):746-51.

[846] Botham SJ, Isaacs D, Hendeson-Smart DJ. Incidence of Apnoea and Bradycardia in Preterm Infants Following DTPw and Hib Immunization: A Prospective Study. *J Paediatr Child Health*. 1997 Oct;33(5):418-21.

[847] Slack MH, Schapira D. Severe Apnoeas Following Immunisation in Premature Infants. *Arch Dis Child Fetal Neonatal Ed*. 1999 Jul;81(1):F67-8.

[848] Cooper PA, Madhi SA, Huebner RE, et al. Apnea and Its Possible Relationship to Immunization in Ex-Premature Infants. *Vaccine*. 2008 Jun 25;26(27-28):3410-3.

[849] Wilsom K, Hawken S. Incidence of adverse events in premature children following 2-month vaccination. *Human Vaccines Immunother*. 2012 May 1;8(5):592-5.

[850] Furck AK, Richter JW, Kattner E. Very low birth weight infants have only few adverse events after timely immunization. *J Perinatology*. 2010;30:118-21.

[851] Gagneur A, Pinquier D, Quach C. Immunization of preterm infants. *Human Vaccines Immunotherap*. 2015 Mar 4;11(11):2556-63.

[852] DeMeo SD, Raman SR, Hornik CP, et al. Adverse Events After Routine Immunization of Extremely Low Birth Weight Infants. *JAMA Pediatr*. 2015 Aug 1;169(8):740–745.

[853] Navar-Boggan AM, Halsey NA, Golden WC, et al. Risk of fever and sepsis evaluations after routine immunizations in the neonatal intensive care unit. *J Perinatol*. 2010 Feb 25;30:604-9.

[854] Natural Health Ed. Newlywed Died of Sepsis after Flu Shot: Discover how to prevent this from happening to you or your loved ones. Available at: https://naturalhealthed.com/newlywed-died-of-sepsis-after-flu-shot/ [Accessed March 7, 2020].

[855] Vaccine Impact. NY State Senator Dies of Sepsis After Receiving Flu Vaccine. Available at: https://vaccineimpact.com/2018/ny-state-senator-dies-of-sepsis-after-receiving-flu-vaccine/ [Accessed March 7, 2020].

[856] Vaxxed II The People's Truth. Vaccines Causing Sepsis Leading to Limb Amputation. Available at: https://vaccine-injury.info/infant-vaccines-causing-sepsis-leading-to-limb-amputation- [Accessed March 7, 2020].

[857] Matzaraki V, Kumar V, Wijmenga C, et al. The MHC locus and genetic susceptibility to autoimmune and infectious diseases. *Genome Biol*. 2017;18(76).

[858] Cruz-tapias P, Castiblanco J, Anaya JM. Autoimmunity: From Bench to Bedside. Chapter 17, HLA Association with Autoimmune Diseases. Available at: https://www.ncbi.nlm.nih.gov/books/NBK459459/ [Accessed February 22, 2020].

[859] Gough SCL, Simmonds MJ. The HLA Region and Autoimmune Disease: Associations and Mechanisms of Action. *Curr Genomics*. 2007 Nov;8(7):453–465.

[860] Grandi N, Tramontano E. Human Endogenous Retroviruses Are Ancient Acquired Elements Still Shaping Innate Immune Responses. *Front Immunol*. 2018;9:2039.

[861] Blomberg J, Ushameckis D, Jern P. Madame Curie Bioscience Database [Internet] Evolutionary Aspects of Human Endogenous Retroviral Sequences (HERVs) and Disease. Available at: https://www.ncbi.nlm.nih.gov/books/NBK6235/ [Accessed March 7 2020].

[862] Miyazawa T. Endogenous Retroviruses as Potential Hazards for Vaccines. *Biologicals*. 2010 May;38(3):371-6.

[863] Grandi N, Tramontano E. HERV Envelope Proteins: Physiological Role and Pathogenic Potential in Cancer and Autoimmunity. *Front Microbiol*. 2018 Mar 14;9(462):1-26.

[864] Sekigawa I, Ogasawara H, Kaneko H. et al. Retroviruses and autoimmunity. *Intern Med*. 2001;40:80–86.

[865] Wucherpfennig KW, Strominger JL. Molecular mimicry in T cell-mediated autoimmunity: viral peptides activate human T cell clones specific for myelin basic protein. *Cell*. 1995;80:695-705.

[866] Benoist C, Mathis D. Autoimmunity provoked by infection: how good is the case for T cell epitope mimicry? *Nature Immunol*. 2001;2:797-801.

[867] Hahn AF. Guillain-Barre syndrome. *Lancet*. 1998;352:635-641.

[868] Reif DM, McKinney BA, Motsinger AA, et al. Genetic Basis for Adverse Events After Smallpox Vaccination. *J Infect Dis*. 2008 Jul 1;198(1):16-22.

[869] Schwann BC, Rozen R. Madame Curie Bioscience Database [Internet]. Methylenetetrahydrofolate Reductase Polymorphisms: Pharmacogenetic Effects. Available at: https://www.ncbi.nlm.nih.gov/books/NBK5968/ [Accessed February 22, 2020].

[870] Sharaki OA, Elgerby AH, Nassat ES, et al. Impact of methylenetetrahydrofolate reductase (MTHFR) A1298C gene polymorphism on the outcome of methotrexate treatment in a sample of Egyptian rheumatoid arthritis patients. *Alexandria J Med*. 2018 Dec;54(4):633-8.

[871] Berkani LM, Rahal F, Allam I, et al. Association of MTHFR C677T and A1298C gene polymorphisms with methotrexate efficiency and toxicity in algerian rheumatoid arthritis patients. *Heliyon*. 2017;3:e00467.

[872] Austin DW, Spolding B, Gondalia S, et al. Genetic Variation Associated with Hypersensitivity to Mercury. *Toxicol Int*. 2014 Sep-Dec;21(3):236–241.

[873] Mosharov E, Cranford MR, Banerjee R. The quantitatively important relationship between homocysteine metabolism and glutathione synthesis by the transsulfuration pathway and its regulation by redox changes. *Biochem*. 2000;39(42):13005–11.

[874] Liu X, Solehdin F, Cohen IL, et al. Population- and family-based studies associate the MTHFR gene with idiopathic autism in simplex families. *J Autism Develop Dis*. 2011;41(7):938–944.

[875] Lordelo GS, Miranda-Videla AL, Akimoto AK, et al. Association between methylene tetrahydrofolate reductase and glutathione S-transferase M1 gene polymorphisms and chronic myeloid leukemia in a Brazilian population. *Genetics Mol Res*. 2012;11(1):1013-26.

[876] Goodbourn S, Didcock L, Randall RE. Interferons: cell signalling, immune modulation, antiviral response and virus countermeasures. *J Gen Virol*. 2000 Oct; 81(Pt 10):2341-2364.

[877] Korachi M, Ceran N, Adaleti R, et al. An association study of functional polymorphic genes IRF-1, IFNGR-1, and IFN-g with disease progression, aspartate aminotransferase, alanine aminotransferase, and viral load in chronic hepatitis B and C. *Int J Infect Dis*. 2013;17:e44-e49.

[878] Luoni G, Verra F, Arca B, et al. Antimalarial antibody levels and IL4 polymorphism in the Fulani of West Africa. *Genes Immun*. 2001;2:411-4.

[879] Michael S, Minhas K, Ishaque M, et al. IL-4 Gene Polymorphisms and Their Association With Atopic Asthma and Allergic Rhinitis in Pakistani Patients. *J Investig Allergol Clin Immunol*. 2013;23(2):107-11.

[880] Vojdani A, Pollard KM, Campbell AW, et al. Environmental Triggers and Autoimmunity. *Autoimmune Dis*. 2014;2014:798029.

[881] Richardson B. The interaction between environmental triggers and epigenetics in autoimmunity. *Clin Immunol*. 2018 Jul;192:1-5.

[882] Javierre BM, Hernando H, Ballestar E. Environmental Triggers and Epigenetic Deregulation in Autoimmune Disease. *Discov Med*. 2011 Dec;12(67):535-45.

[883] Vojdani A. A Potential Link between Environmental Triggers and Autoimmunity. *Autoimmune Dis*. 2014;2014:437231.

[884] Mitchell LA, Tingle AJ, MacWilliam L, et al. HLA-DR class II associations with rubella vaccine-induced joint manifestations. *J Infect Dis*. 1998;177:5–12.

[885] Stanley SL Jr, Frey SE, Taillon-Miller P, et al. The immunogenetics of smallpox vaccination. *J Infect Dis*. 2007;196:212–219.

[886] Feenstra B, Pasternak B, Geller F, et al. Common variants associated with general and MMR vaccine-related febrile seizures. *Nat Genet*. 2014 Dec;46(12):1274-82.

[887] Reif DM, McKinney BA, Motsinger AA, et al. Genetic Basis for Adverse Events After Smallpox Vaccination. *J Infect Dis*. 2008 Jul 1;198(1):16-22.

[888] Shoenfeld Y, Agmon-Levin N, Tomljenovic L. *Vaccines and Autoimmunity*. 2015 Jul 7, Wiley-Blackwell: Hoboken, New Jersey.

[889] Ovsyannikova IG, Vierkant RA, Poland GA. Importance of HLA-DQ and HLA-DP polymorphisms in cytokine responses to naturally processed HLA-DR-derived measles virus peptides. *Vaccine*. 2006 Jun 19;24(25):5381-9.

[890] Poland GA, Ovsyannikova IG, Jacobson RM, et al. Identification of an association between HLA class II alleles and low antibody levels after measles immunization. *Vaccine*. 2001 Nov 12;20(3-4):430-8.

[891] Desombere I, Willems A, Leroux-Roels G. Response to hepatitis B vaccine: multiple HLA genes are involved. *Tissue Antigens*. 1998 Jun;51(6):593-604.

[892] Kruger A, Adams P, Hammer J, et al. Hepatitis B surface antigen presentation and HLA-DRB1*-lessons from twins and peptide binding studies. *Clin Exp Immunol*. 2005 May;140(2):325-32.

[893] Ovsyannikova IG, Jacobson RM, Dhiman N, et al. Human leukocyte antigen and cytokine receptor gene polymorphisms associated with heterogeneous immune responses to mumps viral vaccine. *Pediatrics*. 2008 May;121(5):e1091-9.

[894] Tanjena V, David CS. Association of MHC and rheumatoid arthritis: Regulatory role of HLA class II molecules in animal models of RA - studies on transgenic/knockout mice. *Arthritis Res*. 2000;2(3):205–207.

[895] Kampstra ASB, Toes REM. HLA class II and rheumatoid arthritis: the bumpy road of revelation. *Immunogenetics*. 2017;69(8):597–603.

[896] Gatto M, Agmon-Levin N, Soriano A, et al. Human Papillomavirus Vaccine and Systemic Lupus Erythematosus. *Clin Rheumatol*. 2013 Sep;32(9):1301-7.

[897] Berkovic SF, Harkin L, McMahon JM, et al. De-novo Mutations of the Sodium Channel Gene SCN1A in Alleged Vaccine Encephalopathy: A Retrospective Study. *Lancet Neurol*. 2006 Jun;5(6)488-92.

[898] McIntosh AM, McMahon J, Dibberns LM, et al. Effects of Vaccination on Onset and Outcome of Dravet Syndrome: A Retrospective Study. *Lancet Neurol*. 2010 Jun;9(6):592-8.

[899] Verbeek NE, Jansen FE, Vermeer-de Bondt PE, et al. Etiologies for Seizures Around the Time of Vaccination. *Pediatrics*. 2014 Oct;134(4):658-66.

[900] Pellegrino P, Falvella FS, Perrone V, et al. The first steps towards the era of personalised vaccinology: predicting adverse reactions. *Pharmacogenomics J*. 2015;15:284-7.

[901] Schaefer A, Lim A, Gorman G. Epidemiology of Mitochondrial Disease. Diag Mgt Mitochondrial Disorders. 2019 May 4. Available at: https://link.springer.com/chapter/10.1007/978-3-030-05517-2_4#citeas [Accessed February 22, 2020].

[902] Meyer JN, Hartman JH, Mello DF. Mitochondrial Toxicity. *Toxicol Sci*. 2018 Mar;162(1):15–23.

[903] Xu F, Liu Y, Zhao H, et al. Aluminum Chloride Caused Liver Dysfunction and Mitochondrial Energy Metabolism Disorder in Rat. *J Inorg Biochem*. 2017 Sep;174:55-62.

[904] Mailloux RJ, Lemire J, Appanna VD. Hepatic Response to Aluminum Toxicity: Dyslipidemia and Liver Diseases. *Exp Cell Res*. 2011 Oct 1;317(16):2231-8.

[905] Sharpe MA, Livingston AD, Baskin DS. Thimerosal-Derived Ethylmercury Is a Mitochondrial Toxin in Human Astrocytes: Possible Role of Fenton Chemistry in the Oxidation and Breakage of mtDNA. *J Toxicol*. 2012;2012:373678.

[906] Kahrizi F. Repeated Administration of Mercury Intensifies Brain Damage in Multiple Sclerosis through Mitochondrial Dysfunction. *Iran J Pharm Res*. 2016;15:834-841.

[907] Alvarez-Iglesias V, Mosquera-Miguel A, Cusco I, et al. Reassessing the role of mitochondrial DNA mutations in autism spectrum disorder. *BMC Med Genet*. 2011 Apr 6;12(1):50.

[908] Siddiqui MF, Elwell C, Johnson MH. Mitochondrial Dysfunction in Autism Spectrum Disorders. *Autism Open Access*. 2016 Sep 27;6(5):1000190.

[909] World Health Organization. Mitochondrial diseases and vaccination. Available at: https://www.who.int/vaccine_safety/committee/topics/mitochondrial_diseases/Jun_2008/en/ [Accessed February 22, 2020].

[910] Arvas A. Vaccination in patients with immunosuppression. *Turk Pediatri Ars*. 2014 Sep;49(3):181–185.

[911] Moss W, Lederman H. Immunization of the immunocompromised host. *Clin Focus Prim Immune Def*. 1998 Oct;1(1):1-8.

[912] Tereskerz PM, Hamric Ab, et al. Guterbock TM, et al. Prevalence of Industry Support and Its Relationship to Research Integrity. *Account Res*. 2009 Apr-Jun;16(2):78-105.

[913] Rasmussen K, Bero L, Redberg R, et al. Collaboration Between Academics and Industry in Clinical Trials: Cross Sectional Study of Publications and Survey of Lead Academic Authors. *BMJ*. 2018 Oct 3;363:k3654.

324

914 Farva GA. Preserving Intellectual Freedom in Clinical Medicine. *Psychother Psychosom.* 2009;78(1)::1-5.

915 Borgstein J, Watine J. Feudal lords of science and medicine. *West J Med.* 2001;175:139–140.

916 Friedman LS, Richter ED. Relationship Between Conflicts of Interest and Research Results. *J Gen Intern Med.* 2004 Jan;19(1):51–56.

917 Horton R. The dawn of McScience. 2004. New York Rev Books, 51(4):7–9.

918 Angell M. The truth about drug companies: How they deceive us and what to do about it. 2005. New York: Random House. 336 p.

919 Smith R. Medical Journals Are an Extension of the Marketing Arm of Pharmaceutical Companies. *PLoS Med.* 2005;2(5):e138.

920 Fanelli D. How many scientists fabricate and falsify research? A systemic review and meta-analysis of survey data. *PLoS One.* 2009 May;4(5):e5738.

921 Martinson BC, Anderson MS, de Vries R. Scientists behaving badly. *Nature.* 2005 Jun;435:737-8.

922 Roseman M, Milette K, Bero LA, et al. Reporting of Conflicts of Interest in Meta-Analyses of Trials of Pharmacological Treatments. *JAMA.* 2011 Mar 9;305(10):1008-17.

923 Roseman M, Turner EH, Lexchin J, et al. Reporting of conflicts of interest from drug trials in Cochrane reviews: cross sectional study. *BMJ.* 2012; 345: e5155.

924 Carlowe J. WHO vaccine expert had conflict of interest, Danish newspaper claims. *BMJ.* 2010;340:c201.

925 Age of Autism. Voting Himself Rich: CDC Vaccine Adviser Made $29 Million Or More After Using Role to Create Market. Available at: https://www.ageofautism.com/2009/02/voting-himself-rich-cdc-vaccine-adviser-made-29-million-or-more-after-using-role-to-create-market.html [Accessed February 22, 2020].

926 Hearing before the Committee on Government Reform, House of Representatives, 106th Congress session, June 15, 2000. FACA: CONFLICTS OF INTEREST AND VACCINE DEVELOPMENT-- PRESERVING THE INTEGRITY OF THE PROCESS. Available at: https://www.govinfo.gov/content/pkg/CHRG-106hhrg73042/html/CHRG-106hhrg73042.htm [Accessed February 22, 2020].

927 Hearing before the Committee on Government Reform, House of Representatives, 106th Congress session, June 15, 2000. FACA: CONFLICTS OF INTEREST AND VACCINE DEVELOPMENT-- PRESERVING THE INTEGRITY OF THE PROCESS. Available at: https://www.govinfo.gov/content/pkg/CHRG-106hhrg73042/html/CHRG-106hhrg73042.htm [Accessed February 22, 2020].

928 Levinson DR, Inspector General. CDC'S ETHICS PROGRAM FOR SPECIAL GOVERNMENT EMPLOYEES ON FEDERAL ADVISORY COMMITTEES. Available at: https://oig.hhs.gov/oei/reports/oei-04-07-00260.pdf [Accessed February 22, 2020].

929 DeLong G. Conflicts of Interest in Vaccine Safety Research. *Account Res.* 2012;19(2):65-8.

930 Kaiser Health News. Big Pharma Greets Hundreds Of Ex-Federal Workers At The 'Revolving Door.' Available at: https://khn.org/news/big-pharma-greets-hundreds-of-ex-federal-workers-at-the-revolving-door/ [Accessed February 22, 2020].

931 Kaiser Health News. Big Pharma Greets Hundreds Of Ex-Federal Workers At The 'Revolving Door.' Available at: https://khn.org/news/big-pharma-greets-hundreds-of-ex-federal-workers-at-the-revolving-door/ [Accessed February 22, 2020].

932 Lenzer J. Centers for Disease Control and Prevention: protecting the private good? *BMJ.* 2015;350:h2362.

933 Noble Jr JH. Detecting Bias in Biomedical Research: Looking at Study Design and Published Findings Is Not Enough. Monash Bioeth Rev. 2007 Jan-Apr;26(1-2):24-45.

934 Glick JL. Scientific data audit—A key management tool. *J Account Res.* 1992;2(3):153-68.

935 Ioannidis JPA. Why Most Published Research Findings Are False. *PLoS Med.* 2005 Aug;2(8):e124.

936 Rath B, Muhlhans S, Gaedicke G. Teaching Vaccine Safety Communication to Medical Students and Health Professionals. *Curr Drug Saf.* 2015;10(1):23-6.

937 Kerneis S, Jacquet C, Bannay A, et al. Vaccine Education of Medical Students: A Nationwide Cross-sectional Survey. *Am J Prev Med.* 2017 Sep;53(3):e97-e104.

938 Cao Y, Li L, Feng Z, et al. Comparative genetic analysis of the novel coronavirus (2019-nCoV/SARS-CoV-2) receptor ACE2 in different populations. *Cell Discov.* 2020; 6():11.

939 Moghadas SM, Fitzpatrick MC, Sah P, et al. The implications of silent transmission for the control of COVID-19 outbreaks. *Proc Natl Acad Sci U S A.* 2020 Jul 28;117(30):17513-17515.

[940] University of Utah. Utah Hero Project Announces Phase One Findings. Available at: https://healthcare.utah.edu/publicaffairs/news/2020/07/utah-hero-project-phase-1.php [Accessed September 7, 2020].

[941] Bourouiba L. Turbulent Gas Clouds and Respiratory Pathogen Emissions: Potential Implications for Reducing Transmission of COVID-19. *JAMA*. 2020;323(18):1837-38.

[942] Bourouiba L, Dehandschoewercker E, Bush John WM. Violent expiratory events: on coughing and sneezing. *J Fluid Mech*. 2014;745:537-63.

[943] Bourouiba L. Images in Clinical Medicine: A Sneeze. *New Engl J Med*. 2016;375(8):e15.

[944] Rancourt DG. Masks Don't Work: A Review of Science Relevant to COVID-19 Social Policy. Available at: https://www.rcreader.com/commentary/masks-dont-work-covid-a-review-of-science-relevant-to-covide-19-social-policy [Accessed August 29, 2020].

[945] Abbott BW, Greenhalgh M, St. Clair SI, et al. Making sense of the research on COVID-19 and masks. Available at: https://pws.byu.edu/covid-19-and-masks [Accessed August 29, 2020].

[946] The Centre for Evidence-Based Medicine. COVID-19: What proportion are asymptomatic? Available at: https://www.cebm.net/covid-19/covid-19-what-proportion-are-asymptomatic/ [Accessed August 29, 2020].

[947] Johns Hopkin's University & Medicine. COVID-19 Dashboard by the Center for Systems Science and Engineering (CSSE) at Johns Hopkins University (JHU). Available at: https://coronavirus.jhu.edu/map.html [Accessed August 29, 2020].

[948] Lavezzo E, Franchin E, Ciaverella C, et al. Suppression of a SARS-CoV-2 outbreak in the Italian municipality of Vò. *Nature*. 2020;584:425-9.

[949] Oran DP, Topol EJ. Prevalence of Asymptomatic SARS-CoV-2 Infection. *Ann Intern Med*. 2020 Jun 3:M20-3012.

[950] U.S. Centers for Disease Control and Prevention. COVID-19 Overview and Infection Prevention and Control Priorities in non-US Healthcare Settings. Available at: https://www.cdc.gov/coronavirus/2019-ncov/hcp/non-us-settings/overview/index.html# [Accessed August 29, 2020].

[951] Worldometer. Coronavirus (COVID-19) Mortality Rate. Available at: https://www.worldometers.info/coronavirus/coronavirus-death-rate/ [Accessed August 29, 2020].

[952] U.S. Centers for Disease Control and Prevention. COVID-19 Pandemic Planning Scenarios. Available at: https://www.cdc.gov/coronavirus/2019-ncov/hcp/planning-scenarios.html#box [Accessed August 29, 2020].

[953] CEBM. University of Oxford. Global Covid-19 Case Fatality Rates. Available at: https://www.cebm.net/covid-19/global-covid-19-case-fatality-rates/ [Accessed August 29, 2020].

[954] Bhatia R, Klausner J. Estimation of Individual Probabilities of COVID-19 Infection, Hospitalization, and Death From A County-level Contact of Unknown Infection Status. Available at: https://www.medrxiv.org/content/10.1101/2020.06.06.20124446v2.full.pdf [Accessed August 29, 2020].

[955] CEBM. University of Oxford. Global Covid-19 Case Fatality Rates. Available at: https://www.cebm.net/covid-19/global-covid-19-case-fatality-rates/ [Accessed August 29, 2020].

[956] U.S. Centers for Disease Control and Prevention. People with Certain Medical Conditions. Available at: https://www.cdc.gov/coronavirus/2019-ncov/need-extra-precautions/people-with-medical-conditions.html [Accessed August 29, 2020].

[957] Onder G, Rezza G, Brusaferro S. Case-Fatality Rate and Characteristics of Patients Dying in Relation to COVID-19 in Italy. *JAMA*. 2020;323(18):1775-1776.

[958] U.S. Centers for Disease Control and Prevention. Weekly Updates by Select Demographic and Geographic Characteristics. Provisional Death Counts for Coronavirus Disease 2019 (COVID-19). Available at: https://www.cdc.gov/nchs/nvss/vsrr/covid_weekly/index.htm [Accessed August 29, 2020].

[959] U.S. Centers for Disease Control and Prevention. People at High Risk For Flu Complications. Available at: https://www.cdc.gov/flu/highrisk/index.htm [Accessed August 29, 2020].

[960] U.S. Department of the Health and Human Services, Office of the Assistant Secretary for Planning and Evaluation. CDC—Influenza deaths: Request for correction (RFC). Available at. https://aspe.hhs.gov/cdc-%E2%80%94-influenza-deaths-request-correction-rfc [Accessed August 29, 2020].

[961] Prasso JE, Deng JC. Postviral Complications: Bacterial Pneumonia. *Clin Chest Med*. 2017 Mar; 38(1): 127–138.

[962] Khanal S, Ghimire P, Dhamoon AS. The Repertoire of Adenovirus in Human Disease: The Innocuous to the Deadly. *Biomedicines*. 2018 Mar; 6(1): 30.

[963] Radke JR, Cook JL. Human adenovirus infections: update and consideration of mechanisms of viral persistence. *Curr Opin Infect Dis*. Author manuscript; available in PMC 2019 Feb 8.

[964] Dada MA, Lazarus NG. SUDDEN NATURAL DEATH | Infectious Diseases. *Encyclopedia of Forensic and Legal Medicine*. 2005 : 229–236.

[965] Dada MA, Lazarus NG. SUDDEN NATURAL DEATH | Infectious Diseases. *Encyclopedia of Forensic and Legal Medicine*. 2005 : 229–236.

[966] Feldstein LR, Rose EB, Horwitz SM, et al. Multisystem Inflammatory Syndrome in U.S. Children and Adolescents. *N Engl J Med*. 2020;383:334-6.

[967] Godfred-Cato S, Bryant B, Leung J, et al. COVID-19–Associated Multisystem Inflammatory Syndrome in Children — United States, March–July 2020. *MMWR*. 2020 Aug 14;69(32):1074-80.

[968] Cardi A, Bernabei R, Landi F, et al. Persistent Symptoms in Patients After Acute COVID-19. *JAMA*. 2020;324(6):603-605.

[969] Varatharaj A, thomas N, Ellul MA, et al. Neurological and neuropsychiatric complications of COVID-19 in 153 patients: a UK-wide surveillance study. *Lancet Psych*. 2020 Jun. [Online ahead of print].

[970] Fraser E. Long term respiratory complications of covid-19. *BMJ*. 2020;370.

[971] Puntmann VO, Carerj L, Wieters I, et al. Outcomes of Cardiovascular Magnetic Resonance Imaging in Patients Recently Recovered from Coronavirus Disease 2019 (COVID-19). *JAMA Cardiol*. [Online ahead of print]

[972] The Washington Post. These are the top coronavirus vaccines to watch. Available at: https://www.washingtonpost.com/graphics/2020/health/covid-vaccine-update-coronavirus/ [Accessed August 29, 2020].

[973] Moderna Therapeutics. White Paper, mRNA Vaccines: Disruptive Innovation in Vaccination. Available at: https://www.modernatx.com/sites/default/files/RNA_Vaccines_White_Paper_Moderna_050317_v8_4.pdf [Accessed August 29, 2020].

[974] Iwasaki A, Yaqng Y. The potential danger of suboptimal antibody responses in COVID-19. *Nature Rev Immunol*. 2020;20:339-41.

[975] Cao X. COVID-19: immunopathology and its implications for therapy. *Nature Rev Immunol*. 2020;20:270.

[976] Global Virus Network. Antibody dependent enhancement and SARS-CoV-2. Available at: https://gvn.org/antibody-dependent-enhancement-and-sars-cov-2/ [Accessed August 29, 2020].

[977] Tseng C Te, Sbrana E, Iwata-Yoshikawa N, et al. Immunization with SARS coronavirus vaccines leads to pulmonary immunopathology on challenge with the SARS virus. *PLoS ONE*. 2012;7:35421.

[978] Bolles M, Deming D, Long K, et al. A double-inactivated severe acute respiratory syndrome coronavirus vaccine provides incomplete protection in mice and induces increased eosinophilic proinflammatory pulmonary response upon challenge. *J Virol*. 2011;85:12201–12215.

[979] Yasui F, Kai C, Kitabatake M, et al. Prior immunization with severe acute respiratory syndrome (SARS)-associated coronavirus (SARS-CoV) nucleocapsid protein causes severe pneumonia in mice infected with SARS-CoV. *J Immunol*. 2008;181:6337–6348.

[980] Lv H, Wu NC, Tsang OTY, et al. Cross-reactive Antibody Response between SARS-CoV-2 and SARS-CoV Infections. *Cell Reports*. 2020 Jun 2;31(9):107725.

[981] Mulligan MJ, Lyke KE, Kitchin N, et al. Phase 1/2 Study to Describe the Safety and Immunogenicity of a COVID-19 RNA Vaccine Candidate (BNT162b1) in Adults 18 to 55 Years of Age: Interim Report. Available at: https://www.medrxiv.org/content/10.1101/2020.06.30.20142570v1.full.pdf [Accessed August 29, 2020].

[982] Jackson LA, Anderson EJ, Rouphael NG, et al. An mRNA Vaccine against SARS-CoV-2 — Preliminary Report. *N Engl J Med*. 2020 Jul 14;NEJMoa2022483.

[983] Folegatti PM, Ewer KJ, Aley PK, et al. Safety and immunogenicity of the ChAdOx1 nCoV-19 vaccine against SARS-CoV-2: a preliminary report of a phase 1/2, single-blind, randomised controlled trial. *Lancet*. 2020 Aug 15;396(10249):467-8.

[984] CBS News. AstraZeneca pauses COVID-19 vaccine trial over possible adverse reaction in participant. Available at: https://www.cbsnews.com/news/covid-19-vaccine-trial-oxford-astrazeneca-pauses-participant-may-have-suffered-adverse-reaction/ [Accessed September 9, 2020].

[985] Npr.org. AstraZeneca Resumes Its COVID-19 Vaccine Trials in the U.K. Available at: https://www.npr.org/sections/coronavirus-live-updates/2020/09/12/912281381/astrazeneca-resumes-its-covid-19-vaccine-trials-in-the-u-k [Accessed September 12, 2020].

[986] Logunov DY, Dolzhikova IV, Zubkova OV, et al. Safety and immunogenicity of an rAd26 and rAd5 vector-based heterologous prime-boost COVID-19 vaccine in two formulations: two open, non-randomised phase 1/2 studies from Russia. *Lancet*. 2020 Sep 4. Online ahead of print.

[987] Zhu FC, Guan XH, Li YH, et al. Immunogenicity and safety of a recombinant adenovirus type-5-vectored COVID-19 vaccine in healthy adults aged 18 years or older: a randomised, double-blind, placebo-controlled, phase 2 trial. *Lancet*. 2020 Aug 15;396(10249):479-488.

[988] Zhu PFC, Li PYH, Guan PXH, et al. Safety, tolerability, and immunogenicity of a recombinant adenovirus type-5 vectored COVID-19 vaccine: a dose-escalation, open-label, non-randomised, first-in-human trial. *Lancet*. 2020 Jun 13;395(10240):1845-54.

[989] Raghupathi W, Raghupathi V. An Empirical Study of Chronic Diseases in the United States: A Visual Analytics Approach to Public Health. *Int J Environ Res Public Health*. 2018 Mar; 15(3): 431.

[990] World Health Organization. Obesity and Overweight. Available at: https://www.who.int/news-room/fact-sheets/detail/obesity-and-overweight [Accessed August 29, 2020].

[991] Painter SD, Ovsyannikova IG, Poland GA. The weight of obesity on the human immune response to vaccination. *Vaccine*. 2015 Aug 26;33(36):4422-9.

[992] Tagliabue C, Principi N, Giavoli C, et al. Obesity: impact of infections and response to vaccines. *Eur J Clin Microbiol Infect Dis*. 2016 Mar;35(3):325-31.

[993] Lord JM. The effect of aging of the immune system on vaccination responses. *Hum Vaccin Immunother*. 2013 Jun 1;9(6):1364–1367.

[994] Derhovanessian E, Pawelec G. Vaccination in the elderly. *Microb Biotechnol*. 2012 Mar; 5(2): 226–232.

Index

B

B cells, 116, 179, 249
bacteria, 17, 37, 38, 45, 46, 60, 69-71, 76,
    80, 90, 91, 92, 101, 102, 105,
    108, 112, 119-122, 124, 128, 139,
    140, 169, 171, 178, 182, 183,184,
    189,194, 197, 215, 227-229, 230,
    231, 232, 240, 241, 277
baculovirus, 22, 143, 146, 149, 214, 215, 216
Bell's Palsy, 52, 153, 154, 176, 197, 209,
    236, 237, 238
Bexsero, 231, 232, 233, 235, 236
blood-brain barrier, 23, 31, 34, 41
blood-cerebrospinal fluid barrier, 31
Bordetella parapertussis, 90
Bordetella pertussis, 71, 76, 77, 78, 79, 90
Boostrix, 75, 79, 84, 86, 89
bovine, *see cow*

C

cabbage looper, 22, 214
cancer, 18, 20, 21, 28, 32, 44, 45, 48, 58,
    102, 105, 122, 162, 163, 180-183,
    190, 191, 202, 211-213, 219-220,
    226, 246, 250, 254, 275, 276
cardiorespiratory events, 46, 242-245,
cardiovascular disease, 122, 177, 178, 190
catalase, 253
cellulitis, 87, 89, 90, 126, 152, 153, 176,
    194, 197, 208, 218, 236, 237, 238
Centers for Disease Control & Prevention
    (CDC), 23, 25, 26, 63, 94, 141,
    155, 159, 161, 186, 217, 230,
    237, 262, 264, 275, 276, 277
Cervarix, 35, 213, 214, 215, 217, 218, 220
cetyltrimethylammonium bromide, 38, 145,
    146, 149
chickenpox, 172, 176, 177, 181, 182, 183,
    193-195, 197-202, 239, 279
Chinese hamster ovary, 22
chronic fatigue, 32, 33, 222
Clostridium tetani, 70, 75, 76, 77, 79, 80,
    108, 109
colitis, 40, 188

Comvax, 108, 109, 110, 111
congenital defect (anomaly), 171, 209
congenital heart disease, 167
congenital rubella syndrome, 167, 168, 169,
    171, 172, 176, 191, 196
contaminants, 18, 20-22, 65, 246
coronaviruses, 158, 271-278, 279, 284
Corynebacterium diphtheriae, 69, 70, 75,
    76, 77, 79, 80, 124, 231
COVID-19, 271-288
Cow, 65, 76, 77, 79, 80, 83, 132, 173 174,
    196, 207
cytosine phosphoguanine, 35, 36, 50, 51

D

Daptacel, 75, 76, 78, 79, 81, 85, 87
death, 7, 90, 97, 98, 98, 99, 100, 101, 102,
    103, 105, 107, 112, 117, 122,
    125, 126, 128, 135, 139, 140,
    141, 153, 155, 156, 158, 160,
    163, 169, 170, 175, 176, 183,
    194, 200, 202, 210, 213, 216,
    217, 218, 219, 220, 221, 226,
    229, 230, 238, 245, 272, 275,
    276, 277, 288
Department of Health and Human Services
    (DHS), 262, 263, 276
dehydration, 59, 60, 61, 67, 74, 86, 163, 208
demyelination, 54, 58, 90, 102, 223
developmental delays, 24-28, 31, 55, 160,
    167, 239
diabetes, 28, 46, 112-117, 139, 142, 175,
    190, 191, 246, 252, 254, 275,
    276
diarrhea, 36, 40, 51, 59-62, 63, 66, 67, 87,
    88, 106, 111, 150, 153, 154, 169,
    175, 188, 203, 208, 216, 228,
    234, 235, 236, 274, 278
diphtheria, 69-70, 72-73, 75, 76, 77, 78, 79,
    80, 81, 82, 83, 84, 87, 89, 93, 96,
    97, 102, 103, 116, 124, 125, 231,
    232, 233
DNA, 17-22, 37, 46, 48, 49, 65, 141, 143,
    146, 149, 174, 175, 190, 196,

207, 214, 245-247, 252, 253, 254, 279, 280, 281

DQA genes, 251

DRB genes, 33, 251

DTaP, 23, 26, 28, 41, 69, 75, 77, 79, 91, 92, 96, 101, 102, 108, 124, 134, 179, 242, 250

E

ear infection, 66, 74, 115, 119, 121, 140, 141, 169, 175, 187, 190, 208, 239

eczema, 52, 178, 190, 202, 209, 239

elderly, 74, 87, 107, 112, 121, 122, 123, 127, 128, 138, 140, 155, 158

embryonated chick eggs, 20, 21, 142

encephalopathy, 52, 74, 81, 88, 90, 93, 103, 131, 135, 141, 152, 153, 175, 176, 191, 205, 209

encephalitis, 52, 88, 89, 140, 153, 163, 169, 170, 171, 175, 176, 190, 191, 194, 197, 199, 200, 202, 209

Energix-B, 52

epidemic, 137, 158, 166, 168, 186, 200, 229

eyesight impairment, 128, 202

F

fall armyworm, 22

Facebook, 10

fetal DNA/cells, 18-20, 85, 175, 190, 196

fetus, 17-20, ,168, 173

filamentous hemagglutinin, 71, 76, 77, 78, 81, 82, 83, 84

flu, *see influenza*

Fluad, 35, 141, 143, 144, 150, 152

Fluarix, 141, 143, 145, 150, 152

Flublok, 141, 143, 145, 150, 152

Flucelvax, 141, 143, 146, 150, 152

Fluenz Tetra, 141, 143, 146, 150, 152

FluLaval, 141, 143, 147, 151, 153

FluMist, 141, 143, 147, 151, 153

Fluvirin, 141, 143, 148, 151, 153

Fluzone, 141, 143, 148, 149, 151, 153, 154

Food and Drug Administration (FDA), 21, 24, 26, 259, 262, 263, 264, 265

foreign DNA, 17-20

formaldehyde, 38-39, 49, 50, 51, 76, 77, 78, 79, 80, 81, 82, 83, 84, 85, 108, 109, 110, 132, 133, 145, 147, 148, 149, 207, 231, 232, 233, 234

fulminant hepatitis, 205, 210

functional magnetic resonance imaging, 32

G

Gardasil, 213-218, 219, 220

Gardasil 9, 213-215, 218

gastric bleeding, 131, 135

gastroenteritis, 66, 86, 125, 188, 208, 221, 226

General Practice Research Database, 54

genes (genetics), 19, 22, 30, 33, 48, 55, 57, 94, 95, 137, 223, 240, 245-251, 254, 268, 281

genetic testing, 250

genital warts, 211, 212, 213

German measles, *see rubella*

Glutaraldehyde, 40, 76, 77, 78, 79, 81, 83, 84

Glutathione, 248

glutathione peroxidase, 253

Google, 10

Guillain-Barré syndrome, 52, 54, 58, 81, 87, 89, 90, 101, 103, 126, 142, 152, 153, 154, 176, 197, 209, 218, 224, 236, 237, 238

Guinea pig cells,196

Gulf War syndrome, 34

H

Havrix, 205, 206, 208, 209

Haemophilus influenzae type b, 78, 105-117, 124, 125, 250

Haemophilus influenzae type a, 111-112

Hansenula polymorpha, 49

Headache, 32, 36, 40, 47, 51, 71, 86, 87, 88, 89, 90, 106, 121, 125, 126, 130, 133, 138, 142, 150, 151, 143, 166, 167, 171, 175, 176, 198, 203, 208, 216, 217, 218,

PedvaxHIB, 108, 109, 110, 111
Pentacel, 75, 78, 82, 86, 88, 108, 132
personality disorder, 27
pertactin, 71, 76, 77, 79, 81, 82, 83, 84
pertussis, 69-84, 90, 91, 92, 93, 94, 96, 97,
        98, 102, 103, 111, 113, 116, 183,
        189, 239, 282
phenols, 28, 40-41, 65, 109, 125, 148, 149
physicians, 3, 8, 9, 10, 14, 94, 100, 106,
        161, 225, 259, 268
pneumococcus (pneumococcal infection), 9,
        119-123
Pneumonia, 66, 74, 85, 86, 101, 102, 103,
        105, 106, 107, 117, 119, 120,
        121, 122, 124, 125, 128, 139,
        140, 163, 169, 170, 175, 190,
        194, 197, 200, 202, 239, 277, 284
poliovirus (polio), 20, 22, 77, 78, 79, 82, 83,
        92, 93, 96, 97, 98, 108, 112, 116,
        129-135, 250, 254
polyomavirus simian virus 40 (SV-40), 20-21
polysorbate 80, 41-42, 49, 50, 51, 65, 81,
        82, 83, 84, 85, 124, 125, 144,
        145, 146, 147, 149, 214, 215,
        216, 225, 234, 241
polysorbate 20, 41-42, 146, 149, 206, 207
porcine circoviruses, 21, 65
postherpetic neuralgia, 199-200, 202
postural orthostatic tachycardia syndrome,
        222, 226
pregnancy (pregnant), 133, 141, 160, 161,
        167, 168, 169, 172,191, 196, 213,
        224, 225, 276
premature infants, 23, 28, 111, 240-245
premature ovarian insufficiency, 224-226
premature puberty, 28
Priorix-Tetra, 172, 173, 174, 175, 176, 197
Proquad, 172, 174, 175, 176, 197
pulmonary embolism, 74, 102, 217, 218

Q

Quadracel, 75, 78, 83, 86, 89
QS-21, 35, 36

R

reactive oxygen species (ROS), 253
Recombivax HB, 49, 50, 51, 109
recombinant human albumin, 37, 173, 175
rectal prolapse, 74, 103
rheumatoid arthritis, 33, 54, 57, 58
Rho(D)-immune globulin, 26
Rotarix, 21, 63, 64, 65, 66, 67
RotaTeq, 21, 63, 64, 65, 66, 67, 262
rotavirus, 9, 21, 59-67, 112, 262,
rubella, 101, 112, 165-172, 173, 174, 176,
        182, 183, 187, 189, 191, 201,
        208, 237, 250, 254
rubeola see *measles*

S

S-Adenosyl methionine, 248
Saccharomyces cerevisiae, 49, 77, 206, 214
Sanofi Pasteur (diphtheria/tetanus), 79, 84,
        87, 89, 280, 282
SARS-CoV-1, 272, 284
SARS-CoV-2, 271-288
sclerosing panencephalitis, 170, 176, 190
SCN1a, 94, 250
SCN2a, 94, 250
seizure, 52, 66, 71, 81, 85, 88, 89, 90, 91,
        92-96, 102, 111, 117, 122, 127,
        128, 133, 135, 152, 153, 154,
        162, 163, 170, 176, 177, 187,
        190, 200, 208, 209, 218, 230,
        236, 238, 250, 252
sepsis, 85, 98, 105, 121, 128, 140, 163,
        244-245
septicemia, 119, 227, 228, 229, 230
serotype, 119-120, 121, 123,124, 125, 127,
        227
shingles, 35, 52, 176, 183, 194, 197-201,
        202, 209
single nucleotide polymorphisms (SNPs),
        246-249
smallpox, 20, 246, 250, 251, 257
sodium deoxycholate, 42, 145, 147, 149
sodium taurodeoxycholate, 42, 144, 149
speech disorder, 26, 27